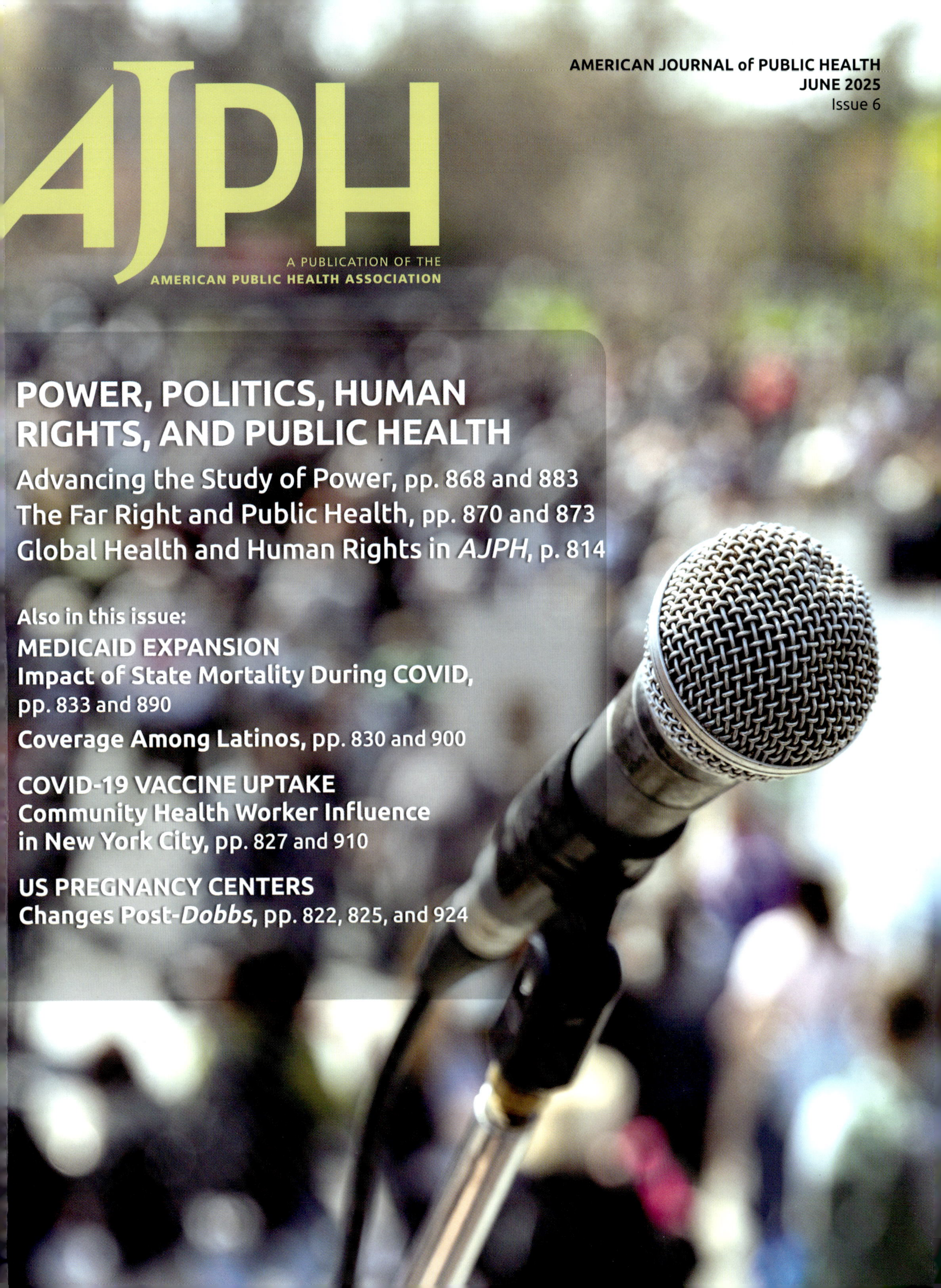

AMERICAN JOURNAL of PUBLIC HEALTH
JUNE 2025
Issue 6

AJPH

A PUBLICATION OF THE
AMERICAN PUBLIC HEALTH ASSOCIATION

POWER, POLITICS, HUMAN RIGHTS, AND PUBLIC HEALTH

Advancing the Study of Power, pp. 868 and 883
The Far Right and Public Health, pp. 870 and 873
Global Health and Human Rights in *AJPH*, p. 814

Also in this issue:

MEDICAID EXPANSION
Impact of State Mortality During COVID, pp. 833 and 890
Coverage Among Latinos, pp. 830 and 900

COVID-19 VACCINE UPTAKE
Community Health Worker Influence in New York City, pp. 827 and 910

US PREGNANCY CENTERS
Changes Post-*Dobbs*, pp. 822, 825, and 924

APHA
AMERICAN PUBLIC HEALTH ASSOCIATION
For science. For action. For health.

AJPH®, published monthly, is the official Journal of the American Public Health Association®, 800 I St NW, Washington, DC 20001-3710; (202) 777- APHA; TDD (202) 777-2500. APHA is a nongovernmental professional society founded in 1872, representing all disciplines and specialties in public health.

The *American Journal of Public Health*® (*AJPH*) (print ISSN: 0090-0036; electronic ISSN: 1541- 0048), first published in 1911, is the official journal of the American Public Health Association® (APHA). The oldest and largest organization of public health professionals in the world, APHA represents approximately 30 000 members from more than 50 occupations of public health.

Submissions: Visit www.editorialmanager.com/ajph or ajph.edmgr.com for online manuscript preparation and submission guidelines. Contributions of original unpublished research, social science analyses, scholarly essays, critical commentaries, departments, and letters to the editor are welcome. Questions? Write ajph.submissions@apha.org or call APHA at (202) 777-2469.

Print plus online subscriptions: Institutional price (print copy with online access for a single institution and all authorized users, regardless of geographic location) varies by size of organization and ranges from $993–$1445 for US organizations, and $1073–$1526 for international organizations (air delivery); multiple campuses not permitted without special arrangement. Details of the tiered pricing system at https://subscriptionoffice.com/pages/apha-landing-page. To order, write apha.subscriptions@apha.org.

Online-only subscriptions: Institutional price for one institution and its authorized users (regardless of geographic location) is $878–$1307. To order, write apha.subscriptions@apha.org. For academic consortia or multisite corporate subscriptions, contact apha.subscriptions@apha.org.

Print-only subscriptions: Institutional price is US $701, $782 international.

Back print issues: A limited number of print issues are for sale. Single copies are US $65, $75 international (air delivery). Shipping included; prepay only. To order, write apha.subscriptions@apha.org.

Reprints: For prices and ordering information on 50 or more reprints, check the Reprints section at www.ajph.org. To order smaller quantities of reprints (rush delivery), use the "Purchase Article" link on the article site itself.

Electronic access: Online articles more than 10 years old are available free for personal use at www.ajph.org. Recent articles are available through pay-per-view: single PDF article for $24, single issue access for 24 hours for $33, or entire site access for 24 hours for $38.

Postal information: Periodicals postage paid at Washington, DC, and additional mailing offices. Postmaster: Send address changes to American Journal of Public Health, 800 I St NW, Washington, DC 20001-3710.

Address changes: Send to AJPH, Membership Department (members) or AJPH Subscriptions (subscribers), APHA, 800 I St NW, Washington, DC 20001-3710. Or write to membership.mail@apha.org (members) or apha.subscriptions@apha.org (subscribers).

Indexes: Publications that index or abstract articles from *AJPH* include the following: Ageline, Assia (Applied Social Science Index and Abstracts), Biological Abstracts, Chemical Abstracts, CINAHL, Criminal Justice Abstracts, EMBASE, EMCare, Environmental Abstracts, e-psyche, ERIC, ETOH (Alcohol and Alcohol Problems Science Database), Excerpta Medica, Food Science and Technology, General Science Index, Grateful Med, Hospital Literature Index, Human Resources Abstracts, International Pharmaceutical Abstracts (IPA), Medline, Physical Education Index, Pollution Abstracts, Psychological Abstracts, PsychINFO, Safety Science Abstracts, Sage Family Studies Abstracts, Sage Human Resources Abstracts, Science Citation Index, SCOPUS, SIIC Data Bases, Social Work Research and Abstracts, and Statistical Reference Index (SRI)/LexisNexis.

AJPH

A PUBLICATION OF THE
AMERICAN PUBLIC HEALTH ASSOCIATION

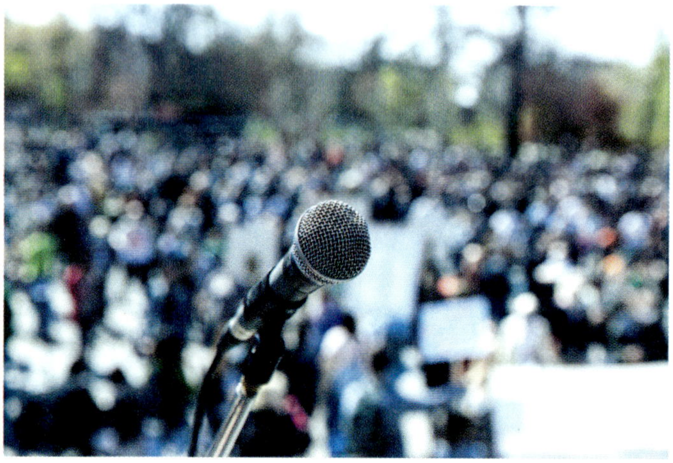

COVER: Advocacy and having your voice heard is a path to power. The microphone, like the theme of this issue, symbolizes the power to mobilize and encourage. Power can be wielded in a variety of ways to effect change and broadcast criticism of antidemocratic policies.

Cover concept and selection by Aleisha Kropf. Photo by well photo/Adobe Stock. Printed with permission.

APHA
AMERICAN PUBLIC HEALTH ASSOCIATION
For science. For action. For health.

Promoting public health research, policy, practice, and education is the *AJPH* mission. As we widen our scope to embrace global issues, we also sharpen our focus to support the needs of public health practitioners. We invite contributions of original unpublished research, opinion and commentary, and letters to the editor.

The *Journal* is printed on acid-free recycled paper.

OPEN ACCESS · ONLINE ONLY · PODCAST · DATA SUPPLEMENT AVAILABLE

EDITOR'S CHOICE

814 Global Health and Human Rights in *AJPH*
L. Ferguson

BOOKS & MEDIA

816 Fostering Epidemiological Theory for Consequential Description and Causal Inference
F. Smit and A. Chiolero

OPINIONS, IDEAS, & PRACTICE

EDITORIALS

819 Health-Focused Arguments for Eliminating Overcrowding in Prisons, Jails, and Other Detention Facilities
J. D. Goldhaber-Fiebert

822 Fake Health Care, Real Crisis: The Continuing Public Health Challenge of Crisis Pregnancy Centers
J. S. Santelli

825 To Curb the Proliferation of Crisis Pregnancy Centers, End State Grant Funding
C. Daniel

827 Don't Wait for the Next Crisis: The Time for Community Health Workers Is Now
A. L. Freeman, D. Pimenova, and N. S. Islam

830 Expanding Medicaid for Undocumented Immigrants: A Path to Better Coverage and Population Health
A. V. Bustamante, M. Chowdhury, and A. N. Ortega

833 Does Medicaid Improve Health?
H. Allen

PERSPECTIVES

835 Medical Providers Require Support and Training for Legislative Testimony About Abortion and High-Risk Pregnancy Care
C. Daniel, G. Riley, A. Raj, and C. Gambala

840 The Public Health Workforce Beyond Government Health Departments: Proposing a New Definition
H. Krasna

845 Wastewater Surveillance: A Rare Bipartisan Opportunity to Strengthen Public Health
J. Auerbach

848 Shuttering the Pregnancy Risk Assessment Monitoring System (PRAMS): A Dangerous Attack on US Mothers and Infants
A. S. Handler, K. Johnson, K. M. Rankin, A. J. Velonis, A. R. James, and M. Kotelchuck

RADICAL HOPE

851 The Master's Tools Will Never Dismantle the House: Reflections on Hope and Equity in Public Health Training
S. Best and K. Wu

854 Passing Out Pamphlets in 8-Inch Heels
A. Wurth

856 Lessons in Grief: Public Health and Healing in Community
L. Tu

EDITORS' CORNER

858 Notes From the Field: An Article Format Appropriate for the Current Times
R. J. Kim-Farley

859 Whose Democracy, and Whose Public Health?
P. Erwin

862 *An American Health Dilemma* 25 Years Later
T. M. Brown

NOTES FROM THE FIELD

864 Passing Policies That Promote Urban Health: Lessons From the CityHealth Project
D. H. Jernigan, K. Forrest, C. Patterson, and B. Castrucci

POWER, POLITICS, AND HUMAN RIGHTS IN PUBLIC HEALTH

868 The Far Right, Authoritarian Power, and Public Health
K. Rochel de Camargo

870 What Can Be Done About the Global Far Right's Threat to Health?
S. L. Greer

RESEARCH & ANALYSIS

POWER, POLITICS, AND HUMAN RIGHTS IN PUBLIC HEALTH

873 Potential Global Effects of the Rise of the Far Right on Public Health
S. March, J. M. Carrasco, Álvaro Flores-Balado, A. Muñoz-Haba, A. Pereira-Iglesias, and Gustavo Andrés Zaragoza on behalf of the APLICA Cooperative

883 Advancing the Study of Power: Opportunities and Priorities for Understanding Population Health Inequities
M. M. Reynolds and S. Galea

POLICY

890 Medicaid Expansion and US Mortality Rates During the COVID-19 Pandemic, 2018–2022
X. Han, K. S. Shi, Q. Fan, P. P. Choudhury, X. Hu, and K. R. Yabroff

900 Medicaid Eligibility Expansion Regardless of Immigration Status and Insurance Coverage Among Latinos Seen in Community Health Centers, 2018–2023
N. Huguet, J. Kaufmann, H. Holderness, J. Erroba, G. Mertes, A. Steeves-Reece, R. Springer, J. Heintzman, and M. Marino

OPEN-THEMED RESEARCH

910 Community Health Worker Influence on COVID-19 Vaccine Uptake in New York City, 2021–2022
M. Miller, B. G. Weiss, Z. M. Sakas, K. E. Parrella, F. Islam, J. L. Watkins, and the COVID-19 Equity Program Team

920 Low HIV Preexposure Prophylaxis Coverage Among Women: Focused, Innovative Strategies Can Increase Use—United States, 2017–2023
K. W. Hoover, W. Zhu, K. L. Hess, P. Spikes, Y-L.A. Huang, J. Wiener, E. K. Dunbar, J. L. Raiford, C. B. Collins, E. A. DiNenno, A. P. Kourtis, J. T. Brooks, R. N. Fanfair, and C. Courtenay-Quirk

AJPH June 2025, Vol. 115, No. 6

924 Crisis Pregnancy Centers in the United States: Post-*Dobbs* Characteristics and Changes
D. N. Lambert, N. Luisi, E. R. Johnson, R. Baugh, and A. Swartzendruber

936 Health Care, Mortality, and Declining Occupancy Rates in California Prisons, 2013–2023
J. L. Adler and W. Chen

945 Cigarette and E-Cigarette Use Among LGBT+ Youths and Young Adults According to Strength of State-Level LGBT+ Equality Protections
E. C. Kierstead, S. N. Yoon, M. L. Iskra, B. A. Schillo, and J. M. Kreslake

BACKMATTER

OTHER DEPARTMENTS

960 Subscription Form

Global Health and Human Rights in *AJPH*

See also Editors' Corner, pp. 858–863.

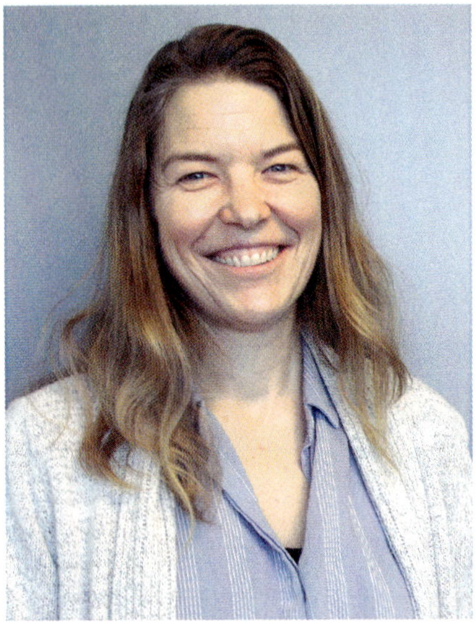

Laura Ferguson, PhD
Institute on Inequalities in Global Health
University of Southern California

Global health is concerned with how the health of everyone, everywhere is affected by an array of local and global forces that transcend national boundaries. In every country, the impacts on health of transnational forces such as climate change, the Internet, trade, and migration defy a response that relies solely on the notion of the nation state. Our world is increasingly interconnected, and, more than ever before, the health of one is dependent on the health of all, across borders and boundaries. Global health provides supra-national structures for addressing these transnational forces as they affect health.

At the same time, around the world, populism, authoritarianism, and statism are on the rise; there is a retreat from multilateralism, science, and public health. Unprecedented mis- and disinformation, alongside ideology-based policies and practices, threaten evidence-based public health. A healthy democracy rests on the assumption that, whatever the chosen priorities, everyone's policies, plans, and actions are grounded in evidence rather than ideology, greed, or self-interest. In the current moment, this assumption does not hold true. The rules of the game have shifted; in places, they have been totally disregarded.

The US public has been betrayed by a leadership campaign based on lies and false promises. This is not unique: the same has occurred in other recent elections around the world. This is an opportune moment for us to learn from other countries who have already grappled with similar challenges as those we now face. What can we learn about promoting and protecting public health from other countries where disinformation campaigns are rife? Where there has also been a political lurch to the right? Where leaders question, or outright reject, the value of science? Where people have been pushing back for years against laws that limit their health and rights?

As we have seen recently in the United States and elsewhere, national laws can discriminate, create barriers to health services, and negatively impact

Continued on page 815...

HISTORY CORNER

16 YEARS AGO

20th Anniversary of the Creation of Brazil's National Health Care System

Throughout its history as an independent nation, Brazil has contended with alternating periods of flourishing democracy and withering authoritarianism, the most recent of the latter being a military dictatorship that lasted from a coup d'état on March 31, 1964, until 1985. During this period, the military rulers restricted civil rights and tampered with electoral processes. . . . The military dictatorship fell without bloodshed in 1985. In 1986 a massive national health conference formally endorsed the proposals of the *Movimento de Reforma Sanitária* (Movement for Sanitary Reform), a mobilization of public health workers, academics, and reformers that was one of the main forces in the struggle for the redemocratization of the country. Their call for a universal health care system had been a rallying cry for the people. . . . After 18 months of hard work and intense political debate, the new constitution was promulgated on October 5, 1988. Besides being a landmark of Brazilian democracy, the new constitution enshrines the principles proposed by the *Movimento de Reforma Sanitária* and marks the beginning of the Brazilian National Health Care System.

From *AJPH*, July 2009, pp. 30–31

AJPH June 2025, Vol. 115, No. 6

health outcomes. Conversely, we have also seen that laws can be used to domesticate international human rights law with the aim of realizing human rights within the national sphere. Human rights are a tool that can be used to promote and protect health. Perhaps because they grew out of conflict and represent a vision of the society that humanity agreed was needed to avoid ever again experiencing the horrors of World War II, human rights can feel particularly relevant during times of crisis. They demand that we interrogate unequal power and privilege; that we seek to understand the historical, political, economic, and social injustices that have created and now perpetuate such inequalities; and that we find ways to redress these wrongs. This is needed now more than ever in my lifetime.

AJPH welcomes submissions that advance public health science and its practical application to the complex challenges of today's world. This includes submissions that help strengthen the evidence base of the links between health and human rights, that seek to highlight how historic and current disregard or violation of rights has detrimentally impacted health and exacerbated inequalities, and that explore how human rights can be used to improve health, reduce inequalities, and provide redress. We also welcome submissions that recognize the interconnection of the United States with the rest of the world and explore how we can apply public health lessons from other countries to our national context, how globalization impacts health here and around the world, and how we can sustainably and equitably collaborate across countries to take on these challenges. We encourage authors to situate American public health within global public health, recognizing the former as part of, and inextricably linked to, the latter. *AJPH*

DOI: https://doi.org/10.2105/AJPH.2025.308086

ORCID iD:
Laura Ferguson https://orcid.org/0000-0002-1340-793X

HISTORY CORNER

85 YEARS AGO

An "American" Health Program

[T]hese approaches toward disease prevention and care for illness are characteristic of, or at least not antagonistic to, the basic essentials American democracy. They involve a minimum degree of compulsion, politicalization, and the kind of collectivism (of which compulsory sickness insurance is an example) that in so many countries has been concomitant with dictatorship. Certainly, it would seem wise and "American" for us to place our chief emphasis on prevention; to do every- thing to maintain and enhance the standards of private medical practice as essential to a democracy; to experiment as fully as possible with voluntary cooperative means for the extension or socialization of medical facilities before introducing the element of compulsion; to use private medical practice and voluntary medical organizations so far as possible, even when employing state subsidies for service to indigents; and exhaustively to explore the extension of public health and medical facilities in the direction of state-salaried medical services before injecting into the American scene a compulsory, political, non-preventive sickness insurance program.

From *AJPH*, September 1940, p. 1026

Fostering Epidemiological Theory for Consequential Description and Causal Inference

Frerik Smit, MPH, MA, and Arnaud Chiolero, MD, PhD

ABOUT THE AUTHORS

Frerik Smit and Arnaud Chiolero are with the Population Health Laboratory, University of Fribourg, Fribourg, Switzerland and the Swiss School of Public Health, Zurich, Switzerland. Arnaud Chiolero is also with the School of Population and Global Health, McGill University, Montreal, QC.

AJPH June 2025, Vol. 115, No. 6

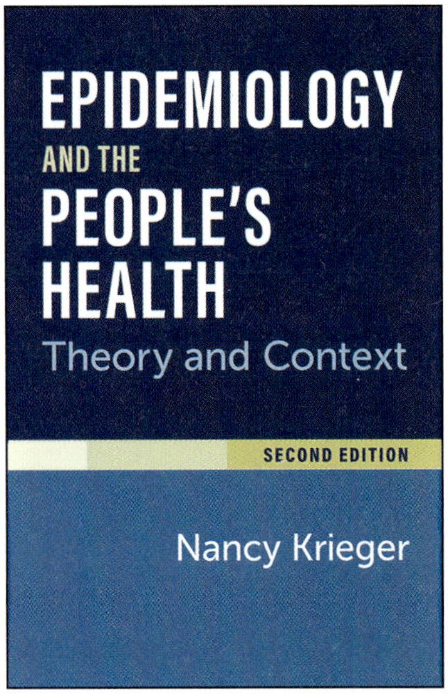

Epidemiology and the People's Health: Theory and Context, 2nd ed.
by Nancy Krieger
New York, NY: Oxford University Press; 2024
520 pp; $45.00
ISBN-10: 0197695558
ISBN-13: 978-0197695555

Public health scientists are increasingly grappling with the rise of misinformation and science denialism—a challenge echoed by Nancy Krieger in the second edition of *Epidemiology and the People's Health: Theory and Context*, in which she writes:

> "Evidence" alone is insufficient to challenge deliberate (and often well-funded) disinformation campaigns that seek to discredit robust scientific findings in conflict with their political and economic agendas.[1(p29)]

More than ever, we need high-quality evidence on the distribution and causes of disease to empower an evidence-based approach to population health. This is the context in which we read the latest edition of Krieger's book, which offers a deep exploration of the history of epidemiological theory and its apparent neglect. Correspondingly, this book raises a compelling question: could more explicit engagement with theory produce higher quality evidence to improve population health?

Krieger's fundamental argument is

> Theoretical clarity about the substantive questions epidemiology poses can improve the odds of generating valid—and potentially useful—knowledge. Theory is essential for formulating, testing, and assessing competing explanations—in other words, for good science. And good science, in turn, is a precondition for science that can make a difference for the good.[1(pxxii)]

Indeed, from a consequentialist perspective, epidemiology aims to produce evidence for improving population health.[2] This calls on health scientists to continuously strive to enhance the value of research through, for example, greater transparency and replication as well as improvements in methodology, peer-reviewing, and reporting.[3,4] Krieger makes the case that theory also plays a pivotal role in improving the quality of epidemiological science, contending that theory should be used

> to frame and interpret previously published data, to generate and guide the testing of new hypotheses, and to produce evidence relevant for both improving the people's health and reducing health inequities.[1(p213)]

THE RISE OF SOCIAL EPIDEMIOLOGY

Krieger recounts epidemiology's historical evolution pertaining to theory, providing a comprehensive timeline of how explanations of population disease patterning have evolved. Following a first chapter dedicated to describing the concepts of scientific and epidemiological theory, in chapter 2 Krieger begins in "ancient Greece in fifth century BCE" (p. 51), where and when the etymology of "epidemiology" can be traced. Chapter 3, subsequently, narrates how epidemiology established itself as a scientific discipline in the 17th to 19th centuries with empirical approaches for understanding disease patterning and etiology. Situated in the first half of the 20th century, chapter 4 outlines how epidemiology evolved in the face of an epidemiological transition in population health from communicable to noncommunicable diseases.

The heart of the book lies in chapters 5 through 7, where Krieger recounts the rise of social epidemiology since the mid-20th century, with epidemiology moving from an emphasis on biomedical and lifestyle perspectives to a growing recognition of the importance of social, political, and ecological contexts. Krieger focuses on three theoretical perspectives, sociopolitical, psychosocial, and ecosocial, arguing:

> These alternative theories demonstrate, it is not only possible but also useful and necessary to analyze health-related biology and behavior in societal, ecological, and historical context, without being constrained by and reduced to the narrow individualistic, reductionist, and ahistorical assumptions of the [biomedical and lifestyle] perspectives.[1(p291)]

Indeed, the rise of social epidemiology has transformed public health and epidemiological research by calling for a shift from "mono-causal thinking" (p. 179) to the multilevel determinants at stake in the full "web of causation" (p. 180). In the eighth and final chapter, Krieger provides case studies of how different choices of epidemiological theory can benefit or harm population health, ultimately concluding that by

> making conscious use of epidemiologic theory . . . we stand a better . . . chance of producing epidemiologic knowledge truly useful for preventing disease, improving the public's health, and advancing health justice.[1(p348)]

DESCRIPTION AND CAUSAL INFERENCE AT EPIDEMIOLOGY'S CORE

Two tasks at the core of epidemiology are description and causal inference, which, respectively, allow the examination of disease distribution according to various factors and for the assessment of the effect of interventions on population health.[5–7] As Krieger recounts (pp. 335–336), causal inference has bourgeoned in recent decades with quantitative data analysis methods, which rely on specific assumptions that can be hard to meet for social epidemiological studies.[8,9] Most notably, this includes the assumption of having a well-defined exposure, which can be a serious problem for many social variables.[8–10] To visualize this issue, inspired by Galea and Hernán's spectrum of hypothetical experiment specificity,[9] Figure 1 depicts how meeting this well-defined exposure assumption becomes ever more daunting as we move from the pervasive biomedical and lifestyle perspectives to the more holistic ecosocial theory. But, for Krieger, "theoretical stances" that place such boundaries on what can or cannot be studied in a causal inference framework "blithely" ignore "the evidence of direct health impacts" of social injustices like racism and sexism (p. 336)—a skepticism at the center of noteworthy intellectual debates.[6,8,10,11]

These limitations of mainstream quantitative causal inference methods place social epidemiologists at a crossroads. On the one hand, the goal is to produce valid and methodologically sound quantitative causal effect estimates. On the other, from a consequential perspective, we cannot exclusively restrict social epidemiological studies to well-defined exposures.[10,11] However, as stated by Kaufman, "There is no point to estimating and reporting a [quantitative effect estimate] if this number does not mean anything precise and objective."[8(p17)] A consequential epidemiologist should therefore seek to, where possible, quantify the causal effects of well-defined exposures while complementarily drawing on other forms of causal reasoning to enhance our knowledge and fill the gaps left by the limitations of mainstream quantitative causal

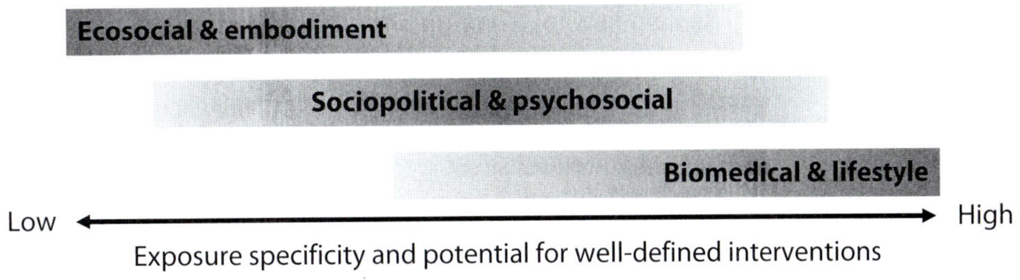

FIGURE 1— Different Epidemiological Theories Along the Spectrum of Exposure Specificity

AJPH June 2025, Vol. 115, No. 6

inference methods.[8,10] This could, as Krieger calls for, include the use of "fresh approaches" that are theoretically driven and conceptualize "disease processes and rates in relation to multiple levels of societally shaped exposures, susceptibility, and resistance across the life-course and trangenerationally."[1(p336)]

APPLYING THEORY IN EPIDEMIOLOGY: A NECESSITY OR A LUXURY?

Krieger lays out how our current understanding of health and its link to societal structures, historical context, and social processes have been theoretically driven and informed through the work of epidemiologists and social scientists alike. However, the consequential question as it pertains to epidemiological research going forward is whether explicit applications of theory throughout the research process is, as Krieger posits, a "practical necessity" (p. 49) for producing valid scientific output "that can make a difference for the good" (p. xxii).

To answer this question, let us take a historical perspective. Above all, the marked improvements in major health outcomes across populations over the past half century reflect, at least in part, the remarkable achievements of public health efforts. This extraordinary progress suggests that, even as theory has been historically neglected in epidemiology, improvements in population health are possible. Concurrently, pervading health inequities indicate that improvements in social epidemiology are needed to offer interventions with far-reaching impacts.[5] Purportedly for Krieger, one solution is fostering epidemiological theory and its explicit use in research, whereas for others the solution lies in reframing research questions to focus on those most likely to provide meaningful answers for policymakers.[5] Rather than being mutually exclusive, these approaches are intertwined.[12] A consequential epidemiologist can, therefore, learn a lot about epidemiological theory from Krieger's book, but they must search beyond for guidance on incorporating theory in their research. AJPH

CORRESPONDENCE

Correspondence should be sent to Frerik Smit, MPH, MA, Population Health Laboratory, University of Fribourg, Route des Arsenaux 41, Fribourg 1700, Switzerland (e-mail: frerik.smit@unifr.ch; social media: #PopHealthLab). Reprints can be ordered at https://www.ajph.org by clicking the "Reprints" link.

PUBLICATION INFORMATION

Full Citation: Smit F, Chiolero A. Fostering epidemiological theory for consequential description and causal inference. *Am J Public Health*. 2025; 115(6):816–818.

Acceptance Date: March 11, 2025.

DOI: https://doi.org/10.2105/AJPH.2025.308117

ORCID iDs:
Frerik Smit https://orcid.org/0009-0007-6034-2300

Arnaud Chiolero https://orcid.org/0000-0002-5544-8510

CONTRIBUTORS

F. Smit drafted the article. A. Chiolero provided critical edits and feedback. Both authors approved the final version of the article.

CONFLICTS OF INTEREST

The authors declare no conflicts of interest.

REFERENCES

1. Krieger N. *Epidemiology and the People's Health: Theory and Context*. 2nd ed. Oxford, UK: Oxford University Press; 2024. https://doi.org/10.1093/oso/9780197695555.001.0001
2. Galea S. An argument for a consequentialist epidemiology. *Am J Epidemiol*. 2013;178(8):1185–1191. https://doi.org/10.1093/aje/kwt172
3. Ioannidis JPA, Greenland S, Hlatky MA, et al. Increasing value and reducing waste in research design, conduct, and analysis. *Lancet Lond Engl*. 2014;383(9912):166–175. https://doi.org/10.1016/S0140-6736(13)62227-8
4. Chiolero A, Tancredi S, Ioannidis JPA. Slow data public health. *Eur J Epidemiol*. 2023;38(12):1219–1225. https://doi.org/10.1007/s10654-023-01049-6
5. Harper S, Strumpf EC. Commentary: social epidemiology questionable answers and answerable questions. *Epidemiology*. 2012;23(6):795–798. https://doi.org/10.1097/EDE.0b013e31826d078d
6. Hernán MA, Hsu J, Healy B. A second chance to get causal inference right: a classification of data science tasks. *Chance*. 2019;32(1):42–49. https://doi.org/10.1080/09332480.2019.1579578
7. Fox MP, Murray EJ, Lesko CR, Sealy-Jefferson S. On the need to revitalize descriptive epidemiology. *Am J Epidemiol*. 2022;191(7):1174–1179. https://doi.org/10.1093/aje/kwac056
8. Kaufman JS. Commentary: causal inference for social exposures. *Annu Rev Public Health*. 2019;40:7–21. https://doi.org/10.1146/annurev-publhealth-040218-043735
9. Galea S, Hernán MA. Win-win: reconciling social epidemiology and causal inference. *Am J Epidemiol*. 2020;189(3):167–170. https://doi.org/10.1093/aje/kwz158
10. VanderWeele TJ. Commentary: on causes, causal inference, and potential outcomes. *Int J Epidemiol*. 2016;45(6):1809–1816. https://doi.org/10.1093/ije/dyw230
11. Krieger N, Davey Smith G. The tale wagged by the DAG: broadening the scope of causal inference and explanation for epidemiology. *Int J Epidemiol*. 2016;45(6):1787–1808. https://doi.org/10.1093/ije/dyw114
12. Berkman LF, Avendano M, Courtin E. Producing change to understand the social determinants of health: the promise of experiments for social epidemiology. *Am J Epidemiol*. 2023;192(11):1835–1841. https://doi.org/10.1093/aje/kwac142

Health-Focused Arguments for Eliminating Overcrowding in Prisons, Jails, and Other Detention Facilities

Jeremy D. Goldhaber-Fiebert, PhD

ABOUT THE AUTHOR

The author is with the Department of Health Policy, Stanford School of Medicine, and the Center for Health Policy, Freeman Spogli Institute at Stanford University, Stanford, CA.

See also Adler and Chen, p. 936.

Living incarcerated in a prison, jail, or detention facility is certainly not intended to be easy, but living in such facilities when they are overcrowded is truly horrific. In this issue of *AJPH*, Adler and Chen (p. 936) report on their analysis of the relationship between the extent of prison overcrowding—prisons with incarcerated populations larger than the designed occupancy—and five health care and health outcomes. They do so by using prison-month level data for 30 California state prisons primarily from 2013 to 2019, generally a period of reduced overcrowding.

The negative health implications of overcrowding are applicable far beyond California's prisons, and hence the potential for decarceration to prevent and mitigate these harms also has broader scope for the more than two million people incarcerated or detained in the United States and the 11 million incarcerated or detained globally.[1] Although there are numerous health-related and non–health-related arguments for eliminating carceral overcrowding, here I focus on those connected to individual and public health.

Crowding in carceral settings is linked to worsened health outcomes via multiple causal mechanisms. These mechanisms include (1) more likely and more rapid spread of infectious diseases for which transmission is density dependent[2]; (2) increased individual stress from crowded conditions, leading to the onset of or worsening of a variety of chronic physical and mental health conditions[3,4]; (3) increased demand for limited health care appointments, reducing access and leading to delays in diagnosis and treatment as well as potentially shorter or lower quality health care visits; and (4) increases in interpersonal conflict, anger, aggression, and violence, leading to increased risks of nonfatal and fatal outcomes.

In their study, Adler and Chen primarily focused on health care access and quality and mortality during incarceration. In the case of health care access and quality, they found that increases in overcrowding generally reduce health care access and that even when access improves at lower levels of overcrowding, healthcare grievances (forms filed by incarcerated people not in agreement with the health care treatment they are receiving) are not significantly diminished. With respect to mortality, they did not find a significant relationship between reductions in overcrowding and reductions in mortality, but their study was not necessarily powered to do so. They did not examine nonfatal health outcomes such as disease incidence or cause-specific mortality for causes more plausibly linked to crowding, nor did they analyze the relationship between overcrowding and infectious disease incidence or mortality during the COVID-19 pandemic period.

From a public health perspective, reducing carceral overcrowding is most important in terms of preventing, mitigating, and controlling infectious disease outbreaks. Although the Adler and Chen study reasonably excluded the COVID-19 pandemic period, numerous studies have documented the greatly increased risk to the health of incarcerated people during this period.[5] In fact, this was the rationale for California decarcerating thousands of people from the state prison system during first six months of the pandemic.[6] Notably, such dynamics are by no means particular to COVID-19.[2] Tuberculosis incidence in both incarcerated populations and the community at large has become much higher with rising prison population sizes and resultant overcrowding.[7,8] Within prisons, jails, and other detention facilities, the size of seasonal spikes in respiratory viruses and the impact of emerging infectious diseases depend on the extent of overcrowding and are amenable to decarceration.

The health effects of overcrowding likely depend on both the intensity of overcrowding, the focus of Adler and Chen's study, and the duration of exposure to overcrowding. For example, risks may be moderately elevated for someone incarcerated for a day in an overcrowded jail, but the extent of risks and harms may be much greater if that same person is incarcerated for several years in a facility at the same level of overcrowding. Such differential effects could arise because it is unlikely that one day of exposure to overcrowded conditions meaningfully alters an individual's ability to access timely and appropriate medical care, whereas residing in a chronically overcrowded situation likely implies backlogs and consequent delays in receipt of care. Long durations of incarceration in overcrowded conditions can also greatly compound the risk of acquiring a transmissible infection.

Furthermore, the chronic stress of being confined in overcrowded conditions for a long period of time may itself be sufficient to harm health or worsen an array of preexisting conditions.[4,5] Thus, when carceral systems formulate and implement decarceration plans, attention should be given to both dimensions of overcrowding.

The size of health benefits achieved through decarceration depends on how decarceration is operationalized. Decarcerating frail or vulnerable people from overcrowded institutions (e.g., older people, those with existing health conditions, young children held in immigration facilities) may result in greater absolute reductions in risk.[9] Unfortunately, older people incarcerated in prisons often are still there because of long sentences for convictions related to more serious criminal offenses. Thus, despite evidence suggesting that recidivism among frail, vulnerable, and elderly people is extremely low, it may be more challenging for systems to release them; moving them to lower density settings may be more feasible. Furthermore, the extent to which overcrowding harms health through increased stress leading to violence or mental health issues elevates the priority of decarcerating additional at-risk groups.

Across the incarcerated population, many people who receive health care for a variety of chronic conditions lack insurance or connections to clinics and providers outside.[10,11] Thus, for those who are decarcerated, redirecting a portion of the expenditures that would have been used to incarcerate them toward transition programs that ensure there are no gaps in care is essential given the evidence that release in the presence of such gaps can carry substantial health risks.[10,11] Better and more timely health care, mental health services, and infection control measures during incarceration, along with linkages to appropriate care upon release, can also address public health concerns about how released individuals might transmit infections acquired while they were incarcerated.[2,7]

The harmful effects of overcrowding and the health benefits of decarceration are generalizable far beyond the prisons of California. They apply to prisons and jails in other states and countries. But they also apply to populations that are increasingly incarcerated before being charged with or convicted of a crime, including people—adults and children alike—whose immigration status is in question. It may soon be the case that many more such individuals, per shifts in Trump administration policy, will be held for longer periods in Immigration and Customs Enforcement detention facilities with consequent increases in health risks, as was witnessed during the COVID-19 pandemic.[12]

Eliminating overcrowding is not the only measure required to ensure reasonable access to health care and improve health outcomes among incarcerated people. Yet, regardless of one's view of incarceration, the body of evidence shows that incarcerating people in overcrowded facilities impedes their access to health care, exposes them to increased risks, and harms their health in numerous ways; it is simply cruel and unjustifiable. AJPH

CORRESPONDENCE

Correspondence should be sent to Jeremy D. Goldhaber-Fiebert, PhD, 615 Crothers Way, Encina Commons, Stanford, CA 94305 (e-mail: jeremygf@stanford.edu). Reprints can be ordered at http://www.ajph.org by clicking the "Reprints" link.

PUBLICATION INFORMATION

Full Citation: Goldhaber-Fiebert JD. Health-focused arguments for eliminating overcrowding in prisons, jails, and other detention facilities. *Am J Public Health*. 2025;115(6):819–821.

Acceptance Date: February 19, 2025.

DOI: https://doi.org/10.2105/AJPH.2025.308089

ORCID iD:

Jeremy D. Goldhaber-Fiebert https://orcid.org/0000-0002-4007-5192

ACKNOWLEDGMENTS

I thank Paul H. Wise and Jason R. Andrews for helpful conversations related to this work.

CONFLICTS OF INTEREST

The author notes no conflicts of interest.

REFERENCES

1. Fair H, Walmsley R. (2024) World prison population list. Available at: https://www.prisonstudies.org/sites/default/files/resources/downloads/world_prison_population_list_14th_edition.pdf. Accessed January 30, 2025.
2. Weyant C, Lee S, Andrews JR, Alarid-Escudero F, Goldhaber-Fiebert JD. Dynamics of respiratory infectious diseases in incarcerated and free-living populations: a simulation modeling study. *Med Decis Making*. 2023;43(1):42–52. https://doi.org/10.1177/0272989X221115364
3. Rosengren A, Hawken S, Ôunpuu S, et al. Association of psychosocial risk factors with risk of acute myocardial infarction in 11 119 cases and 13 648 controls from 52 countries (the INTERHEART study): case-control study. *Lancet*. 2004;364(9438):953–962. https://doi.org/10.1016/S0140-6736(04)17019-0
4. Schmidt MV, Sterlemann V, Muller MB. Chronic stress and individual vulnerability. *Ann N Y Acad Sci*. 2008;1148(1):174–183. https://doi.org/10.1196/annals.1410.017
5. Sugie NF, Turney K, Reiter K, et al. Excess mortality in US prisons during the COVID-19 pandemic. *Sci*

Adv. 2023;9(48):eadj8104. https://doi.org/10.1126/sciadv.adj8104

6. California Department of Corrections and Rehabilitation. Actions to reduce population and maximize space. Available at: https://www.cdcr.ca.gov/covid19/frequently-asked-questions-expedited-releases. Accessed January 30, 2025.
7. Liu YE, Mabene Y, Camelo S, et al. Mass incarceration as a driver of the tuberculosis epidemic in Latin America and projected effects of policy alternatives: a mathematical modelling study. *Lancet Public Health.* 2024;9(11):e841–e851. https://doi.org/10.1016/S2468-2667(24)00192-0
8. Martinez L, Warren JL, Harries AD, et al. Global, regional, and national estimates of tuberculosis incidence and case detection among incarcerated individuals from 2000 to 2019: a systematic analysis. *Lancet Public Health.* 2023;8(7):e511–e519. https://doi.org/10.1016/S2468-2667(23)00097-X
9. Miller KEM, Shen K, Yang Y, Williams BA, Wolff JL. Prevalence of disability among older adults in prison. *JAMA Netw Open.* 2024;7(12):e2452334. https://doi.org/10.1001/jamanetworkopen.2024.52334
10. Aminawung JA, Puglisi LB, Roy B, Horton N, Elumn JE, Lin HJ, Bibbins-Domingo K, Krumholz H, Wang EA. Cardiovascular disease risk factor control following release from carceral facilities: a cross-sectional study. *J Am Heart Assoc.* 2024;13(18):eJAHA2024035683T. https://doi.org/10.1161/JAHA.124.035683
11. Borschmann R, Mortality After Release from Incarceration Consortium (MARIC) Collaborators, Kinner SA. Rates and causes of death after release from incarceration among 1 471 526 people in eight high-income and middle-income countries: an individual participant data meta-analysis. *Lancet.* 2024;403(10438):1779–1788. https://doi.org/10.1016/S0140-6736(24)00344-1
12. Weyant C, Meyer JP, Bromberg D, Beyrer C, Altice FL, Goldhaber-Fiebert JD. Decarceration and COVID-19 infections in US immigration and customs enforcement detention facilities: a simulation modeling study. *Lancet Reg Health Am.* 2024;42:100971. https://doi.org/10.1016/j.lana.2024.100971

Fake Health Care, Real Crisis: The Continuing Public Health Challenge of Crisis Pregnancy Centers

John S. Santelli, MD, MPH

ABOUT THE AUTHOR

John S. Santelli is with the Department of Population and Family Health, Mailman School of Public Health and Department of Pediatrics, Vagelos College of Physicians and Surgeons, Columbia University, New York, NY.

See also Daniel, p. 825, and Lambert et al., p. 924.

"'When I use a word,' Humpty Dumpty said in rather a scornful tone, 'it means just what I choose it to mean—neither more nor less.'"

—*Lewis Carroll*[1]

The work of the public health community today is increasingly upended by disinformation, resistance to science, legal reversals, and poor political leadership. Overcoming these ongoing challenges demands an understanding of scientific concepts and data, of social and political forces that shape public policy, and of the human rights principles that should guide public health practice. One such ongoing challenge is the public health response to so-called crisis pregnancy centers (CPCs). In this issue of *AJPH*, Lambert and her courageous academic colleagues (p. 924) provide the latest update on the ongoing challenges to public health created by CPCs in the United States.

CPCs, operated by conservative Evangelical and Catholic (antiabortion) organizations, attempt to dissuade pregnant persons from abortion through disinformation and coercion.[2] They mimic women's health care facilities by providing free pregnancy testing, sexually transmitted infection testing, and ultrasounds, but not contraception. Although they provide these limited medical services, they are commonly not subject to state regulation. Although CPCs do not provide information about or referrals for abortion, they use deceptive names like "pregnancy care center," "your options medical," "center for pregnancy choices," and "caring choices pregnancy help"[3]—names that suggest that CPCs are abortion clinics or comprehensive reproductive care centers. CPCs target college students, people of color, and people with low incomes, enticing vulnerable people to continue an unwanted pregnancy.[4]

The first CPCs were founded around 1970 as states began to liberalize their state abortion laws; growth accelerated after *Roe v Wade* (410 US 113 [1973]) was decided.[5] Federal support came in 2000 as part of new funding for abstinence-only until-marriage "education." As early as 2002, the Guttmacher Institute[5] noted the effort of conservative lawmakers to use taxpayer dollars to fund CPCs. In 2012, the American Public Health Association (APHA) took a principled position against CPCs, warning, "CPCs often engage in techniques that are coercive, threatening, misleading, and aggressive."[4] Other health and medical groups followed with similar critiques, including a joint statement from the Society for Adolescent Health and Medicine and the North American Society for Pediatric and Adolescent Gynecology,[6] the American College of Obstetricians and Gynecologists,[7] and the American Medical Association.[8] These continuing concerns become more acute as access to abortion care has been derailed in the post-*Roe* world. More recently, Project 2025 has proposed shifting funding in the Teen Pregnancy Prevention program toward sexual risk avoidance (i.e., abstinence-only) approaches, which are supported by proponents of CPCs.[9]

CPCs fail to meet the ethical standards of medicine and public health regarding complete information and nonjudgmental care.[4,6–8] They do not provide nonjudgmental counseling about pregnancy options. In fact, they purposely limit information about abortion and provide misinformation and disinformation about the "dangers" of abortion to coerce women to continue a pregnancy. Thus, CPCs violate women's rights to medically accurate and comprehensive information.

The very existence of CPCs is founded on a misconception about how women make decisions about an unwanted pregnancy. The Turnaway Study, which examined abortion decision-making, demonstrated that almost all women seeking abortion care have already made their decision about pregnancy termination before seeking health care.[10] Very limited research has examined the specific impact of CPCs on pregnancy decision-making. A 2018 study of 114 abortion and 269 prenatal patients in southern Louisiana found that few women (< 6%) had visited a CPC, and very few (n = 3) prenatal patients reported that the CPC had an impact on their decision.[2]

CPCs have been supported by an increasingly conservative US Supreme Court. In *National Institute of Family & Life Advocates v Becerra* (585 US 755 [2018]), the court ruled in favor of CPCs and against the state of California, which had required licensed CPCs to provide information about abortion services.[11] In this case, the court seemed more concerned about the free speech rights of CPCs than the disclosure of complete or medically accurate information to patients. Of course, the court also overturned the national right to abortion in the *Dobbs v Jackson Women's Health Org*. (142 S. Ct. 2228 [2022]), decision; we do not know what will come next. The 1973 *Roe v. Wade* case was built on a series of Supreme Court decisions providing rights to contraception (*Griswold v Connecticut* [381 US 479] in 1965 and *Eisenstadt v Baird* [405 US 438] in 1972) and rights to privacy in reproductive health care (*Griswold*); these may now be threatened. The court may be poised to return women to the 19th century by reinstating Comstock chastity laws (from the Comstock Act of 1873 [18 USC §1461]), which forbid the interstate trade (via US mail) of obscene, lewd, or lascivious material, including pornography and contraception and abortion items.[12]

The helpful new article from Lambert et al. describes the status of CPCs in the United States in the period before and after the *Dobbs* decision. In 2024, following the repeal of *Roe v Wade* in the 2022 *Dobbs* decision, 2633 brick-and-mortar CPCs were operating in the United States. This was an increase of 3.3% from 2021. By contrast, in 2023 the Guttmacher Institute reported that there were 765 brick-and-mortar abortion clinics, a decrease of 5% from 2020.[13] CPCs are found in all 50 states. Growth in CPCs has occurred in every region of the country but is greatest in conservative regions such as the South and the Midwest. Overall, 72% of CPCs provide nondiagnostic pregnancy ultrasounds, and 4% claim to provide unproven "abortion reversal" treatment. States that provide taxpayer funding for CPCs, not surprisingly, show greater growth in the number of CPCs.

So, what should the public health community do? Lambert et al. provide a series of sensible recommendations based on their new findings and previous research. Likewise, the APHA and other professional health associations such as the Society for Adolescent Health and Medicine, the North American Society for Pediatric and Adolescent Gynecology, the American College of Obstetricians and Gynecologists, and the American Medical Association provide authoritative guidance. Here is a composite list of recommendations:

1. People in public health must understand that CPCs are neither a medical model nor a public health model of care. CPCs violate basic public health and medical ethics and fail to meet the basic principles of health care practice.
2. CPCs should not be licensed by state regulators unless they provide medically accurate information about pregnancy and abortion. That appears to be impossible for them—given their belief systems.
3. CPCs should not be funded by state governments or the US federal government.
4. CPCs should not be allowed to provide abstinence-only until-marriage programs in public schools or any other instruction.
5. Public health should demand truth in labeling. If the Supreme Court is going to support the free speech rights of CPCs, state governments should provide corrective information on their own Web sites about the services CPCs provide and the disinformation they promote. A good number of states and cities are already doing this.[3]
6. The APHA, working with partners, should implement a communication campaign to educate the US public about the dangers of CPCs.

Although CPCs have been a problem for decades, they are particularly painful at a time when access to abortion and other reproductive care is being limited. Barriers to real health care may push people to CPCs. There is an urgent need to educate health professionals and the public about the fake health care provided by CPCs. AJPH

CORRESPONDENCE

Correspondence should be sent to John Santelli, MD, MPH, Professor, Columbia University, Population and Family Health, 60 Haven Ave, B2, New York, NY 10032 (e-mail: js2637@columbia.edu). Reprints can be ordered at https://www.ajph.org by clicking the "Reprints" link.

PUBLICATION INFORMATION

Full Citation: Santelli JS. Fake health care, real crisis: the continuing public health challenge of crisis pregnancy centers. *Am J Public Health*. 2025;115(6): 822–824.

Acceptance Date: March 10, 2025.

DOI: https://doi.org/10.2105/AJPH.2025.308111

ORCID iD:
John S. Santelli https://orcid.org/0000-0003-2768-1910

ACKNOWLEDGMENTS

The author wishes to express deep gratitude to Laura Lindberg, PhD, Andrea Swartzendruber, PhD, MPH, and Debbie Malden, DPhil, for their helpful suggestions on drafts of this editorial.

CONFLICTS OF INTEREST

The author has no conflicts of interest to report.

REFERENCES

1. Carroll L. *Through the Looking-Glass, and What Alice Found There.* New York, NY: Penguin Classics; 2003.
2. Kimport K, Kriz R, Roberts SCM. The prevalence and impacts of crisis pregnancy center visits among a population of pregnant women. *Contraception.* 2018;98(1):69–73. https://doi.org/10.1016/j.contraception.2018.02.016
3. Crisis Pregnancy Center. Map. Available at: https://crisispregnancycentermap.com. Accessed March 2, 2025.
4. American Public Health Association. Regulating disclosure of services and sponsorship of crisis pregnancy centers. November 1, 2011. Available at: https://www.apha.org/policies-and-advocacy/public-health-policy-statements/policy-database%E2%80%8C/2014/07/22/08/33/regulating-disclosure-of-services-and-sponsorship-of-crisis-pregnancy-centers. Accessed March 2, 2025.
5. Lin V, Dailard C. Crisis pregnancy centers seek to increase political clout, secure government subsidy. *Guttmacher Rep Public Policy.* 2002;5(2):4–6.
6. Society for Adolescent Health and Medicine; North American Society for Pediatric and Adolescent Gynecology. Crisis pregnancy centers in the US: lack of adherence to medical and ethical practice standards. *J Adolesc Health.* 2019;65(6):821–824. https://doi.org/10.1016/j.jadohealth.2019.08.008
7. American College of Obstetricians and Gynecologists. Issue brief: crisis pregnancy centers. October 2022. Available at: https://www.acog.org/-/media/project/acog/acogorg/files/advocacy/issue-briefs/crisis-pregnancy-centers.pdf?rev=57762c9dbc624161b1b21018417e2011&hash=25CDF1171054215CCD197C06A6D0940A. Accessed March 2, 2025.
8. American Medical Association. Truth and transparency in pregnancy counseling centers. 2024. Available at: https://policysearch.ama-assn.org/policyfinder/detail/pregnancy?uri=%2FAMADoc%2FHOD.xml-0-3697.xml. Accessed February 28, 2025.
9. Heritage Foundation. Project 2025. Available at: https://www.project2025.org/policy. Accessed March 6, 2025.
10. Foster DG. *The Turnaway Study: Ten Years, a Thousand Women, and the Consequences of Having—or Being Denied—an Abortion.* New York, NY: Simon and Schuster; 2021.
11. Parmet WE, Berman ML, Smith JA. The Supreme Court's crisis pregnancy center case—implications for health law. *N Engl J Med.* 2018;379(16):1489–1491. https://doi.org/10.1056/NEJMp1809488
12. Goldberg M. Trump's allies say they'll enforce the Comstock Act. Believe them. *New York Times.* June 21, 2024. Available at: https://www.nytimes.com/2024/06/21/opinion/trump-comstock-act-abortion.html. Accessed March 4, 2025.
13. Guttmacher Institute. Abortion in the United States. June 2024. Available at: https://www.guttmacher.org/fact-sheet/induced-abortion-united-states. Accessed February 28, 2025.

To Curb the Proliferation of Crisis Pregnancy Centers, End State Grant Funding

Clare Daniel, PhD

ABOUT THE AUTHOR

Clare Daniel is with the Newcomb Institute, Tulane University, New Orleans, LA.

See also Santelli, p. 822, and Lambert et al., p. 924.

Crisis pregnancy centers (CPCs), sometimes referred to as "unregulated pregnancy centers" or "antiabortion pregnancy centers," emerged in the late 1960s as a way for antiabortion activists to interact directly with people experiencing an unplanned pregnancy.[1] Over the past 50 years, they have proliferated and become a key component of the antiabortion movement, employing a multitude of tactics, including deception, aimed at preventing and stigmatizing abortion.[2,3] Often designed to appear as medical clinics and attract women considering a pregnancy termination, CPCs tend to be located near abortion clinics or reproductive health facilities[4] and near college campuses,[5] and, in recent years, they have targeted communities of color.[6] Despite often receiving public funding, they are largely unregulated and have drawn heavy criticism from reproductive health advocates related to health, safety, mis- and disinformation, and data privacy.

Although CPCs have been a public health concern for decades, the 2022 *Dobbs v Jackson Women's Health Organization* (*Dobbs*)—the US Supreme Court decision that overturned *Roe v Wade* (*Roe*)—has made the question of whether states should fund or regulate CPCs even more pressing. Before *Dobbs* was decided, when states variably regulated abortion but could not ban it, evidence indicated that abortion access was important to maternal and infant health.[7,8] In the two and a half years since *Dobbs* was decided, evidence has mounted that banning abortion is correlated with increased fertility and infant mortality rates, affecting disadvantaged populations disproportionately.[9,10] Simultaneously, antiabortion legislatures have increased public funding for CPCs in the name of strengthening resources for needy families,[11] and antiabortion advocates are emphasizing CPCs as an important part of the post-*Dobbs* support system for people experiencing an unplanned pregnancy.[12]

Given these shifts, the study in this issue of *AJPH* by Lambert et al. (p. 924) provides a much-needed analysis of the changing CPC landscape since the overturning of *Roe*. As the first study to examine changes in the number of CPCs and the health-related services they offer, it shows a nationwide increase in CPCs of more than 3% from 2021 to 2024. Importantly, Lambert et al. look at how the specific characteristics of each state may be correlated with an increase in CPCs. The authors accounted for whether states had abortion bans and restrictions, whether they had a Republican governor, and whether CPCs receive public funding through tax breaks or grant programs. The only statistically significant factor associated with a higher rate of increase in the number of CPCs was having an enacted grant program. According to Lambert et al., 18 states have grant programs funding CPCs.

These grant programs, commonly referred to as "alternatives to abortion" programs, are often funded through state tax revenue and federal Temporary Assistance to Needy Families funds distributed to states for the purposes of alleviating poverty through direct support to low-income families. Reproductive health advocates have decried these programs, arguing that they misuse public funds, funneling them toward unregulated, deceptive, and harmful religious organizations. Although other sources of support exist for CPCs, such as tax breaks and incentives, the study by Lambert et al. suggests that grant programs may be the most important factor and thus the most effective target of reform efforts for those concerned about the proliferation of these centers. Moreover, the authors note that some of the 18 states with grant programs do not have abortion bans or restrictions. These states, such as Wisconsin and Kansas, may be particularly conducive to such reform.

Although Lambert et al. provide crucial insight into the changing landscape of CPCs, noting that they proliferate in "red" and "blue" states alike and that the number of CPCs is greater than the number of local health departments nationally, several questions remain about the role that CPCs play in reproductive health and reproductive politics in the post-*Dobbs* United States. Research has shown that CPCs contribute to a delay in abortion care and prenatal care, which likely contributes to poor maternal health outcomes. However, to date, there appear to be no studies that address the question of what direct effect, if any, CPCs have on maternal health. More research is also needed to understand the client experience and how it might vary across geographies and demographics.

For instance, given that CPCs target vulnerable women, are touted as a source of support for them, and sometimes represent the most accessible and affordable option, research should address the following questions: What specifically do clients receive or learn through their engagements with CPCs? How accurate is the information they receive? How prevalent are CPCs' deceptive tactics, and what are the effects of these tactics? What care, if any, do clients get and from whom? What data do CPCs collect on their clients, and what do they do with it? Do CPCs assist clients with accessing health insurance? Do they screen for intimate partner violence? Do they provide active referrals to mental health care and social services, such as assistance with housing, food insecurity, childcare, employment, and education? Are services delivered equitably across region, race, ethnicity, sexuality, gender identity, and religion?

Although some research has studied the client experience, more comprehensive and updated data are crucial for assessing how reproductive health advocates and practitioners should contend with CPCs in the post-*Dobbs* context, whether through attempts to regulate, defund, educate the public, or other means. Lambert et al. have provided an important starting point in what will hopefully be a significant increase in attention to CPCs by public health researchers moving forward. AJPH

CORRESPONDENCE

Correspondence should be sent to Clare Daniel, Newcomb Institute, 43 Newcomb Pl, Tulane University, New Orleans, LA 70118 (e-mail: cdaniel5@tulane.edu). Reprints can be ordered at https://www.ajph.org by clicking the "Reprints" link.

PUBLICATION INFORMATION

Full Citation: Daniel C. To curb the proliferation of crisis pregnancy centers, end state grant funding. *Am J Public Health*. 2025;115(6):825–826.

Acceptance Date: March 10, 2025.

DOI: https://doi.org/10.2105/AJPH.2025.308113

ORCID iD:

Clare Daniel https://orcid.org/0000-0002-5360-599X

ACKNOWLEDGMENTS

I thank Tulane University's Newcomb Institute for supporting this research. I am also grateful to Anita Raj and the *AJPH* associate editor for their valuable comments.

CONFLICTS OF INTEREST

The author has no competing interests to disclose.

REFERENCES

1. Haugeberg K. *Women Against Abortion: Inside the Largest Moral Reform Movement of the Twentieth Century*. Urbana, IL: University of Illinois Press; 2017. https://doi.org/10.5406/illinois/9780252040962.001.0001
2. Warren E, Kissling A, Norris AH, Gursahaney PR, Bessett D, Gallo MF. "I felt like I was a bad person . . . which I'm not": stigmatization in crisis pregnancy centers. *SSM Qual Res Health*. 2022;2:100059. https://doi.org/10.1016/j.ssmqr.2022.100059
3. Frasik C, Jordan C, McLeod C, Flink-Bochacki R. A mystery client study of crisis pregnancy center practices in New York State. *Contraception*. 2023;117:36–38. https://doi.org/10.1016/j.contraception.2022.08.004
4. Swartzendruber A, Luisi N, Johnson ER, Lambert DN. Spatial analyses of crisis pregnancy centers and abortion facilities in the United States, 2021 (pre-*Dobbs*): cross-sectional study. *JMIR Public Health Surveill*. 2024;10:e60001. https://doi.org/10.2196/60001
5. Luisi N, Lambert D, Johnson E, Swartzendruber A. Proximity of crisis pregnancy centers to colleges and universities in the United States, 2021. *J Adolesc Health*. [Epub ahead of print February 19, 2025; S1054-139X(25)00036-9]. https://doi.org/10.1016/j.jadohealth.2025.01.007
6. Kelly K, Gochanour A. Racial reconciliation or spiritual smokescreens? Blackwashing the crisis pregnancy center movement. *Qual Sociol*. 2018;41:423–443. https://doi.org/10.1007/s11133-018-9392-0
7. Vilda D, Wallace ME, Daniel C, Evans MG, Stoecker C, Theall KP. State abortion policies and maternal death in the United States, 2015–2018. *Am J Public Health*. 2021;111(9):1696–1704. https://doi.org/10.2105/AJPH.2021.306396
8. Karletsos D, Stoecker C, Vilda D, Theall KP, Wallace ME. Association of state gestational age limit abortion laws with infant mortality. *Am J Prev Med*. 2021;61(6):787–794. https://doi.org/10.1016/j.amepre.2021.05.022
9. Bell SO, Franks AM, Arbour D, et al. US abortion bans and fertility. *JAMA*. [Epub ahead of print February 13, 2025; e2428527]. https://doi.org/10.1001/jama.2024.28527
10. Gemmell A, Franks AM, Anjur-Dietrich S, et al. US abortion bans and infant mortality. *JAMA*. [Epub ahead of print February 13, 2025; e2428517]. https://doi.org/10.1001/jama.2024.2851
11. O'Donoughue J. Tax credit approved for donors to Louisiana anti-abortion centers. *Louisiana Illuminator*. July 2, 2023. Available at: https://lailluminator.com/2023/07/02/anti-abortion-centers. Accessed March 25, 2025.
12. Luthra S. Even at March for Life, abortion opponents don't talk about a national ban. *The 19th*. January 19, 2024. Available at: https://19thnews.org/2024/01/march-for-life-dc-anti-abortion-rally. Accessed February 28, 2025.

Don't Wait for the Next Crisis: The Time for Community Health Workers Is Now

Amy L. Freeman, PhD, MPH, Dina Pimenova, MPH, and Nadia S. Islam, PhD

ABOUT THE AUTHORS

The authors are with the Department of Population Health and the Community Health Worker Research and Resource Center, New York University (NYU) Grossman School of Medicine, New York, NY. Nadia Islam is also with the NYU–City University of New York (CUNY) Prevention Research Center.

See also Miller et al., p. 910.

For community health workers (CHWs) and advocates of the CHW profession, it is always affirming to read about a successful program where CHWs demonstrate, again, that they are incredibly effective at addressing health care disparities and providing a bridge to care for disconnected communities.[1] CHWs fill an essential role in our country's fragmented and complex health care system, and, as many have noted, this reality was made much more visible during the COVID-19 pandemic.[2–4] As we brace for the fallout from the current administration's reckless attacks on federal agencies, and particularly on the Department of Health and Human Services, the National Institutes of Health, and the Centers for Medicare and Medicaid Services, it is precisely now, when we are not in a public health emergency, that we need to advocate for and dedicate resources to building and strengthening the CHW workforce and connections between local health departments, health care providers, and community-based organizations (CBOs).

COMMUNITY HEALTH WORKER IMPACT AT THE COMMUNITY LEVEL

CHW approaches have been demonstrably cost-effective,[5] and there is a strong body of literature indicating that CHWs improve a range of health outcomes at the individual level.[6] However, our national conversation on the impact of CHW efforts has been stymied by this individual-level focus. In fact, CHW advocates highlight that CHWs' rootedness in a community and ability to engender neighborhood and community-level change through their knowledge and connectedness to trusted community resources are key qualities to their success. The article by Miller et al. in this issue of *AJPH* (p. 910) adds important and timely evidence of CHWs' ability to modify health behaviors and provide access to needed care at the community level. In this way, the authors are responsive to calls from researchers, advocates, and clinicians to conduct evaluations that embrace real-world complexity, particularly in the context of the CHW workforce.[7]

PARTNERSHIPS LEADING TO INCREASED VACCINE UPTAKE

While the role of CHWs in expanding vaccination coverage has long been prominent in low-resource countries, their potential to play an important role in providing vaccine education and addressing vaccine hesitancy in the United States came to the fore during the COVID-19 pandemic. The unique analysis by Miller et al. provides compelling evidence of population health–level effects of a CHW-mediated intervention aimed at changing vaccination behaviors. Considering where we are in the United States with waning vaccination rates and increased public health mis- and disinformation, these findings should provide us with a sense of both hope and urgency.

As the authors underscore, early in the pandemic, the historical effects of systemic racism and health inequities quickly manifested themselves in the data that emerged showing acute racial and geographic disparities in COVID-19 mortality and vaccine uptake. In response, the New York City (NYC) Health Department launched a program deploying CHWs to communities hardest hit by the disease, which were primarily in Black and Latino neighborhoods. By embedding culturally competent CHWs within trusted CBOs, Miller et al. describe the importance of CHWs' ability to build on existing relationships to forge connections in communities and provide timely, culturally responsive information about COVID-19 transmission, testing and treatment, and vaccination. In the span of 1 year, they found that in the neighborhoods targeted, vaccination rates increased from 44% to 76%. Their findings indicate that a CHW intervention designed to change community health behaviors was successful in reaching the people for whom it was intended and had an impact on changing vaccination behaviors of the population targeted as a whole.

Miller et al. demonstrate the ways in which CHWs were effective at increasing vaccination uptake during a crisis, by building trust, providing culturally competent information, and meeting community members where they were, addressing whatever concerns were most important to them. The authors also note that the referrals CHWs made to other health and social services were a key component of the trust-building process. Not surprisingly, other researchers have found that providing supportive services alongside vaccination efforts can lead to increased acceptance and uptake.[4,8] Given the expanding measles outbreak and the increasing threat of avian influenza, local health departments and health care systems should prioritize their partnerships with CBOs and continue to support the work of CHWs to improve vaccine uptake and prevent community outbreaks while also addressing community members' social needs.

Partnerships between local health departments and CBOs to implement CHW programs, like the one detailed by Miller et al., represent a promising model that has the advantage of pairing public health expertise with CHWs' local leadership and CBOs' deep and trusted community relationships to generate a place-based approach where targeted CHW efforts are most needed. Their findings indicate that these partnerships have the potential for significant impact, not just at the individual level but on a larger population health scale than previously understood. As the authors and others have noted, we learned from the pandemic that investing in these relationships and maintaining community partnerships makes good public health sense, and it is important to support this work not only during times of crisis.[2,9]

SUSTAINABLE INVESTMENT IN COMMUNITY HEALTH WORKERS

This work, of course, requires stable financial resources. Calls to create sustainable funding mechanisms for the CHW workforce are not new but have grown louder in recent years and have been met with some significant successes. Advocacy groups, including the National Association of Community Health Workers (NACHW), Partners In Health United States, and statewide CHW associations, among many others, are at the forefront of this call, providing resources to help organizations and states understand what funding options exist and examples of successful strategies.[10,11] Many states now cover CHW services through their Medicaid State Plan Amendments or 1115 Waivers,[12] and advocates are pushing for changes to these mechanisms from a "fee-for-service" to a "shared risk" model,[13] so that more focus can be placed on preventive services and quality-of-care metrics.

While much of the advocacy has focused on traditional Medicaid as the most sustainable source of funding, there have been reliable community-engaged grant-funded structures at both the federal and state levels that are essential to supporting CBOs, federally qualified health centers, and other safety net settings, as well as academic–clinical–CBO partnerships. Initiatives such as the National Institutes of Health Community Engagement Alliance and, in New York State, the Perinatal and Infant Community Health Collaboratives are specifically designed to address health disparities by supporting community-based research and partnerships, with the CHW workforce engaged as key partners across these initiatives.[14,15] This type of funding enables CHWs to work in the community, spending time developing relationships and meeting people where they live, which is generally not feasible as part of a fee-for-service model. Other federal funding mechanisms, whether through the Centers for Disease Control and Prevention, Health Resources and Services Administration, or Congressional Appropriations, are all viable mechanisms for directing resources to support a community-based CHW workforce.

When it comes to efforts aimed at changing health behaviors at the population level, including vaccine uptake, Miller et al. have demonstrated that embedding CHWs in trusted CBOs is a successful strategy for reaching specific communities. These findings should help fuel our determination to continue advocating for CHWs and similar evidence-based, community-engaged strategies to improve health disparities. The progress in recent years garnering greater support for the CHW workforce is undeniable, and now is the time to push the needle further. AJPH

CORRESPONDENCE

Correspondence should be sent to Amy Freeman, Department of Population Health, NYU Grossman School of Medicine, 9th Floor, 180 Madison Ave, New York, NY 10016 (e-mail: amy.freeman@nyulangone.org). Reprints can be ordered at https://www.ajph.org by clicking the "Reprints" link.

PUBLICATION INFORMATION

Full Citation: Freeman AL, Pimenova D, Islam NS. Don't wait for the next crisis: the time for community health workers is now. *Am J Public Health*. 2025; 115(6):827–829.

Acceptance Date: March 15, 2025.

DOI: https://doi.org/10.2105/AJPH.2025.308126

ORCID iDs:
Amy L. Freeman https://orcid.org/0000-0002-3496-6247

Dina Pimenova https://orcid.org/0009-0000-6701-4229

Nadia S. Islam https://orcid.org/0000-0003-1470-2073

CONTRIBUTORS

All authors contributed equally to the conceptualization, writing, and review of this editorial.

ACKNOWLEDGMENTS

A. Freeman and D. Pimenova are supported by NYU Langone Hospitals' Community Health Improvement funding. A. Freeman is also partly supported by a grant from the New York Health Foundation. N. Islam's time is supported in part by the National Institutes of Health (NIH; grant R01DK11048), the NIH National Institute on Minority Health and Health Disparities (NIMHD; grant R01MD018528), the Centers for Disease Control and Prevention (grant U48DP001904), the National Institute of Diabetes and Digestive Kidney Diseases (grant 1U2CDK137135), the National Heart Lung and Blood Institute (grant 1UG3HL15310), and the NIH National Center for the Advancement of Translational Science (grant UL1TR0001445).

Note. The views expressed are those of the authors and do not necessarily represent the official position of the funding organizations.

CONFLICTS OF INTEREST

The authors have no conflicts of interest to disclose.

REFERENCES

1. Cosgrove S, Moore-Monroy M, Jenkins C, et al. Community health workers as an integral strategy in the REACH US program to eliminate health inequities. *Health Promot Pract*. 2014;15(6):795–802. https://doi.org/10.1177/1524839914541442
2. Peretz PJ, Islam N, Matiz LA. Community health workers and Covid-19—addressing social determinants of health in times of crisis and beyond. *N Engl J Med*. 2020;383(19):e108. https://doi.org/10.1056/NEJMp2022641
3. Ibe CA, Hickman D, Cooper LA. To advance health equity during COVID-19 and beyond, elevate and support community health workers. *JAMA Health Forum*. 2021;2(7):e212724. https://doi.org/10.1001/jamahealthforum.2021.2724
4. Compton WM, Hooper MW, Hodes RJ, Pérez-Stable EJ. Lessons from COVID-19 testing research: the power of rapid response. *Am J Public Health*. 2024;114(suppl 5):S343–S346. https://doi.org/10.2105/AJPH.2024.307653
5. Kangovi S, Mitra N, Grande D, Long JA, Asch DA. Evidence-based community health worker program addresses unmet social needs and generates positive return on investment: a return on investment analysis of a randomized controlled trial of a standardized community health worker program that addresses unmet social needs for disadvantaged individuals. *Health Aff (Millwood)*. 2020;39(2):207–213. https://doi.org/10.1377/hlthaff.2019.00981
6. Kim K, Choi JS, Choi E, et al. Effects of community-based health worker interventions to improve chronic disease management and care among vulnerable populations: a systematic review. *Am J Public Health*. 2016;106(4):e3–e28. https://doi.org/10.2105/AJPH.2015.302987
7. Edwards ST, Park B. Health care hotspotting—a randomized controlled trial. *N Engl J Med*. 2020;382(22):2172–2173. https://doi.org/10.1056/NEJMc2001920
8. Nawaz S, Moon KJ, Anagbonu F, Trinh A, Escobedo L, Montiel GI. Evaluation of the COVID-19 vaccination campaign *¡Ándale! ¿Qué Esperas?* in Latinx communities in California, June 2021–May 2022. *Public Health Rep*. 2024;139(1 suppl):44S–52S. https://doi.org/10.1177/00333549231204043
9. Chokshi DA. People and places for the future of public health. *JAMA Health Forum*. 2021;2(3):e210423. https://doi.org/10.1001/jamahealthforum.2021.0423
10. Rush C, Mason T. *Sustainable Financing of Community Health Worker Employment: Key Options for States to Consider*. National Association of Community Health Workers. 2023. Available at: https://nachw.org/wp-content/uploads/2023/12/sustainable-financing-of-community-health-worker-employment.pdf. Accessed March 3, 2025.
11. Camaliche A, Marshall M, Lofton S, Tripoli S. *Charting the Course for Community Health Workers: Identifying Challenges and Opportunities to Secure Medicaid Reimbursement for CHWs in State Medicaid Programs*. Families USA. 2024. Available at: https://familiesusa.org/wp-content/uploads/2024/10/CHW-Listening-Sessions-9-27-24.pdf. Accessed March 3, 2025.
12. National Academy for State Health Policy. State community health worker policies. State trackers. January 11, 2024. Available at: https://nashp.org/state-tracker/state-community-health-worker-policies. Accessed March 3, 2025.
13. Chen AT, Smith DO, Ojikutu BO, Auerbach J. The community as a full partner: a new model for public health. *Health Aff (Millwood)*. 2024;43(6):805–812. https://doi.org/10.1377/hlthaff.2024.00033
14. Rodriguez Espinosa P, Vázquez E, AuYoung M, et al. Partnering with community health workers to address COVID-19 health inequities: experiences of the California Alliance Against COVID-19. *Am J Public Health*. 2024;114(suppl 1):S45–S49. https://doi.org/10.2105/AJPH.2023.307471
15. Larson R, Hussain S, Chau MM, et al. The power of partnership: NYCEAL collaborations with health agencies and mobile vaccination vans. *Am J Public Health*. 2024;114(suppl 1):S92–S95. https://doi.org/10.2105/AJPH.2023.307455

Expanding Medicaid for Undocumented Immigrants: A Path to Better Coverage and Population Health

Arturo Vargas Bustamante, PhD, MPP, Marvin Chowdhury, MPP, and Alexander N. Ortega, PhD

ABOUT THE AUTHORS

Arturo Vargas Bustamante and Marvin Chowdhury are with the Department of Health Policy and Management, Fielding School of Public Health, University of California, Los Angeles. Alexander N. Ortega is with the Thompson School of Social Work & Public Health, University of Hawaii at Manoa.

See also Huguet et al., p. 900.

AJPH June 2025, Vol. 115, No. 6

Immigrants are essential to the US economy and society, but they are often excluded from public benefits that ensure equitable access to health care. They make up more than one third of the workforce in certain industries, help local labor markets adapt to shortages, and contribute to public coffers through taxation.[1] Nonetheless, many immigrants lack comprehensive health coverage and are disproportionately more likely to be uninsured than are citizens.[2] Undocumented immigrants face even worse health inequities, with half of the undocumented adult population being uninsured compared with a quarter of documented immigrants and 8% of citizens.[3]

Lack of health insurance coverage is especially pronounced among Latinos, who make up roughly three quarters of the undocumented population and have consistently had the highest uninsured rate of any racial/ethnic group.[4] These disparities stem from federal policies that exclude immigrants from Medicaid and Medicare or impose eligibility barriers and waiting periods, such as the five-year delay for "lawfully present" immigrants seeking federally funded Medicaid. Access to health insurance is essential not only for individual health and well-being but also for economic productivity and the financial protection of households.

Before the 2000s, circular or temporary migration helped ease health care demand, as many aging immigrants returned to their home countries.[2] However, between 2000 and 2024, immigrants became more likely to settle in the United States and are aging faster than US-born adults.

FULL-SCOPE MEDICAL EXPANSION

To support California's growing population of aging uninsured immigrants, the state expanded full-scope Medi-Cal (its Medicaid program) in May 2022 to provide coverage to undocumented immigrant adults aged 50 years and older. "Full scope" refers to the comprehensive health care coverage that includes a wide array of services, going beyond just emergency care, and encompassing medical, dental, mental health, vision, and substance use disorder services. This state-funded initiative circumvents federal restrictions on Medi-Cal funding. California had previously expanded full-scope Medi-Cal to all children (0–18 years) in 2015 and to young adults (19–25 years) in 2020. The final expansion, which covers undocumented adults aged 26 to 49 years, took effect in 2024. With this expansion, all income-eligible adults, regardless of documentation status, can enroll in full-scope Medi-Cal.[5]

As of January 2025, 14 states (CA, CO, CT, IL, MA, ME, MN, NJ, NY, OR, RI, UT, VT, WA) and Washington, DC, provide coverage for children, two states (NJ, VT) provide coverage for pregnant individuals, six states (CA, CO, IL, MN, OR, WA) provide coverage for adults, and one state (NY) provides coverage for adults aged 65 years and older, regardless of documentation status.[6]

CALIFORNIA VERSUS OREGON

In this issue of *AJPH*, Huguet et al. (p. 900) compared the impact of state-level Medicaid expansions in California and Oregon, which in 2021 offered coverage to adults aged 50 years and older regardless of documentation status. The authors used a difference-in-difference design with electronic health records from community health centers to determine changes in reported rates of Medicaid, privately insured, and uninsured visits likely resulting from these policies.

Because they were unable to determine immigration status from the data, they focused on Latinos, who represent a significant portion of the immigrant population. Their main findings indicate that the policies led to increases in Medicaid-insured visits and decreases in uninsured visits, which aligns with the policies' intent. In addition, the authors used language preference as an indirect measure of citizenship status and found positive results. Some Spanish-speaking citizens in the study may have already qualified for Medicaid, potentially weakening the measured effect. These findings suggest that the connection between Medicaid enrollment and coverage outcomes may be even stronger. The study offers insights for state governments on the effects of such policies and the potential coverage gains, particularly for those aged 50 years and older.

Huguet et al. highlight that the effect was more pronounced among Spanish-preferring Latinos, suggesting that addressing this population's mistrust of health care could improve take-up. The findings are consistent with recent studies that have identified access to care barriers, such as delays and worse experiences of care, among Spanish-preferring Latinos.[7,8] Additionally, the effects of Medicaid expansion were strongest in its third year, indicating that policy implementation and enrollment awareness took some time to materialize. Medicaid expansion policies for undocumented immigrants may still face challenges, such as those related to language, technology access, funding restrictions, eligibility awareness, and restrictive immigration policies (e.g., the "public charge" rule and increased deportations).[9]

An important finding in the study is that, despite increases in Medicaid enrollment in both states following Medicaid expansion, the uninsured rate did not decrease to zero. Some community health center users may have been above the federal poverty line eligibility and thereby ineligible for Medicaid regardless of the expansion. Additionally, take-up among the Latino community may not have been optimal. This could be because of factors such as anti-immigrant rhetoric in the United States, perceived discrimination and mistrust of health care, and fears of detection and deportation regardless of state law.

MEDICAID EXPANSION

The findings of Huguet et al. underscore the urgent need for state policies that expand Medicaid regardless of documentation status. The uninsured rate for Spanish-preferring individuals aged 50 years and older in states without the eligibility expansion was estimated to be approximately 42% to 49% between the pre- and postamendment periods, which is alarmingly high. This issue is particularly salient now, as anti-immigrant rhetoric is more prevalent than ever, which further increases distrust in health care and exacerbates health inequities among immigrant populations.

Medicaid expansions for undocumented immigrants are beneficial for states that implement them. From a population health perspective, research has shown a link between increased health coverage and better health outcomes.[10] Expansions would improve health outcomes among immigrants and reduce the inequities they face. Additionally, immigrants have lower coverage costs than do their US-born counterparts, suggesting little risk of increasing costs.[11] Lastly, and most importantly, from a human rights perspective, health care is a fundamental right. Medicaid expansion policies support all of these goals, and states should continue to implement them.

Even in California and Oregon, implementation variation across counties could have contributed to lower enrollment in Medicaid or access to and utilization of health care in community health centers. When implementing these policies, states should be mindful of immigrant mistrust of the government. They should design outreach strategies and messaging that address fears arising from mis- and disinformation about the program's intent.[5]

As undocumented immigrants in the United States age, their need to access the health care system will increase. Nevertheless, they remain ineligible to enroll in Medicare and are likely to continue being ineligible in the foreseeable future, despite many having contributed to the tax base during their productive lives. If current trends persist, as undocumented immigrant populations age, they will have to rely on health insurance options offered by state and local governments, such as Medicaid-like programs and safety net facilities.

Medicaid faces potential cuts in 2025, which could destabilize state finances and leave many, including undocumented immigrants recently enrolled in Medicaid-like programs, without coverage. A sudden cut in Medicaid funding could strain the financial stability of community health centers and increase demand from uninsured individuals. As policymakers debate Medicaid funding, the article by Huguet et al. highlights that preserving and expanding coverage of Medicaid-like programs to undocumented immigrants benefits the community. AJPH

CORRESPONDENCE

Correspondence should be sent to Arturo Vargas Bustamante, PhD, Professor, Department of Health Policy & Management, UCLA Fielding School of Public Health, 650 Charles E. Young Dr South, Room 31-245, Los Angeles, CA 90095 (e-mail: avb@ucla.edu). Reprints can be ordered at https://www.ajph.org by clicking the "Reprints" link.

PUBLICATION INFORMATION

Full Citation: Bustamante AV, Chowdhury M, Ortega AN. Expanding Medicaid for undocumented immigrants: a path to better coverage and population health. *Am J Public Health*. 2025;115(6):830–832.

Acceptance Date: March 18, 2025.

DOI: https://doi.org/10.2105/AJPH.2025.308131

ORCID iDs:

Arturo Vargas Bustamante https://orcid.org/0000-0003-0414-5015

Marvin Chowdhury https://orcid.org/0009-0007-5273-6019

Alexander N. Ortega https://orcid.org/0000-0001-6861-6993

CONTRIBUTORS

All authors contributed to writing this editorial.

ACKNOWLEDGMENTS

This editorial was supported by the National Institute on Minority Health and Health Disparities, National Institutes of Health (NIH; award R01MD018727).

Note. The content is solely the responsibility of the authors and does not necessarily represent the official views of the NIH.

CONFLICT OF INTERESTS

The authors have no conflicts of interest to disclose.

REFERENCES

1. Sherman A, Trisi D, Stone C, Gonzales S, Parrot S. Immigrants contribute greatly to US economy, despite administration's "public charge" rule rationale. Available at: https://www.cbpp.org/research/poverty-and-inequality/immigrants-contribute-greatly-to-us-economy-despite-administrations. Accessed February 20, 2025.
2. Bustamante AV, Chen J, Beltrán FL, Ortega AN. Health policy challenges posed by shifting demographics and health trends among immigrants to the United States. *Health Aff (Millwood)*. 2021;40(7):1028–1037. https://doi.org/10.1377/hlthaff.2021.00037
3. Kaiser Family Foundation. Key facts on health coverage of immigrants. January 15, 2025. Available at: https://www.kff.org/racial-equity-and-health-policy/fact-sheet/key-facts-on-health-coverage-of-immigrants. Accessed February 20, 2025.
4. Ortega AN, Chen J, Roby DH, Mortensen K, Rivera-González AC, Bustamante AV. Changes in coverage and cost-related delays in care for Latino individuals after elimination of the Affordable Care Act's individual mandate. *JAMA Netw Open*. 2022;5(3):e221476. https://doi.org/10.1001/jamanetworkopen.2022.1476
5. Bustamante AV, Beltrán FL, Cuadros NN, Zeng XL, González SR. Implementation lessons from the 2022 Medi-Cal expansion to undocumented adults aged fifty and above. July 13, 2023. Available at: https://latino.ucla.edu/research/lessons-2022-adult-medical-expansion. Accessed February 20, 2025.
6. Pillai A, Pillai D, Artia S. State health coverage for immigrants and implications for health coverage and care. Available at: https://www.kff.org/racial-equity-and-health-policy/issue-brief/state-health-coverage-for-immigrants-and-implications-for-health-coverage-and-care. Accessed February 20, 2025.
7. Bustamante AV, Melgoza E, Ismail A, Majano R, Félix Beltrán L. Bridging language barriers: access to primary care for Medicaid Managed Care patients with limited English proficiency in three metropolitan areas. *Health Aff Sch*. 2025;3(2):qxaf025. https://doi.org/10.1093/haschl/qxaf025
8. Melgoza E, Ismail A, Félix-Beltrán L, Majano R, Bustamante AV. A qualitative mystery shopper study that de(codes) the experiences of English and Spanish-speaking patients who call to schedule a first-time primary care appointment in the Los Angeles, Houston, and New York metropolitan statistical areas. *SSM Qual Res Health*. 2025;7:100525. https://doi.org/10.1016/j.ssmqr.2025.100525
9. Bustamante AV, Félix-Beltrán L, Nwadiuko J, Ortega AN. Avoiding Medicaid enrollment after the reversal of the changes in the public charge rule among Latino and Asian immigrants. *Health Serv Res*. 2022;57(suppl 2):195–203. https://doi.org/10.1111/1475-6773.14020
10. Lopez Mercado D, Rivera-González AC, Stimpson JP, et al. Undocumented Latino immigrants and the Latino health paradox. *Am J Prev Med*. 2023;65(2):296–306. https://doi.org/10.1016/j.amepre.2023.02.010
11. Zallman L, Woolhandler S, Touw S, Himmelstein DU, Finnegan KE. Immigrants pay more in private insurance premiums than they receive in benefits. *Health Aff (Millwood)*. 2018 Oct;37(10):1663–1668. https://doi.org/10.1377/hlthaff.2018.0309

Does Medicaid Improve Health?

Heidi Allen, MSW, PhD

ABOUT THE AUTHOR

Heidi Allen is an associate professor in the School of Social Work at Columbia University in the City of New York.

See also Han et al., p. 890.

This perennial policy question has resurfaced, particularly after the US House of Representatives recently passed a budget blueprint tasking the committee overseeing Medicaid and Medicare with cutting $880 billion over the next 10 years.[1] This issue was also a focal point during state deliberations on whether to adopt Medicaid expansions under the Affordable Care Act (ACA). Since the ACA's passage in 2015, 40 states and the District of Columbia have expanded Medicaid, with a few adopting it through citizen ballot initiatives, while 10 states have not.[2] Because of the staggered implementation of Medicaid expansion, Medicaid is far more studied than other forms of coverage. Whether this focus is fair or not is debatable,[3] but Medicaid skeptics often cite research my colleagues and I conducted 15 years ago—the Oregon Health Insurance Experiment (OHIE)—as evidence against expansion. More recently, some have used this research to justify targeting Medicaid spending[4] to offset the continuation of the 2017 tax cuts, which disproportionately benefit higher-income Americans.

The OHIE leveraged an Oregon lottery in 2008 to allocate 10 000 Medicaid slots, allowing us to estimate the causal impact of Medicaid on uninsured nonelderly adults. Our findings showed that, compared with being uninsured, Medicaid increased health care utilization across all types of care, improved self-reported health, reduced clinical depression, and improved financial stability.[5] However, we found no statistically significant differences in blood sugar control, high blood pressure, or cholesterol.[6] Mortality is a rare event among nonelderly adults (0.8% of our control sample died during the study period), and while our non–statistically significant point estimates suggested a reduction in mortality attributable to Medicaid, the wide confidence intervals indicated that we lacked the power to draw any conclusions.[5]

One key takeaway from the OHIE is that Medicaid did what insurance is supposed to do: it increased access to care and protected the finances of low-income adults. Although we did not observe improvements in specific metrics like diabetes or blood pressure control, the improvements we did see in self-reported health are significant and offer a broader picture of Medicaid's impact. Increases in health care utilization are suggestive of better long-term health outcomes, but more research was needed. Fortunately, this is not the end of the causal empirical basis for understanding the relationship between Medicaid and health outcomes.

MEDICAID'S IMPACT ON MORTALITY

In the past 15 years, several rigorous studies have been conducted with sufficient power to detect population-level health improvements associated with Medicaid—most importantly, its effects on mortality. For instance, Sommers et al. found a 6.1% relative reduction in mortality when comparing a 10-year cohort of individuals in three Medicaid expansion states compared with neighboring states without expansion.[7] Miller et al. linked large-scale federal survey data with administrative death records and similarly estimated a 9.4% reduction in mortality related to Medicaid expansion.[8] Wherry and Meyer used a regression discontinuity approach from a Medicaid expansion that only applied to children born after a certain date and found a 13% to 20% reduction in mortality rates among Black adolescents later in life.[9]

A timely and rigorous study in this issue of *AJPH* further strengthens this accumulating body of evidence, focusing on Medicaid's role during the COVID-19 pandemic. In just under two weeks at the start of the pandemic, 9 million Americans filed for unemployment, and employment trends did not return to normal until 2022.[10] In the United States, employment is closely tied to both income and health insurance. This poses a unique test of Medicaid as part of the safety net.

In their study, reported in this issuer of *AJPH*, Han et al. (p. 890) used data from the National Center for Health Statistics and the National Cancer Institute's Surveillance, Epidemiology, and End Results (SEER) Program Mortality database to compare mortality trends in Medicaid expansion versus nonexpansion states during the pandemic. They found that while all-cause mortality increased among adults aged 20 to 64 years during the pandemic, the rise was slower in Medicaid expansion states than in nonexpansion states. Specifically, they found that Medicaid expansion was associated with a net decrease of 31.8 deaths per 100 000 person-years following the pandemic, compared with mortality rates in nonexpansion states. This difference in trends was statistically significant overall and for deaths related to chronic illnesses like heart and liver disease, though similar non–statistically significant trends were observed for 11 of 14 major causes of death. The protective effect of Medicaid was consistent across age, sex, and race.

POLICY CONSIDERATION FOR LIFE-SAVING POTENTIAL OF MEDICAID

This study is significant for several reasons. First, because Medicaid expansions are funded at 90% by the federal government, and the federal government can run deficits while most states are constitutionally required to maintain a balanced budget, the program was able to grow in response to the increased need caused by rising unemployment. This was not the case in nonexpansion states, where Medicaid eligibility remained limited.[11] Current Republican proposals to change the federal share of Medicaid expansion could place additional pressure on states during times of economic insecurity, such as public health emergencies, national recessions, or natural disasters. In fact, 12 states have "trigger laws" that could end Medicaid expansion if the federal cost-sharing parameters change.[12]

Second, consider a counterfactual scenario in which Medicaid work requirements were in place during the COVID-19 pandemic. Low-income Americans who became uninsured when they lost their jobs would have been further penalized by these requirements. This study suggests that if COVID-19 did not claim their lives, chronic diseases and other health issues could have. Third, this study highlights the benefits of continuous Medicaid coverage, which was especially relevant during the pandemic when re-enrollment requirements were paused and people did not churn off and on the program because of minor fluctuations in income or the administrative burden of reapplying.

Finally, it is important to consider that mortality before the age of 65 years is considered premature—13 years below the US life expectancy and more than 15 years below that of the United Kingdom, a country with a universal health insurance scheme.[13] Excess mortality because of uninsurance represents more than a decade of time lost with family and loved ones. With 10 states still refusing to expand Medicaid and the program under significant legislative threat, this research serves as a reminder that Medicaid is a crucial part of the public health safety net and, quite literally, saves lives. AJPH

CORRESPONDENCE

Correspondence should be sent to Heidi Allen, 1255 Amsterdam Ave, New York, NY 10027 (e-mail: ha2332@columbia.edu). Reprints can be ordered at https://www.ajph.org by clicking the "Reprints" link.

PUBLICATION INFORMATION

Full Citation: Allen H. Does medicaid improve health? *Am J Public Health*. 2025;115(6):833–834.

Acceptance Date: March 15, 2025.

DOI: https://doi.org/10.2105/AJPH.2025.308124

CONFLICTS OF INTEREST

H. Allen reports no conflicts of interest related to this editorial.

REFERENCES

1. To make their numbers work, Republicans must slash health spending. *The Economist*. February 27, 2025. Available at: https://www.economist.com/united-states/2025/02/27/to-make-their-numbers-work-republicans-must-slash-health-spending?giftId=ac99cd9f-833e-4754-a56d-3c3d061f1307&utm_campaign=gifted_article. Accessed March 7, 2025.
2. KFF. Status of state Medicaid expansion decisions. February 12, 2025. Available at: https://www.kff.org/status-of-state-medicaid-expansion-decisions. Accessed March 7, 2025.
3. Allen HL. Medicaid's heavy lift. *Milbank Q*. 2019;97(4):935–938. https://doi.org/10.1111/1468-0009.12433
4. Critics of Medicaid point to a rigorous study conducted 15 years ago. *The Economist*. February 27, 2025. Available at: https://www.economist.com/united-states/2025/02/27/critics-of-medicaid-point-to-a-rigorous-study-conducted-15-years-ago. Accessed March 7, 2025.
5. Finkelstein A, Taubman S, Wright B, et al. The Oregon Health Insurance Experiment: evidence from the first year. *Q J Econ*. 2012;127(3):1057–1106. https://doi.org/10.1093/qje/qjs020
6. Baicker K, Taubman SL, Allen HL, et al. The Oregon experiment—effects of Medicaid on clinical outcomes. *N Engl J Med*. 2013;368(18):1713–1722. https://doi.org/10.1056/NEJMsa1212321
7. Sommers BD, Baicker K, Epstein AM. Mortality and access to care among adults after state Medicaid expansions. *N Engl J Med*. 2012;367(11):1025–1034. https://doi.org/10.1056/NEJMsa1202099
8. Miller S, Johnson N, Wherry LR. Medicaid and mortality: new evidence from linked survey and administrative data. *Q J Econ*. 2021;136(3):1783–1829. https://doi.org/10.1093/qje/qjab004
9. Wherry LR, Meyer BD. Saving teens: using a policy discontinuity to estimate the effects of Medicaid eligibility. *J Hum Resour*. 2016;51(3):556–588. https://doi.org/10.3368/jhr.51.3.0913-5918R1
10. Bhatia A, Cabreros I. 30 charts that show how Covid changed everything in March 2020. *New York Times*. March 10, 2025. Available at: https://www.nytimes.com/interactive/2025/03/09/upshot/covid-lockdown-five-year-charts.html. Accessed March 10, 2025.
11. Shafer PR, Anderson DM, Whitaker R, Wong CA, Wright B. Association of unemployment with Medicaid enrollment by social vulnerability in North Carolina during COVID-19. *Health Aff (Millwood)*. 2021;40(9):1491–1500. https://doi.org/10.1377/hlthaff.2021.00377
12. Tolbert J, Bell C, Rudowitz R. Medicaid expansion is a red and blue state issue. KFF. November 27, 2024. Available at: https://www.kff.org/medicaid/issue-brief/medicaid-expansion-is-a-red-and-blue-state-issue. Accessed March 17, 2025.
13. Bloomberg American Health Initiative. 2024 Life Expectancy Report. Available at: https://americanhealth.jhu.edu/2024-life-expectancy-report. Accessed March 8, 2025.

Medical Providers Require Support and Training for Legislative Testimony About Abortion and High-Risk Pregnancy Care

Clare Daniel, PhD, Grace Riley, MPH, Anita Raj, MS, PhD, and Cecilia Gambala, MD

ABOUT THE AUTHORS

Clare Daniel and Anita Raj are with the Newcomb Institute, Tulane University, New Orleans, LA. Grace Riley is a medical student at Rush Medical College, Rush University, Chicago, IL. Cecilia Gambala is with the School of Medicine, Tulane University, New Orleans, LA.

In 2022, the US Supreme Court set a landmark decision in *Dobbs v Jackson Women's Health* that ended federal protections for abortion rights and resulted in abortion bans that target medical providers for criminalization.[1] Since then, advocates and legislators in abortion-ban states have leveraged the testimony of medical providers in legislative debates related to abortion and high-risk pregnancy. Examination of these testimonies is limited, but our recent analysis of provider testimonies in the 2023 Louisiana legislative session reveals important insights and recommendations for supporting provider engagement in legislative testimony, as well as the need for further research to inform how to effectively engage providers in policy debates around these laws.

Louisiana has been at the forefront of creating highly restrictive and punitive legislation for abortion patients and providers, both before and after *Dobbs*. Louisiana's current abortion legislation, in effect as of 2022, bans abortion in all cases except to save the pregnant person's life or when the fetus is deemed "medically futile." The law contains penalties for providers of up to 15 years in prison and up to $200 000 in fines.

We identified three bills in the 2023 Louisiana legislative session related to the abortion ban that dealt significantly with the patient and provider relationship and provider penalties in cases of abortion and high-risk pregnancy care. Each bill sought to improve providers' ability to care for pregnant patients under the abortion ban: HB 461 amends vague language relative to exceptions to the state abortion ban, HB 522 reduces penalties associated with the state abortion ban, and HB 598 amends the state abortion ban to add clarity around serious pregnancy complications.

We examined the debate transcripts, obtained from videos of the debates that are publicly available, using a critical discourse analysis methodology to understand how language is used in such debates to promote specific understanding of and approaches to social issues.[2–4] We examined medical providers' testimony (including 10 physicians and one nurse practitioner) for and against each bill, and we evaluated the providers' characteristics, the language and arguments they used, and legislators' questions and responses.

WHAT PROVIDERS ARE TESTIFYING AND WHAT IS THEIR ROLE?

In each debate, a relatively large portion of those who testified orally or were quoted in oral testimony were clinicians (HB 461: four of 12; HB 522: five of 10; HB 598: five of seven), highlighting how legislators and advocates valued their testimony. A greater number of providers testified in support of each of these bills than in opposition. The total time spent by providers testifying in support of these bills was 49 minutes and 19 seconds, as compared with 7 minutes and 14 seconds spent by providers testifying in opposition.

Providers who testified for versus against these bills differed in terms of qualifications and demographic characteristics (Table 1). Of the six medical providers in support of the bills, all had active relevant Louisiana licenses and were employed providers at the time of their testimony. All six were women, and three were providers of color. Of the five who testified or were quoted in opposition, two did not an have active Louisiana medical license and three were not employed as a medical provider at the time. Four of these providers were men and all five were White.

AJPH June 2025, Vol. 115, No. 6

TABLE 1— Provider Characteristics and Qualifications: New Orleans, Louisiana, January–October 2024

	Medical Provider	Bill(s)	Gender	Race	Provider Specialty	Active Louisiana Medical License	Employed as a Health Provider	Parish	Type of Facility Where Provider Works/Worked	No. of Abortion News Quotes (June 2022–June 2023)
Testified in support[a]	Provider A, MD	HB 461, HB 522, HB 598	Female	White	OB/GYN	Yes	Yes	Orleans	Teaching hospital	15
	Provider B, MD	HB 461, HB 598	Female	White	Emergency medicine	Yes	Yes	Orleans	Local health department and teaching hospital	23
	Provider C, MD	HB 522	Female	Asian Indian	OB/GYN	Yes	Yes	East Baton Rouge	Teaching hospital	0
	Provider D, MD	HB 522	Female	White	Emergency medicine	Yes	Yes	Orleans	Teaching hospital	0
	Provider E, FNP-C	HB 598	Female	Black	Family medicine	Yes	Yes	Orleans	Outpatient clinic	1
Quoted in support	Provider F, MD	HB 461	Female	Black	OB/GYN	Yes	Yes	Ouachita	State health department and outpatient clinic	1
Testified against	Provider G, MD	HB 522	Female	White	OB/GYN	Yes	Yes	East Baton Rouge	Non-teaching hospital	5
	Provider H, MD	HB 522	Male	White	OB/GYN	Yes	No	Lafayette	Non-teaching hospital and outpatient clinic	2
Quoted against	Provider I, MD	HB 461	Male	White	OB/GYN	No	No	Jefferson	Teaching hospital	3
	Provider J, MD	HB 598	Male	White	OB/GYN	Yes	Yes	Lafayette	Outpatient clinic	20
	Provider K, MD	HB 598	Male	White	OB/GYN	No	No	N/A	Teaching hospital	≥50

Note. OB/GYN = obstetrics/gynecology.
[a]Most providers testified in person at the legislature, but in a few cases, providers submitted statements to be read by a proxy. In these cases, we note whether providers were being quoted in support or quoted against.

Many of the providers had repeatedly publicly established their positions on the topic of abortion, meaning that legislators may have been familiar with their stances before they even spoke. This familiarity may mean that the testimonies serve more to reinforce existing beliefs than to sway undecided lawmakers, highlighting the polarized nature of the abortion debate.[5]

Legislators often struggle to understand the nuanced medical terminology and the specific circumstances under which providers operate. We also found that providers speaking in support of these bills sometimes addressed issues not directly targeted by the bill at hand. This may have been due to providers' misunderstanding of the specific bill, or it may have been unintentional digression; in either case, however, it seemed to create a misalignment between how legislators and providers who were otherwise allied described the current law and its implications, leading to misunderstanding, confusion, or skepticism.

WHAT ARE THEY SAYING ABOUT PREGNANCY?

The testimonies from providers supporting these bills reveal a pattern of contradictions regarding the clarity and interpretation of the legislation, further complicated by the inherent uncertainty in medical prognoses and diagnoses.[6] In contrast to the providers testifying in opposition to these bills, those testifying in support emphasized the uniqueness of each medical situation and the necessity for physician discretion and expert judgment. However, they also made conflicting claims about the clarity of existing laws.

For instance, in this exchange during the debate around HB 522, provider A emphasizes medical uncertainty and the uniqueness of each pregnancy:

> Representative 4: Personal experience, I have my middle son, he's in his 30s now. About halfway through the pregnancy, we were advised that he had certain conditions. One doctor told us he had certain conditions which he would not survive, hydrocephaly, among other things. And guess what? Against the recommendations of the doctor, we did not have an abortion. One doctor, he survived, and guess what? He's fine. . . but if we had listened to one doctor's advice, we would have aborted a healthy son. Is that something you might?
>
> Provider A: No, that is nothing that I ever would want—to put a patient in that situation, but I think what's important is to be able to present all of the information and to say, these are the possibilities in medicine. We often say there's no 0% or 100%. Unfortunately, things are just almost never as black and white as that. And if I present all the possibilities of what could happen, both in good outcomes, like in your son, but also in bad outcomes, I think that the patient needs to decide.

However, earlier in that same debate, provider A stated:

> I can't speak for every single one of my colleagues, but we do not want to be in a criminalization environment, having that over our heads when we're in the exam room with our patients, when we're making these decisions that have to be made in very short split second intervals to save a life or to make the correct decision so that you don't cause any harm to the patient that's in front of you. And I think that for myself, I've been very lucky. I've had a lot of lawyers going over the laws, and I know exactly what I can and can't do within the laws.

The idea that each pregnancy is unique and that providers must assess the probability of morbidities or mortality was discussed in the first example as an argument for why the current law is inadequate in terms of protecting the lives of pregnant patients. However, the second example, although it deals with a different medical issue, suggests that an appropriate amount of physician education on the current law can clarify the legality of care in every situation, which undermines the claim that the bill is necessary to add clarity to the law.

These conflicting statements also highlight a deeper issue: the principle that medical diagnosis and treatment inherently involve uncertainty.[7] As provider A noted, there are rarely absolute certainties in medicine. This fundamental aspect of medical practice means that providers must often make decisions based on probabilities and the best available information.[8] The inability to be 100% certain in any medical diagnosis complicates the legal landscape for abortion care. For instance, according to Louisiana's abortion ban, a licensed physician can use "reasonable medical judgment" to determine whether a procedure is medically necessary to "prevent the death or substantial risk of death due to a physical condition, or to prevent the serious, permanent impairment of a life-sustaining organ of a pregnant woman."[9] With imprisonment as a potential consequence for violation of the law, the question of what "reasonable" means and who defines it can become a source of great fear and anxiety among physicians, compromising care for pregnant patients.[10,11]

WHAT ARE THEY SAYING ABOUT THE FETUS AND LIFE?

Medical providers on both sides of the debates frequently used fetal personhood terminology, such as referring to a fetus as a baby or child, reinforcing legislators' "pro-life" beliefs.[12,13] Although providers speaking in support of the legislation used this terminology fewer times per minute, they referred to a fetus as a baby or child 11 times throughout the bill testimonies, in comparison with only three times among those in opposition.

For instance, a provider speaking in support of HB 461 stated that "At 20 weeks of pregnancy, I was in severe pain, carrying the baby and two watermelon-sized cysts." Likewise, according to a different provider speaking in support of HB 522:

> Patients come to me who have been turned away at other hospitals bleeding profusely in a miscarriage process that there's no way to save the pregnancy. Unfortunately, there's nothing you can do; this woman is hemorrhaging, but the baby still had a heartbeat, so they did nothing to help her.

In both of these cases, providers used the term "baby" instead of "fetus" and in the second example the provider used the term "heartbeat" instead of the more accurate "cardiac activity." The use of fetal personhood language arguably further entrenches the focus on fetal rights rather than facilitating a clearer understanding of the medical nuances involved in pregnancy care and abortion legislation.

LIMITATIONS AND RECOMMENDATIONS

Medical provider testimony is invaluable for legislatures considering abortion-related bills. Providers may be more willing to engage in this time-consuming process given the impact of these bills on their patients' health and on their medical practice. This analysis suggests that medical providers are taking the time to testify on these bills.

The insights from our research should be considered in light of certain limitations. Louisiana is an exceptionally conservative state on the issue of abortion, so our findings may not be generalizable to all other states. We also identified three debates, and this legislative space continues to evolve as states grapple with restrictions that are legislatively supported but are compromising care and resulting in loss of providers.[11] Furthermore, each of the three bills failed, impeding our ability to determine how physician testimony can aid in the passage of bills that are supportive of abortion access.

Despite these limitations, our research illuminates some points that may by useful at a time of rapid legislative activity surrounding providers' roles and potential culpability in states with abortion bans. We found that providers are willing to testify despite hectic work schedules and the need, for many, to travel to legislative sites outside of their own city. More training and support may be needed for these providers to facilitate success but also simply to sustain efforts for providers to speak out against their criminalization when they are implementing evidence-based care. Further research is needed to understand how provider testimony functions in other state contexts and over time in Louisiana as well as the role of advocates in recruiting and preparing providers for testimony. Nonetheless, we offer the following recommendations to support provider engagement in legislative testimony on abortion:

1. Advocates and providers should be aware that legislators may value providers' expert testimony and that lawmakers on all sides of abortion debates can be open to provider expertise on how to support patients and high-risk pregnancies.
2. Legislators and advocates should be educated on the importance of prioritizing the testimony of employed providers, who manage difficult work schedules to provide this testimony, over retired or unemployed providers who may be more available but less aware of the current impact of these bans.
3. Efforts should be made to recruit new providers to testify publicly on the issue of abortion, as legislators may be more open to new voices and especially residents of their districts.
4. Providers could benefit from in-depth preparation to ensure that:
   a. Their messages emphasize known outcomes of abortion bans such as delayed care and the likelihood of maternal complications and maternal and infant death.
   b. They have an opportunity in advance of their testimony to discuss the proposed bill with key legislators or advocates to understand what major points

are needed for legislator clarity on the potential ramifications of the proposed bill.

c. They are comfortable and in agreement with terminology that is aligned with medical understandings of the processes of pregnancy rather than, for instance, using fetal personhood language. Evidence indicates that fetal personhood language drives antiabortion sentiment, whereas a focus on medical expertise may drive support for abortion access.[12,14] Clarity on optimal language for a lay audience may be helpful for providers seeking to communicate with legislators about abortion access or restrictions. AJPH

CORRESPONDENCE

Correspondence should be sent to Clare Daniel, Newcomb Institute, 43 Newcomb Pl, Tulane University, New Orleans, LA 70118 (e-mail: cdaniel5@tulane.edu). Reprints can be ordered at https://www.ajph.org by clicking the "Reprints" link.

PUBLICATION INFORMATION

Full Citation: Daniel C, Riley G, Raj A, Gambala C. Medical providers require support and training for legislative testimony about abortion and high-risk pregnancy care. *Am J Public Health*. 2025;115(6):835–839.

Acceptance Date: January 17, 2025.

DOI: https://doi.org/10.2105/AJPH.2025.308035

ORCID iDs:

Clare Daniel https://orcid.org/0000-0002-5360-599X

Grace Riley https://orcid.org/0009-0009-8434-6378

Cecilia Gambala https://orcid.org/0009-0002-6123-6466

CONTRIBUTORS

All of the authors collaborated on the conceptualization of the project. C. Daniel and G. Riley provided the original outline for the article, completed the initial writing, obtained the data, devised the coding scheme, and verified coding through validation checks. A. Raj and C. Gambala contributed to the drafting and revision of the article.

ACKNOWLEDGMENTS

We thank Tulane University's Center for Public Service and Newcomb Institute for supporting this research. We are grateful to the anonymous reviewers and the *AJPH* editor-in-chief for their valuable comments.

CONFLICTS OF INTEREST

The authors report that there are no competing interests to disclose.

REFERENCES

1. Guttmacher Institute. State bans on abortion throughout pregnancy. Available at: https://www.guttmacher.org/state-policy/explore/state-policies-abortion-bans. Accessed September 22, 2024.
2. Evans-Agnew RA, Johnson S, Liu F, Boutain DM. Applying critical discourse analysis in health policy research: case studies in regional, organizational, and global health. *Policy Polit Nurs Pract*. 2016;17(3):136–146. https://doi.org/10.1177/1527154416669355
3. Dalglish SL, Khalid H, McMahon SA. Document analysis in health policy research: the READ approach. *Health Policy Plan*. 2021;35(10):1424–1431. https://doi.org/10.1093/heapol/czaa064
4. Isaacs A. An overview of qualitative research methodology for public health researchers. *Int J Med Public Health*. 2014;4(4):318–323. https://doi.org/10.4103/2230-8598.144055
5. Peterson M. The limits of social learning: translating analysis into action. *J Health Polit Policy Law*. 1997;22(4):1077–1114. https://doi.org/10.1215/03616878-22-4-1077
6. Han PKJ, Strout TD, Gutheil C, et al. How physicians manage medical uncertainty: a qualitative study and conceptual taxonomy. *Med Decis Making*. 2021;41(3):275–291. https://doi.org/10.1177/0272989X21992340
7. Malterud K, Guassora AD, Reventlow S, Jutel A. Embracing uncertainty to advance diagnosis in general practice. *Br J Gen Pract*. 2017;67(659):244–245. https://doi.org/10.3399/bjgp17X690941
8. Guileyardo JM. Probability and uncertainty in clinical and forensic medicine. *Proc Bayl Univ Med Cent*. 2015;28(2):247–249. https://doi.org/10.1080/08998280.2015.11929244
9. Louisiana State Legislature. Human Life Protection Act, R.S. 40:1061. Available at: https://legis.la.gov/legis/Law.aspx?d=97020. Accessed September 22, 2024.
10. Schultz A, Smith C, Johnson M, Bryant A, Buchbinder M. Impact of post-*Dobbs* abortion restrictions on maternal-fetal medicine physicians in the Southeast: a qualitative study. *Am J Obstet Gynecol MFM*. 2024;6(7):101387. https://doi.org/10.1016/j.ajogmf.2024.101387
11. Center for Reproductive Rights. Criminalized care: how Louisiana's abortion bans endanger patients and clinicians. Available at: https://reproductiverights.org/louisiana-abortion-bans-criminalized-care-report. Accessed September 22, 2024.
12. Halva-Neubauer G, Zeigler S. Promoting fetal personhood: the rhetorical and legislative strategies of the pro-life movement after Planned Parenthood v. Casey. *Fem Formations*. 2010;22(2):101–123. https://doi.org/10.1353/ff.2010.0011
13. Bueno X, LaRoche KJ, Crawford BL, Turner RC, Lo WJ, Jozkowski KN. Do fetal development markers influence attitudes toward abortion legality? *Soc Currents*. 2023;10(2):107–120. https://doi.org/10.1177/23294965221137830
14. Hawbaker A, Paiz JY, Crawford BL, Turner RC, Jozkowski KN. Medicine and abortion: public trust in medical authority and Americans' acceptance of legal abortion. *SSM Qual Res Health*. 2023;4:100361. https://doi.org/10.1016/j.ssmqr.2023.100361

The Public Health Workforce Beyond Government Health Departments: Proposing a New Definition

Heather Krasna, PhD, EdM, MS

ABOUT THE AUTHOR

The author is with the Mailman School of Public Health, Columbia University, New York, NY.

AJPH June 2025, Vol. 115, No. 6

Who makes up the public health workforce? Without a clear definition, it is impossible to know how many people make up the workforce, whether there are enough of them to provide essential public health services, whether the workers are paid appropriately, whether essential workers have been replaced by temporary staff, and ultimately whether our nation will be protected from future health calamities.

Although the public health workforce is acknowledged to be much broader, research on the workforce focuses almost exclusively on local, state, tribal, or territorial governmental health departments.[1] Previous constructs of the public health workforce in the United States have acknowledged that individuals in many sectors contribute to public health,[2,3] including "those who work for official public health agencies at all levels of government, community-based and voluntary organizations with a health promotion focus, the public health-related staff of hospitals and health care systems, and a range of others in private industry, government, and the voluntary sector."[3]

In other countries including the United Kingdom, the public health workforce is described differently, with the "core" workforce[4] comprising both government and academia, and a "wider" workforce[5] defined as "non–health sector professionals including actors from other sectors whose decisions and actions positively affect health."[6] Other definitions of the public health workforce have been used in different countries; for example, some studies have defined the workforce as based on employer type alone (e.g., employees of a local health center), by the functions that workers perform (e.g., workers who perform public health functions), or by the workers' previous training (e.g., workers with a public health degree).[7]

One study in the Netherlands included workers who performed specific functions for more than half an hour per week, and a study in Hawaii incorporated a conceptual definition of a public health worker as "anyone who works with groups and/or communities to protect, promote, or advance health/wellness."[7(p4)] Public health in the United States is considered an intersectional field comprising different occupations and sectors, and more than 70 different occupations have been identified within the governmental public health workforce alone.[8] Focusing only on occupation or job function is not a feasible way to define the workforce; calculating the number of nurses overall, for example, does not provide information on the number of public health nurses.[9] However, there are certain occupations (e.g., occupational health specialists) that arguably should be included as public health occupations, even if few of those in the profession work in health departments.

This article proposes a new, intersectional definition of the public health workforce in the United States. The core workforce, in alignment with past definitions, would continue to consist of those employed in government health departments but would include federal, territorial, and tribal health departments in the enumeration. The "wider" public health workforce, however, would be defined as those workers, irrespective of industry, sector, or occupation, for whom 50% or more of their work directly contributes to the Centers for Disease Control and Prevention's 10 Essential Public Health Services[10] or the Foundational Public Health Services.[11]

RATIONALE FOR A NEW DEFINITION

This definition creates a framework for enumerating those who contribute to public health, beyond the current workforce definition, while illuminating the unique role of government. Using this broader definition, researchers can begin to gain a fuller picture of the contributions to public health from sectors beyond government. By naming specific occupations and sectors as part of the public health workforce, those engaged in advocating for public health can include new parties in alliances and coalitions.

In addition, by examining the extent to which certain public health services or functions that had previously been exclusively delivered by government agencies are now outsourced to other sectors such as contractors and consulting firms, researchers can begin to assess whether taxpayer investments in public health activities would perhaps be better spent on hiring permanent government agency staff. Finally, public health academic institutions can begin assessing whether they are meeting their mandate to "educate the educators, practitioners and researchers as well as to prepare public health leaders and managers"[12(p9)] according to whether their graduates actually enter the public health workforce or whether they are "misemployed"[13] in health care, for-profit enterprises, or even in sectors that do not contribute to public health.

NEW DEFINITION BASED ON SERVICES PROVIDED

If public health is defined as "the science and art of preventing disease, prolonging life and promoting health through the organized efforts and informed choices of society, organizations, public and private, communities and individuals"[14(p205)] and "public health workers are defined as all those responsible for providing the essential services of public health regardless of the organization in which they work,"[15(p2)] then we create a broader definition of public health workers by delineating the essential services of public health and then asking who delivers these services.

Rather than enumerating workers by industry or sector, or even by occupation, the new definition would thus propose a more intersectional approach, "reverse engineering" the definition and enumeration of the workforce by assessing which workers contribute to each of the 10 Essential Public Health Services[10] and the Foundational Public Health Services.[11] According to the Centers for Disease Control and prevention, "[t]he 10 Essential Public Health Services provide a framework for public health to protect and promote the health of all people in all communities."[10] Although the Foundational Public Health Services are meant to apply specifically to government health departments and to "define a minimum package of public health capabilities and programs that no jurisdiction can be without,"[11] they could similarly be used to assess which workers contribute to these services beyond government agencies.

ROADMAP FOR IMPLEMENTING THE DEFINITION

To implement this definition, researchers could use an existing crosswalk between the 10 Essential Public Health Services and the Foundational Public Health Services.[16] Similar frameworks have been used in previous research. For example, the Local Public Health System Assessment in Mobilizing for Action through Planning and Partnerships defines "local public health systems" as all entities, agencies, and organizations that affect the health of the public and contribute to essential public health services.[17]

Next, researchers can match the Essential Public Health Services and the Foundational Public Health Services to occupations or job functions and the types of organizations (including those in the government, nonprofit, and for-profit sectors) where the work of the employees might contribute to these services. One way to identify types of organizations conducting each type of service or function would be a brief keyword search of Indeed.com, a large-scale job board. For example, the author conducted a search in November 2022 and assessed which organizations were currently hiring individuals to conduct these services, a method used in other studies.[18]

Each of the 10 Essential Public Health Services and the Foundational Public Health Services are listed in Appendix A (available as a supplement to the online version of this article at http://www.ajph.org), with brief descriptions of the sectors that are most likely to contribute to these services. Appendix B (available as a supplement to the online version of this article at http://www.ajph.org) presents a preliminary schema matching of the 10 Essential Public Health Services and the Foundational Public Health Services, with occupations and organizations within and outside health departments. Each of the Essential Public Health Services is likely to include a different mix of workers and sectors.

For example, Essential Public Health Service 2 is to "investigate, diagnose, and address health problems and hazards affecting the population." Most of this work is conducted by government agencies, including health departments but also emergency management agencies, environmental protection or public works departments, and department of transportation staff who prevent injuries through road safety. Protection from environmental health hazards is provided by food inspectors at the Food and Drug Administration, lead prevention specialists from the Healthy Homes Program of the Departments of Housing and Urban Development, and health specialists at the Nuclear Regulatory Commission. Maternal and child health services are provided in health departments but also via school-based health programs, by health teachers, and by child protection services departments.

Nonprofits contribute by implementing tobacco cessation programs, providing health education, and offering early childhood development and reproductive health services. Researchers at universities and think tanks, workers in Federally Qualified Health Centers who provide sexually transmitted infection testing and counseling, hospitals providing newborn screening, and community-based nonprofits that offer nutrition counseling all contribute to Essential Public Health Service 2.

Furthermore, we can include corporations such as pharmaceutical and biotechnology firms that manufacture vaccines, retail pharmacies that provide vaccinations and testing, personal protective equipment manufacturers, high-efficiency particulate air filter companies, and syringe manufacturers; environmental health contractors and consultants; tobacco cessation programs offered by health insurance corporations; and specific occupations such as infection preventionists, environmental health specialists, nutritionists, toxicologists, occupational health specialists, emergency preparedness professionals, exercise and fitness instructors, and occupational medicine physicians.

SOURCES OF INFORMATION FOR FUTURE RESEARCH

Beginning to define who contributes to essential or foundational public health services is only a first step; implementing these definitions to examine the broader public health workforce is far more challenging. Even enumerating the local, state, tribal, and territorial governmental health department workforce has been challenging. Much of the data for nonprofit or private sector organizations are proprietary, such as the number of workers at for-profit consulting firms with public health–related contracts. There are also problems associated with overcounting workers who may be in a related profession but whose work does not contribute to public health and challenges related to double counting workers who are categorized according to their occupation but also their work setting.

Because the definition of the wider public health workforce in this framework is intersectional, sources of data are diverse. Although data on federal agencies are relatively simple to find through the FedScope database,[19] information on nonprofit organizations requires detailed research involving analyses of publicly available 990 tax returns, which include data on numbers of workers.[20] When a particular occupation is included, data can be found through the US Department of Labor.[8]

Other Local and State Departments

Many of the same challenges in enumerating or researching local and state health departments are likely to pertain to other departments in local and state governments, in that the Department of Labor does not separately count staff in initiatives such as school-based health programs. If data were available, maternal and child health services provided by public schools and administrations for children and families could be enumerated. In addition, prorated numbers of staff in departments of transportation, aging, substance use disorder and mental health, education, planning, and development should be included. Central administrative staff who provide support to health departments, such as those in communications, human resources or civil service departments, departments of budget, and legal support, could be counted, as could those in the judicial system who administer health-related legislation and elected officials at the state and local levels who deal with public health issues, including board of health members, city council members, and legislative branch staff.

Nonprofit Sector

Data on the number of individuals working in public health–related nonprofits could be gathered by analyzing the 990 tax returns of nonprofit organizations from data sets such as Candid.org.[20] Each nonprofit has a publicly visible 990 tax return that lists its number of staff members. By reviewing tax returns, one could estimate the number of public health workers in nonprofit organizations.

Hospitals and Health Care

Hospitals and health clinics contribute to the Essential Public Health Services by providing disease surveillance data, conducting newborn screenings, ensuring compliance with health regulations, and providing screening and preventive care. Researching these workers would require identifying the job titles of individuals who report data to health departments or prorating the amount of time health care providers spend on prevention and patient education. Professional association information could be used to assess certain occupations within health care.

Academia

Academic institutions of public health support Essential Public Health Service 8. Estimates of the number of faculty and staff working within certain schools and programs of public health can be found through associations such as the Association of Schools and Programs of Public Health,[21] with additional research on nonmember institutions. A "prorated" number of faculty and staff at other schools, such as schools of nursing, medicine, social work, and engineering, might be counted as part of the public health workforce.

Contractors and Consulting Firms

Creating a full picture of the number of individual staff in the private sector who support the Essential Public Health Services would require gathering budgetary information from federal and other government grants and contracts given to third-party contractors and data regarding the number of staff who work in, for example, the health-related "public sector practices" of consulting firms. A Freedom of Information Act request could reveal proprietary data.

Publicly traded corporations' staff numbers can be found through Securities and Exchange Commission Form 10K,[22] but privately owned corporations present further challenges for research. Although the number of workers within the specific for-profit firms that provide contract-based work to health departments is likely to be proprietary information, key informant interviews of company leaders might be used to discern these data. Another indirect method to gather a rough estimate of staff numbers is through advanced searches on social media platforms such as LinkedIn.com.

Occupation-Specific information

Although the Department of Labor's Bureau of Labor Statistics gathers extensive information on different occupations,[23,24] it does not provide sufficient granularity to determine which individuals in a certain occupation work in health departments as opposed to other local or state government agencies. Some occupations may be clearly focused on public health because of the nature of the occupation, whereas others are more likely to provide individual services, making it difficult to discern which should be included in the broader public health workforce without conducting further research such as surveys or focus groups. To avoid double counting of staff in the broader public health workforce, care would need to be taken to ensure that staff who have already been counted through sector-based enumerations are not included.

CONCLUSION

Because government still provides the core of public health services, it is essential to focus research efforts on public health workers in health departments; a new enumeration is now available.[25] It is important to be clear that many services cannot or should not be outsourced, and tracking the degree to which essential public health services have been delegated to contractors is a crucial aspect of workforce research. But it is also important to monitor the partners beyond health departments that implement much of the work that keeps our nation healthy.

Significant new research would be needed to begin enumerating the broader workforce, and still more would be needed to determine whether certain functions are provided with better quality or lower cost by permanent "core" workforce staff as opposed to the wider workforce. AJPH

CORRESPONDENCE

Correspondence should be sent to Heather Krasna, PhD, EdM, MS, 722 W 168th St, New York, NY 10032 (e-mail: hk2778@cumc.columbia.edu). Reprints can be ordered at https://www.ajph.org by clicking the "Reprints" link.

PUBLICATION INFORMATION

Full Citation: Krasna H. The public health workforce beyond government health departments: proposing a new definition. *Am J Public Health*. 2025;115(6):840–844.

Acceptance Date: January 28, 2025.

DOI: https://doi.org/10.2105/AJPH.2025.308050

ORCID iD:
Heather Krasna https://orcid.org/0000-0002-4820-9773

ACKNOWLEDGMENTS

The concepts outlined in this article were presented at the 2022 American Public Health Association Annual Meeting and Expo.

I gratefully acknowledge the input on the original presentation by Katarzyna Czabanowska at Maastricht University.

CONFLICTS OF INTEREST

The author reports no conflicts of interest.

REFERENCES

1. Beck AJ, Boulton ML, Coronado F. Enumeration of the governmental public health workforce, 2014. *Am J Prev Med*. 2014;47(5):S306–S313. https://doi.org/10.1016/j.amepre.2014.07.018

2. Gebbie KM. *The Public Health Work Force: Enumeration 2000.* Washington, DC: US Department of Health and Human Services; 2000.
3. Tilson H, Gebbie KM. The public health workforce. *Annu Rev Public Health.* 2004;25:341–356. https://doi.org/10.1146/annurev.publhealth.25.102802.124357
4. Centre for Workforce Intelligence. Mapping the core public health workforce. Available at: https://assets.publishing.service.gov.uk/media/5a74e93bed915d502d6cbfe6/CfWI_Mapping_the_core_public_health_workforce.pdf. Accessed September 1, 2022.
5. The wider public health workforce: the next major public health workforce. *Perspect Public Health.* 2016;136(1):13–15. https://doi.org/10.1177/1757913915618312
6. World Health Organization. Roadmap to professionalizing the public health workforce in the European Region. Available at: https://apps.who.int/iris/handle/10665/351526?search-result=true&query=%29%E2%80%8E.+Roadmap+to+professionalizing+the+public+health+workforce+in+the+European+Region&scope=&rpp=10&sort_by=score&order=desc. Accessed September 1, 2022.
7. Watts RD, Bowles DC, Ryan E, Fisher C, Li IW. No two workforces are the same: a systematic review of enumerations and definitions of public health workforces. *Front Public Health.* 2020;8:588092. https://doi.org/10.3389/fpubh.2020.588092
8. Krasna H, Venkataraman M, Robins M, Patino I, Leider J. Standard occupational classification codes: gaps in federal data on the public health workforce. *Am J Public Health.* 2024;114(1):48–56. https://doi.org/10.2105/AJPH.2023.307463
9. Gebbie K, Merrill J, Sanders L, Gebbie EN, Chen DW. Public health workforce enumeration: beware the "quick fix." *J Public Health Manag Pract.* 2007;13(1):72–79. https://doi.org/10.1097/00124784-200701000-00012
10. Centers for Disease Control and Prevention. Public health system and the 10 Essential Public Health Services. Available at: https://www.cdc.gov/publichealthgateway/publichealthservices/essentialhealthservices.html. Accessed November 17, 2019.
11. Public Health National Center for Innovations. Foundational Public Health Services: building a strong foundation of public health infrastructure. Available at: https://phnci.org/national-frameworks/fphs. Accessed December 25, 2020.
12. Institute of Medicine. *Who Will Keep the Public Healthy?: Educating Public Health Professionals for the 21st Century.* National Academies Press; 2002.
13. Krasna H. *Public Health Graduates in the United States: Employment Outcomes and Employer Demand.* Maastricht University; 2021.
14. Gatseva PD, Argirova M. Public health: the science of promoting health. *J Public Health.* 2011;19(3):205–206. https://doi.org/10.1007/s10389-011-0412-8
15. Gebbie K, Merrill J, Tilson HH. The public health workforce. *Health Aff (Millwood).* 2002;21(6):57–67. https://doi.org/10.1377/hlthaff.21.6.57
16. De Beaumont Foundation. Public Health National Center for Innovations T. The Futures Initiative: the 10 Essential Public Health Services aligning the 10 Essential Public Health Services and the Foundational Public Health Services. Available at: https://phnci.org/uploads/resource-files/EPHS-Alignment-EPHSvsFPHS.pdf. Accessed October 9, 2022.
17. Erwin PC, Hamilton CB, Welch S, Hinds B. The local public health system assessment of MAPP/The National Public Health Performance Standards Local Tool: a community-based, public health practice and academic collaborative approach to implementation. *J Public Health Manag Pract.* 2006;12(6):528–532. https://doi.org/10.1097/00124784-200611000-00005
18. Krasna H, Czabanowska K, Jiang S, et al. The future of careers at the intersection of climate change and public health: what can job postings and an employer survey tell us? *Int J Environ Res Public Health.* 2020;17(4):1310. https://doi.org/10.3390/ijerph17041310
19. Office of Personnel Management. FedScope: federal workforce data. Available at: https://www.fedscope.opm.gov. Accessed August 25, 2019.
20. GuideStar. Nonprofit reports and 990 forms for donors, grantmakers, and businesses. Available at: https://www.guidestar.org. Accessed September 1, 2022.
21. Association of Schools and Programs of Public Health. About ASPPH. Available at: https://www.aspph.org/about. Accessed May 5, 2022.
22. Terrell E. Research guides: doing company research. Available at: https://guides.loc.gov/company-research/public. Accessed January 8, 2023.
23. Bureau of Labor Statistics. Occupational Outlook Handbook. Available at: https://www.bls.gov/ooh. Accessed August 21, 2022.
24. O*NET. O*NET home page. Available at: https://www.onetonline.org. Accessed August 21, 2020.
25. Leider JP, Balio CP, Hogg-Graham R, et al. Enumeration 2024: what we now and what we wish we knew about the governmental public health workforce in a COVID-19 recovery landscape. *Am J Public Health.* 2025;115(5):707–715. https://doi.org/10.2105/AJPH.2024.307960

Wastewater Surveillance: A Rare Bipartisan Opportunity to Strengthen Public Health

John Auerbach, MBA

ABOUT THE AUTHOR

John Auerbach is with ICF, Reston, VA.

The number of human cases of H5N1 bird flu continues to rise, in some instances resulting in serious illness. This reinforces the stakes involved in infectious disease data gathering. To assist in capturing as much timely information as possible, the Centers for Disease Control and Prevention (CDC) has utilized not only its well-established means of collecting information—such as its emergency room–based sentinel surveillance—but also a relatively new tool, wastewater surveillance (WWS). Although WWS has demonstrated its current and potentially greater future utility, including globally,[1] it is at a critical juncture. Without support for expanding its current footprint, enhancing training and support to state and local health officials, and, most importantly, ensuring it has sustainable funding, it is unlikely to fulfill its promise as a widespread tool in the United States. The increased use of WWS has the distinction of being supported by policymakers on both sides of the aisle, offering hope that its usage might become more routine.

In July 2020, Houston, Texas, was one of the early adopters of WWS as part of its efforts to combat the COVID-19 pandemic. By analyzing samples from its 38 wastewater treatment plants, the city found it could detect surges in virus levels up to two weeks before clinical cases spiked. This early warning system enabled officials to effectively allocate resources, implement targeted interventions, and provide timely information to the public. Today, Houston's program tracks other infectious diseases like respiratory syncytial virus (RSV) and seasonal influenza.

Houston is far from alone. The CDC's National Wastewater Surveillance System covers approximately 45% of the US population. In rural West Virginia, event-specific surveillance helped manage and isolate COVID-19 at large gatherings, such as a Boy Scouts of America Jamboree that attracted tens of thousands of scouts. The Cherokee Nation has utilized specialized sequencing equipment to differentiate and address the varied strains of pathogens detected in wastewater. Both Minneapolis, Minnesota, and Tempe, Arizona, used WWS for monitoring opioids and other drugs in the communities connected to sewer systems. In Linn County, Iowa, officials transitioned from using federal contractors to analyze wastewater to building local laboratory capacity to monitor a range of pathogens including COVID-19, influenza A and B, and RSV.

These examples highlight WWS's adaptability to different needs and settings, from densely populated urban centers to underpopulated rural and frontier communities. Yet WWS isn't available in all parts of the country. And where it does exist, there are markedly different approaches to the pathogens and substances being monitored and to the use of the data for decision-making.

To better understand both the promise and challenges of WWS, in October 2024, ICF, a global leader in public health, convened a focus group with 13 state, local, and tribal public health leaders who had varying experiences with WWS. They represented municipalities that differed dramatically in terms of size, demographics, and red and blue politics. They differed also in the nature of their experience with WWS. Yet, overwhelmingly, they held similar views regarding WWS: it is a valuable complement to traditional surveillance.

The health officials in the focus group universally saw WWS as a unique way to monitor community health by sampling what flows through our sewers. They appreciated the value of population-level data collection as a complement to the data gathered from clinical surveillance of individual cases of illness. And they highlighted that its value went beyond infectious diseases. Many cited examples where it helped them track markers of a wide range of emerging threats, enabling targeted, proactive interventions.

BARRIERS TO WIDESPREAD USE

Despite the potential of WWS, the participants highlighted that its use faces challenges that must be addressed for it to thrive in their locales and across the nation. These included the following:

1. Funding shortfalls. Federal funding for wastewater surveillance dropped sharply after the pandemic. Although hundreds of millions of COVID-19 one-time-only dollars supported it and other innovative surveillance methods developed during the pandemic, no new money has been provided in the current funded federal budget. Without sustainable investment, many local programs are concerned about its continued availability. They are reluctant to hire specialized staff or pull busy epidemiologists into targeted training if future support is uncertain.
2. Data complexity. Wastewater data are inherently complex and require different skills for analysis. Conventional surveillance involves individual cases, either human or animal. But WWS provides community-level information regarding the presence of a pathogen. Elevated levels of H5N1 in a sewer could reflect animal cases, contaminated raw milk poured down the drain, or human cases. The focus group members reported difficulties in interpreting findings and aligning them with clinical data. They underscored the need for improved analytical tools and training.
3. Lack of standardization. Each public health official relayed how each had tailored their WWS programs to their specific local needs. Although understandable, this flexibility led to inconsistencies in which pathogens were monitored as well as the methods for testing. It also hampered the ability to compare data across jurisdictions or analyze national trends.

Other barriers local health departments may face include the refusal of local watershed plants to participate in the WWS processes and the possible disinclination of nongovernmental WWS efforts to share their data.

RECOMMENDATIONS FOR THE FUTURE

The officials proposed a variety of ways to fully unlock the potential of wastewater surveillance in three general areas:

1. Sustain long-term funding. As mentioned, stable funding is essential for maintaining and expanding WWS. To date, most funding has come from the federal government, although some has also come from local or state governments and the private sector. Focus group members hoped that federal, state, and local governments would see the long-term value of this investment and assure municipalities that such support would continue in the future. Some highlighted the potential value of public–private partnerships—for example, with universities—that might result in supplemental resources.
2. Develop national standards. Focus group members hoped the CDC would have the resources and authority to oversee efforts to create uniform protocols for testing and data interpretation. A standardized core set of monitored pathogens and metrics for such monitoring—with some built-in flexibility when varied conditions call for it—would enable better comparison and trend analysis. For example, given the current concerns, perhaps all federally funded WWS sites should be required to monitor for the H5N1 bird flu.
3. Invest in training and technology. Focus group members cited the need for training on multiple fronts. Local laboratories need support to build capacity, epidemiologists need training regarding the interpretation of findings, and public health leaders need support in understanding how best to respond to varied WWS findings.

These recommendations were largely in alignment with other noteworthy efforts to understand and support WWS, such as the findings of the National Academies of Sciences, Engineering, and Medicines reports[2] and the Rockefeller Foundation report[3] on WWS use in pandemic response and the CDC's own experiences.[4]

A RARE POINT OF AGREEMENT

Despite the wide variation in the social, economic, and political conditions of their municipalities, the health officials in the focus group all agreed on the value of WWS. Members of Congress on both sides of the aisle have also seen the potential of WWS to strengthen traditional surveillance systems and help communities prepare for and respond to current and future threats to the public.

The consensus is clear. WSS is more than an innovative idea—it is a transformative approach to public health. By acting now to secure funding and address the existing challenges, we can ensure healthier, more resilient communities nationwide. Although the focus right now is on the H5N1 bird flu, the next infectious disease threat may be more dangerous to the public. We want the very best tools to prepare and respond. This includes wastewater surveillance. AJPH

CORRESPONDENCE

Correspondence should be sent to John Auerbach, Senior Vice President, Health, ICF, 1902 Reston Metro Plaza, Reston, VA 20190 (e-mail: john.auerbach@icf.com). Reprints can be ordered at https://www.ajph.org by clicking the "Reprints" link.

PUBLICATION INFORMATION

Full Citation: Auerbach J. Wastewater surveillance: a rare bipartisan opportunity to strengthen public health. *Am J Public Health*. 2025;115(6):845–847.

Acceptance Date: February 26, 2025.

DOI: https://doi.org/10.2105/AJPH.2025.308103

ORCID iD:
John Auerbach https://orcid.org/0000-0002-8064-5196

CONFLICTS OF INTEREST

The author has no conflicts of interest to report.

REFERENCES

1. European Union Drugs Agency. Wastewater analysis and drugs—a European multi-city study. 2024. Available at: https://www.euda.europa.eu/publications/html/pods/waste-water-analysis_en. Accessed February 26, 2025.
2. National Academies of Sciences, Engineering, and Medicine. *Increasing the Utility of Wastewater-Based Disease Surveillance for Public Health Action: A Phase 2 Report.* Washington, DC: National Academies Press; 2024. https://doi.org/10.17226/27516
3. Keshaviah A, Karmali RN, Vohra D, Huffman T, Hu XC, Diamond MB. *The Role of Wastewater Data in Pandemic Management.* Washington, DC: Mathematica; 2022.
4. Honein MA, Olsen SJ, Jernigan DB, Daskalakis DC. Challenges and opportunities for wastewater monitoring of influenza viruses during the multistate outbreak of highly pathogenic avian influenza A(H5N1) virus in dairy cattle and poultry. *Am J Public Health.* 2024;114(12):1309–1312. https://doi.org/10.2105/AJPH.2024.307860

Shuttering the Pregnancy Risk Assessment Monitoring System (PRAMS): A Dangerous Attack on US Mothers and Infants

Arden S. Handler, DrPH, Kay Johnson, MPH, EdM, Kristin M. Rankin, PhD, Alisa J. Velonis, PhD, MPH, Arthur R. James, MD, and Milton Kotelchuck, PhD, MPH

ABOUT THE AUTHORS

Arden S. Handler is professor emeritus with the University of Illinois School of Public Health, Chicago. Kay Johnson leads Johnson Policy Consulting, Hinesburg, VT. Kristin M. Rankin is with the University of Illinois School of Public Health Division of Epidemiology and Biostatistics, Chicago. Alisa J. Velonis is with University of Illinois School of Public Health Division of Community Health Sciences, Chicago. Arthur R. James is retired from the Ohio State University Wexner Medical Center and Nationwide Children's Hospital, Columbus. Milton Kotelchuck is with Harvard Medical School and Mass General Hospital for Children, Boston, MA.

AJPH June 2025, Vol. 115, No. 6

With the implementation of Project 2025 by the current Trump administration, we are witnessing a draconian and unprecedented assault on the field of public health, with potentially devastating consequences for all US women, children, and families. A recent direct attack on maternal and infant health appeared in our e-mails on Sunday, February 23, 2025, alerting us to the shuttering of the US Pregnancy Risk Assessment Monitoring System (PRAMS) on January 31, 2025.[1] PRAMS, initiated in 1987 by the Centers for Disease Control and Prevention (CDC), is the quintessential maternal and infant health data collection system. Built on previous surveys,[2] PRAMS reaches out to a sample of women in each state who recently gave birth and asks them about their health (e.g., chronic conditions, weight), behaviors (e.g., smoking, breastfeeding), insurance status, and experiences with the health care system just prior to, during, and after pregnancy; the survey also asks about the health of their newborns. PRAMS surveys are linked to birth certificate information for individual participants, allowing a fuller picture of maternal and infant health status. In the most recent cycle, 46 states, the District of Columbia, New York City, the Northern Mariana Islands, and Puerto Rico participated in PRAMS, representing jurisdictions that cover 81% of all live births in the United States.

Information generated through PRAMS is used daily by state and local health departments, policymakers, maternal and child health (MCH) advocates, and MCH researchers to understand the myriad factors associated with maternal and infant health experiences and outcomes, such as opioid use, maternal depression, and preterm delivery.[3] PRAMS also helps us understand reasons for the shamefully high rates of maternal and infant deaths in the United States, particularly for Black, Brown, and Indigenous women and infants. Finally, PRAMS allows us to examine the role and impact of health care interventions and strategies (e.g., Back to Sleep, breastfeeding promotion, Medicaid expansion, use of doulas). In other words, PRAMS data are essential for understanding how daily experiences, health care, insurance coverage, and practice and policy innovations affect maternal and infant health.

Given the fundamental importance of these data to our ability to protect the health of women, infants, and families, why was PRAMS survey data collection frozen nationwide on January 31? Our understanding from both the Talking Points Memo[1] and our conversations with colleagues is that the Trump administration's effort to scrub all so-called "diversity, equity, and inclusion" and lesbian, gay, bisexual, transgender, and queer (LGBTQ) programs and language from our current national discourse has led to the current PRAMS survey (phase 9, started in 2023) being targeted for including "problematic" language. This includes questions about gender and sexual orientation and others focused on racial discrimination and the social drivers of health. Other questions may be targeted as well. Those in charge appear to believe that when you "erase" issues and deny the visibility of individuals, those issues and individuals no longer exist.

PRAMS is not a federal program that needs to be "downsized," in the parlance of the current administration. In fact, it is a federal–state partnership in which states are in the lead with support from the federal government.[4] All participating states and jurisdictions include a national set of core questions in their surveys but are also able to select additional questions that address issues most salient to their own state populations. This state-specific focus has led to state-specific successes. For example, the West Virginia Division of Perinatal and Women's Health used PRAMS data to make the connection that increasing access to contraceptive services could be an upstream strategy for reducing the number of infants experiencing neonatal opioid withdrawal syndrome. Similarly, New Jersey state officials used PRAMS data to "explore factors associated with infant mortality and provide information to support community-based approaches to reduce mortality among Black infants."[5]

PRAMS is not a stagnant system. It collects data in real time. When new issues emerge that affect the health and well-being of mothers and infants, PRAMS steps up and steps in. Witness the H1N1 Influenza and Seasonal Flu supplement, 2009; the Zika Supplement Questionnaire, 2016–2017; and the Maternal COVID-19 Experiences, 2020 supplement. PRAMS is also being creatively used by several states to conduct longitudinal follow-up on the subsequent health of toddlers and their parents.

Although leaders in the field—and now, the PRAMS website—anticipate an April 2025 restart to data collection, the looming Reductions in Force (RIF) by federal agencies cause us to question the likelihood of this timeline. If the current phase 9 survey is rewritten, new approvals from the CDC institutional review board and Office of Management and Budget will likely be needed, a process that can take many months. Meanwhile, as PRAMS data collection appears to be indefinitely on hold, state health departments will likely be forced to make personnel and resource decisions that could limit their ability to resume collecting PRAMS data, should the program be allowed to restart. Part of what makes PRAMS data so powerful is the number of states that currently participate; the loss of even a few jurisdictions could reduce the utility of these data.

So, what does the potential of a complete shuttering of PRAMS at the federal level mean for mothers and infants? Who will suffer if PRAMS is discontinued or significantly altered? What happens when a data set that has been part and parcel of state MCH planning and programming, and has been used by multiple epidemiologists and researchers for almost 40 years to answer the most important and basic questions about maternal and infant health, no longer exists or is significantly changed?

On a very basic level, if PRAMS is completely shut down at the federal level, going forward, state health departments as well as many MCH advocates and researchers may not have access to the most comprehensive maternal and infant data available in the United States. This will leave a tremendous gap in what we do and do not know about the pressing concerns of the day, particularly those affecting low-income, disabled, and Black, Brown, and Indigenous mothers and infants. Without such data, states will be seriously hampered as they try to tackle issues such as homelessness in pregnancy, the effects of home visiting strategies on postpartum mental health, the extent to which mothers are receiving education about maternal morbidity and mortality warning signs, and so much more. In addition, with questions about gender, sexual orientation, racial discrimination, and social drivers of health potentially removed from the PRAMS survey, we will have missed the opportunity to understand the unique prenatal and postpartum health needs and experiences of the LGBTQ population and the effects of racism and issues such as food insecurity and transportation on maternal and infant health.

We cannot claim for certain that more women and infants will die if PRAMS is not restarted, but we can say without question that a key source of data that can be turned into information for action to improve maternal and infant health and well-being will be lost. The United States—the richest nation in the world—currently experiences some of the worst health outcomes for mothers and infants. Without accurate, up-to-date information on the health and experiences of expectant and new mothers, we will be further stymied in our ability to ensure that Black women don't continue to die at almost three times the rate of White women, and Black infants don't continue to die at more than twice the rate of White infants.

If PRAMS is completely discontinued at the federal level, some states may try to continue the program given its critical importance to understanding the health and well-being of their maternal and infant populations. States such as California that do not participate in PRAMS might serve as a model. For several historical reasons, the PRAMS-like California Maternal and Infant Health Assessment (MIHA) system has been implemented by the California Department of Public Health (CDPH) since the late 1990s, using federal funds from the Title V Maternal and Child Health Block Grant and the Special Supplemental Nutrition Program for Women, Infants and Children (WIC).[6] Importantly, MIHA represents a collaboration between the CDPH and the University of California, San Francisco. Although the funding sources for MIHA will likely also be under strain in the current climate, hopefully this data system will not be collateral damage. In addition to state–university partnerships as a way to continue data collection, if PRAMS efforts at the federal level are discontinued or eliminated, several national MCH nonprofits and university partners are well-positioned to support collaboration and linkage across states.

Removing the essential information that PRAMS has provided for almost 40 years flies in the face of our collective goal of supporting families and ensuring their ability to have healthy infants. To prevent further risk to the health of all mothers and infants, MCH epidemiologists, advocates, and researchers must educate legislators and other partners in their states about the importance of PRAMS and join together to press the CDC to permit states to continue their 2025 PRAMS activities and to provide full support for the PRAMS data collection system going forward. AJPH

CORRESPONDENCE

Correspondence should be sent to Arden Handler, DrPH, Professor Emeritus, University of Illinois School of Public Health Community Health Sciences, 1603 W. Taylor, Chicago, IL 60612 (e-mail: handler@uic.edu). Reprints can be ordered at https://www.ajph.org by clicking the "Reprints" link.

PUBLICATION INFORMATION

Full Citation: Handler AS, Johnson K, Rankin KM, Velonis AJ, James AR, Kotelchuck M. Shuttering the Pregnancy Risk Assessment Monitoring System (PRAMS): a dangerous attack on US mothers and infants. *Am J Public Health*. 2025;115(6):848–850.

Acceptance Date: March 4, 2025.

DOI: https://doi.org/10.2105/AJPH.2025.308107

ORCID iDs:

Kay Johnson https://orcid.org/0000-0002-8347-955X

Alisa J. Velonis https://orcid.org/0000-0002-9787-979X

Milton Kotelchuck https://orcid.org/0000-0002-2667-0227

CONTRIBUTORS

A. S. Handler conceptualized and prepared the initial draft. K. Johnson and M. Kotelchuck provided historical context and contributed to the content of the initial draft. K. M. Rankin, A. J. Velonis, and A. R. James contributed to writing and editing. All authors were involved in responding to the reviewers' comments and preparing the revised article.

ACKNOWLEDGMENT

We gratefully acknowledge the dedication of Centers for Disease Control and Prevention and state public health agency staff who have made PRAMS the quintessential data system for maternal and infant health.

CONFLICTS OF INTEREST

The authors have no conflicts to disclose.

REFERENCES

1. Marshall J. Why PRAMS got shuttered. Talking Points Memo. February 23, 2025. Available at: https://talkingpointsmemo.com/edblog/why-prams-got-shuttered. Accessed February 23, 2025.
2. Kotelchuck M. Pregnancy Risk Assessment Monitoring System (PRAMS): possible new roles for a national MCH data system. *Public Health Rep*. 2006;121(1):6–10. https://doi.org/10.1177/003335490612100105
3. Ghandour RM. The Pregnancy Risk Assessment Monitoring System (PRAMS): current strengths and opportunities for growth. *Am J Public Health*. 2018;108(10):1303–1304. https://doi.org/10.2105/AJPH.2018.304662
4. Shulman HB, D'Angelo DV, Harrison L, Smith RA, Warner L. The Pregnancy Risk Assessment Monitoring System (PRAMS): overview of design and methodology. *Am J Public Health*. 2018;108(10):1305–1313. https://doi.org/10.2105/AJPH.2018.304563
5. Centers for Disease Control and Prevention. PRAMS data to action success stories. Last updated May 15, 2024. Available at: https://www.cdc.gov/prams/php/success-stories-data-to-action/index.html. Accessed February 25, 2025.
6. California Dept of Public Health. Maternal and Infant Health Assessment (MIHA). Last updated February 12, 2025. Available at: https://www.cdph.ca.gov/Programs/CFH/DCMAH/MIHA/Pages/default.aspx. Accessed March 2, 2025.

The Master's Tools Will Never Dismantle the House: Reflections on Hope and Equity in Public Health Training

Sunshine Best, MPH, DrPH(c), and Kimberly Wu, MPH, PhD(c)

ABOUT THE AUTHORS

Sunshine Best and Kimberly Wu are with the Social, Behavioral, and Population Sciences Department, Celia Schott Weatherhead School of Public Health and Tropical Medicine, Tulane University, New Orleans, LA.

Public health academic institutions are overdue for an evolution to remain relevant and meet the mission of protecting our collective health. During a global pandemic, we witnessed the impact of crumbling health care systems. We continue to grapple with what it means to recover and forge ahead while honoring the pain of the loss and destruction of the past years. We are at a juncture to regroup, reflect, and refine our vision for public health. This must include clarifying the purpose of public health, to center the lived experiences of communities affected by unjust policies and practices.

Building radical hope requires the reclamation of hope as a dynamic process, as a capacity latent within each one of us in the face of difficulties and exigencies. The vehicle for hope must be action, fueled by justice and the curiosity to question, urging us to reimagine new paths forward. Toward a hopeful reimagining of a diverse and thriving public health workforce, we offer observations of fundamental barriers in training. Addressing inequities within public health graduate education requires a multifaceted approach that acknowledges the impact of systemic disparities on both students and institutions to foster an environment where hope can be actualized.

ECONOMIC INEQUITIES IN PUBLIC HEALTH

A recent study into the experience of governmental public health workers found significant differences in annual wages between individuals identifying as a person of color (earning $4000 less annually) and their White peers.[1] The same study raised a significant gender wage gap of $3000 for women.[1] Data from the Center for Economic Policy Research found that Black women face the highest average student loan balances compared with all other groups.[2] In 2022, 43.3% of Black women with some college or higher degrees had student loans—double the rate among White women (19.9%) and almost triple that of White men (15.7%).[2] Students of color are also disproportionately affected by the mental health stress related to taking on increased student loan debt.[3] How can public health institutions expect to champion diversity without addressing such pressing inequalities in access to public health training and education?

Tuition costs have risen sharply during the pandemic,[4] while salaries in public health careers remain low.[5] This has led many public health graduates to feel disillusioned with their academic investment. According to recent studies, the median level of student loan debt for completing a public health degree is $33 366. However, the median earnings one year after graduation are about $80 000 for graduates with doctoral degrees and $33 000 for graduates with bachelor's degrees.[6] The persistence of inequities leaves few pathways to economic mobility for those outside the privileged elite.

Higher education, often perceived as a means of increasing human capital, is increasingly viewed as a "sieve more than a ladder"[7]—reproducing inequality across generations. As academic institutions become more entrepreneurial, financial motivations play a significant role in perpetuating these inequities.[8] Academic capitalism allows us to understand higher education's shift from creating scholarship and learning as a public good to generating knowledge as a commodity to be monetized.[9] Academic research institutions driven by philanthropy, grants, and tuition dollars incentivize a system that prioritizes legacy and high-socioeconomic-status students who can afford to be there.[10] As a result, these institutions also risk perpetuating social inequity rather than addressing the structural injustices within their walls.

LIVED EXPERIENCES UNCOVER INSTITUTIONAL GAPS

Coauthor Sunshine Best often draws from her experiences navigating inequities in pursuing her public health graduate studies. Having aged out of foster care, where higher education was neither normalized nor accessible, she recognized the value of earning a degree through her observations in the workforce. Inspired by her diverse experiences growing up, she was drawn to improving the quality of life for those often overlooked by society. Her background provided a unique context that allowed her to gain insights often missed by those without adverse childhood experiences during her pursuit of bachelor's, master's, and doctoral degrees. As a foster care alumnus, Sunshine has faced significant academic disparities, particularly in pursuing advanced degrees. She chooses transparency in discussing her childhood experiences, which included brief periods of homelessness, food scarcity, and financial struggles. These experiences have shaped her worldview and values, driving her determination to improve public health by leveraging her lived experiences to foster change.

Sunshine's journey in public health higher education has been marked by challenges, including the financial strain of living on a tight budget, which makes networking difficult. As a Black woman in a predominantly White, wealthy, private institution, she often feels stigmatized and unwelcomed. Foster care alumni rarely experience homophily—a sense of community among peers with shared traits—in graduate school. This led Sunshine to understand that she had more in common with the populations being studied than with those conducting the research.[6] Instead of viewing her as an outsider, let's consider how institutions can embrace the experiences of students like Sunshine to inform equitable change for every student. Despite the aspirations that drew Sunshine into higher education, she faces the harsh realities of discrimination, pay inequity, and the burden of ever-increasing, near-predatory student loan systems.[11]

BARRIERS WITHIN INSTITUTIONS

Research shows that public health universities can perpetuate health inequities through their hiring and admissions practices. The *International Journal for Equity in Health* highlights how superficial diversity and inclusion strategies often uphold systemic inequities by focusing on representation without addressing the underlying power dynamics in academia. This tokenism allows academic institutions to appear progressive without making meaningful changes to the structures that disadvantage marginalized groups, while maintaining a culture distanced from the health disparities in their communities.[12] By prioritizing academic reputation and research "success" over the translation of that research to address political, corporate, structural, and social determinants of health in their regions, academic institutions shirk opportunities to invest in local change.

Diversity must go beyond increasing non-White representation. Diversity also involves recognizing the importance of uplifting lived experiences when addressing health inequities. Individuals with lived experiences bring a unique worldview shaped by personal histories, allowing them to understand context and construct meaning differently than those with purely academic or professional perspectives. Whether a research study is qualitative or quantitative, lived experiences can offer insights into a wide range of fields of study.

RECOMMENDATIONS FOR INSTITUTIONS

To effectively shape future educational and health policies, it's essential to understand education as it actively shapes opportunities throughout individuals' early lives. This requires expanding our view of education beyond mere degree attainment to consider the long-term processes that influence health and perpetuate inequities. Education should be reconceptualized not only as a means to social success and good health, but also as a system that challenges and corrects inequity across generations. Researchers and practitioners should integrate historical, social, and policy contexts into their work, grants, and curricula. Furthermore, enrolling and supporting students and faculty with lived experiences not only enriches these efforts but also fosters a sense of hope, as it demonstrates a commitment to understanding and addressing health inequities through shared knowledge and authentic perspectives.

Health equity has become a watchword for many public health academic institutions, leading to an increase in courses and research on its relevance for populations and systems.[13] Institutions have a responsibility to bridge research and practice by implementing initiatives that demonstrate their commitment to addressing systemic issues, setting examples for their students and within their communities. To address the entrenched inequities within public health education, it is vital to embrace hope not as a passive sentiment but as a proactive practice.

HOPE AS AN ACTIVE AND TRANSFORMATIVE PROCESS

Hope, in this context, involves actively reimagining and reconstructing the pathways that lead to a more inclusive and equitable public health workforce. Hope is learning from our differences, making them our strengths, and fashioning new tools and practices that can truly "dismantle the master's house" and "bring about genuine change."[14] As Audre Lorde argued, the "master's tools" can never be used to dismantle the oppressive structures that created them, but by centering marginalized voices—particularly of those who have been systematically excluded from leadership in public health institutions—we can create new foundations for authentic change. Institutions must prioritize lived experiences—especially from marginalized communities in roles of leadership, faculty, and well-supported graduate students—to dismantle systemic barriers and incubate a groundswell of organic and meaningful change.

Public health institutions have an opportunity to deepen their impact and enhance research by integrating lived experiences into program design, policy development, and cultivating interdependent community partnerships. Hope, when coupled with intentional collective action, can transform educational practices, inspire systemic change, and ultimately nurture a public health system that is truly representative and responsive to the needs of all communities. By embedding values of inclusivity and equity in its core, public health can evolve into a field that not only addresses disparities but actively resists reproducing them, inspiring a shift toward justice and genuine societal transformation. In this way, hope is only as meaningful as the actions—and the impact—that follow. AJPH

CORRESPONDENCE

Correspondence should be sent to Sunshine Best, 1440 Canal St, New Orleans, LA 70112 (e-mail: sbest2@tulane.edu). Reprints can be ordered at https://www.ajph.org by clicking the "Reprints" link.

PUBLICATION INFORMATION

Full Citation: Best S, Wu K. The master's tools will never dismantle the house: reflections on hope and equity in public health training. *Am J Public Health*. 2025;115(6):851–853.

Acceptance Date: November 20, 2024.

DOI: https://doi.org/10.2105/AJPH.2024.307953

ORCID iDs:
Sunshine Best https://orcid.org/0000-0002-2018-3815

Kimberly Wu https://orcid.org/0000-0003-0638-3199

CONTRIBUTORS

Both authors conceptualized the topic and wrote and edited the manuscript.

ACKNOWLEDGMENTS

Thank you Katherine Theall for your feedback.

CONFLICTS OF INTEREST

There are no conflicts of interest to disclose.

REFERENCES

1. Sellers K, Leider JP, Gould E, et al. The state of the US governmental public health workforce, 2014–2017. *Am J Public Health*. 2019;109(5):674–680. https://doi.org/10.2105/AJPH.2019.305011
2. Curchin E. Student loan debt is common across all race and gender groups, especially for black women. Center for Economic and Policy Research. January 2024. Available at: https://www.cepr.net/student-loan-debt-is-common-across-all-race-and-gender-groups-especially-for-black-women. Accessed July 12, 2024.
3. Jackson V, Williams B. How black women experience student debt. April 2022. Available at: https://edtrust.org/wp-content/uploads/2014/09/How-Black-Women-Experience-Student-Debt-April-2022.pdf. Accessed July 9, 2024.
4. Moody J. Tuition held steady during the pandemic, but now it's climbing. *High Ed*. May 2022. Available at: https://www.insidehighered.com/news/2022/05/13/tuition-held-steady-during-pandemic-now-its-climbing. Accessed July 10, 2024.
5. Ma K. Public health position available: Low pay. Promise of burnout and harassment. Master's preferred. Bulletin of the Atomic Scientists. September 2023. Available at: https://thebulletin.org/2023/09/public-health-position-available-low-pay-promise-of-burnout-and-harassment-masters-preferred. Accessed July 9, 2024.
6. Tait M, Burke E, Leshan T, Casalotti A, Krasna H, Leider JP. Federal student loan debt in public health and the opportunities for loan repayment programs. *Public Health Rep*. 2024;139(4):512–518. https://doi.org/10.1177/00333549231223712
7. Zajacova A, Lawrence EM. The relationship between education and health: reducing disparities through a contextual approach. *Annu Rev Public Health*. 2018;39(1):273–289. https://doi.org/10.1146/annurev-publhealth-031816-044628
8. Slaughter S, Rhoades G. *Academic Capitalism and the New Economy*. Baltimore, MD: Johns Hopkins University Press; 2009. https://doi.org/10.56021/9780801879494
9. Cantwell B, Kauppinen I, eds. *Academic Capitalism in the Age of Globalization*. Baltimore, MD: Johns Hopkins University Press; 2014. https://doi.org/10.1353/book.49259
10. Chetty R, Deming DJ, Friedman JN. *Diversifying Society's Leaders? The Determinants and Causal Effects of Admission to Highly Selective Private Colleges*. Cambridge, MA: National Bureau of Economic Research; 2023.
11. Blake S. Student loan borrower owes $300,000: "the system is predatory." *Newsweek*. March 14, 2024. Available at: https://www.newsweek.com/texas-father-parent-plus-loans-predatory-aid-1879423. Accessed July 10, 2024.
12. Shahram SZ. Five ways "health scholars" are complicit in upholding health inequities, and how to stop. *Int J Equity Health*. 2023;22(1):15. https://doi.org/10.1186/s12939-022-01763-9
13. Plamondon KM, Dixon J, Brisbois B, et al. Turning the tide on inequity through systematic equity action-analysis. *BMC Public Health*. 2023;23(1):890. https://doi.org/10.1186/s12889-023-15709-5
14. Lorde A. The master's tools will never dismantle the master's house. In: Bereano NK, Lorde A, eds. *Sister Outsider: Essays and Speeches*. Berkeley, CA: Crossing Press; 1984:110–114. https://collectiveliberation.org/wp-content/uploads/2013/01/Lorde_The_Masters_Tools.pdf.

Passing Out Pamphlets in 8-Inch Heels

Alexandra Wurth

ABOUT THE AUTHOR

Alexandra Wurth is in the MPH program at the University of South Dakota, Vermillion.

I was living in Portland, Oregon, working full time after having dropped out of an art degree program. I was broke and searching for meaning. That is how I found myself auditioning at a local gentleman's club. I realized quickly that I would be able to pay my rent with this career, however taboo it was to my friends and family. But there was a part of me that wondered if I could pursue an old dream of working in health care. I applied to work for a sexual health clinic just outside of town. I spent my days in a clinic setting, clad in scrubs, educating patients about birth control, taking patient vitals, and giving pregnancy test results. I picked up a volunteer shift as the assistant to the peer-led sex-ed program. But in the evenings, I took the tram back into Portland to change out of my scrubs and into sparkly, sequin-covered outfits, and 8-inch heels.

I realized quickly I was among beautiful, strong, and intelligent women during my night shifts, but many of them were lacking an education on their own bodies and sexual health. I began to bring pamphlets to the strip club from the clinic and facilitated sexual health sessions in the back of the dressing room. We sat, half-naked, hair done, makeup glimmering, and discussed birth control options, vaginal discharge, and how to make an appointment to get tested for sexually transmitted infections. I passed out condoms and quickly became a source of knowledge for these women. I made sure I wasn't giving medical advice, and encouraged them, if they had specific questions, to make an appointment at the clinic. I became good friends with many of the women I worked with, and some of those friendships remain today.

I continued to work in a variety of strip clubs for three years before moving to Iowa, where I completed my undergraduate degree. I later pursued my master's degree in public health. Dancing in those clubs led me to go into public health. I'd be lying if I said that the best education I received and gave wasn't in the back of those poorly lit dressing rooms, and that I didn't quickly come to realize the gaps in our health system, and to understand that some people get left behind.

Although I was simply a nude dancer, I was still participating in sex work. And although the form of sex work I participated in was legal, it was and remains taboo. I had many friends who participated in other forms of sex work, all on their own accord, and I learned then how the health care system is also made to shame them and often not meet their many needs. Sex work is work. Sex workers aren't lurking around on dark corners or in alleyways, and they are deserving of a health system that supports them and meets them where they are.

Where someone works determines the safety of their work environment. People are quick to say that sex work is dangerous but don't seem to make the same statement about enlisting in the military or working as an electrician. All jobs have risks, but some come without worker's compensation or even health insurance. Sure, a full-service sex worker (a term used by the sex worker community to describe someone who performs sex acts in exchange for money) may have higher risks, such as vaginal or urinary tract infections, but a working registered nurse has a higher risk of a poke from a dirty needle. There are protections to be taken in both cases, but only one offers to pay for the associated medical costs.

If we want equity in health care and public health, we need to have hard and uncomfortable conversations, asking questions such as "How can we prevent HIV and other sexually transmitted infections among sex workers?" and "How can we ensure sex workers have the resources they need to remain healthy?" The good news: there is hope. I have hope for the sex worker community and all of its advocates. I also have hope for public health, because I know other people like me believe in equity, even when it feels hard or unorthodox. I have hope that there are other stories, just like mine, being written as you read this, and that people exist who want to make change for those who are often forgotten.

In public health, we talk about prevention (preventative care, and prevention against disease, injury, and illness), but we often forget to look directly at the people we are trying to protect and ask them what they need to be healthy. Sex workers are often left out of conversations about their well-being. Instead, we do what we think is best without consulting them. We need to work alongside sex workers and meet them where they are, even if that means a lone stripper takes it upon herself to pass out pamphlets about chlamydia in a dingy dressing room. I have hope that organizations that are knowledgeable about sex work could dispense information on needed resources. These could be found in public bathrooms, libraries, strip clubs, clinics, and more, to get key information to the people who need it most. I have hope that we as public health professionals can start having dialogue (including vulnerable populations in the conversation) on how to best meet the needs of the community. I have hope that the sex worker community will thrive with support from public health efforts, because the community is resilient. I have hope because I personally know sex workers who are working to unionize, working to radicalize their communities, and working to educate about sex worker–friendly organizations and resources. I have hope because I know there are people out there, like myself, doing the work on the ground. We as public health professionals just need to join the conversation.

I've since traded my heels for sneakers, and I don't find myself in the mirror applying fake lashes or glittery eyeshadow as often, but I haven't forgotten my roots. I know that because of sex workers, I have become a better woman, and I will carry their stories with me through the public health field and everywhere after. AJPH

CORRESPONDENCE

Correspondence should be sent to Alexandra Wurth, 3447 Concordia Dr, Sioux City, IA 51104 (e-mail: Alexandra.wurth@coyotes.usd.edu). Reprints can be ordered at https://www.ajph.org by clicking the "Reprints" link.

PUBLICATION INFORMATION

Full Citation: Wurth A. Passing out pamphlets in 8-inch heels. *Am J Public Health*. 2025;115(6): 854–855.

Acceptance Date: November 20, 2024.

DOI: https://doi.org/10.2105/AJPH.2024.307954

ORCID iD:
Alexandra Wurth https://orcid.org/0009-0004-9255-4322

CONFLICTS OF INTEREST

The author declares no conflicts of interest.

Lessons in Grief: Public Health and Healing in Community

Lucy Tu, AB

ABOUT THE AUTHOR

Lucy Tu is with the Centre for Socio-Legal Studies, Oxford University, Oxford, UK.

When we learn about loss in public health, it is often as an abstraction. We read and talk about the millions of people affected by poor health care systems, but they remain faceless statistics, their emotions and stories out of reach. In spring 2024, hoping to bridge this gap in my work in reproductive and maternal health care, I began meeting with a Boston, Massachusetts–based support group for parents who have lost their children during pregnancy or infancy. At their biweekly sessions, attendees discuss what to do with old maternity clothes, or ask how to handle questions from well-meaning coworkers and family. There is no cost to join, attendance commitment, or strict timeline. It is simply a space for those in grief to gather.

I first visited the group to share community-based resources for postpartum depression and miscarriage recovery as part of a local reproductive health outreach program. But my paltry pamphlets and rehearsed speech felt hollow in a room filled with such raw, honest mourning, and I left that initial meeting believing I had done little to help. Instead of stepping away, though, I asked to attend the next session, wanting to better understand the group's health care experiences. Over the following months, my ideas about effective public health and the meaning of community-building transformed.

In the United States, maternal and reproductive health care has long been riddled with fault lines. Most advocates know the studies well enough to recite their grim findings: the US pregnancy-related mortality rate is double the average of other high-income countries and has worsened over the past two decades.[1,2] Over 80% of these deaths are preventable.[3] Our country's infant mortality rate also surpasses that of other high-income nations, with stark disparities for babies born to Black and American Indian/Alaska Native parents.[2] These poor health outcomes stem from entrenched socioeconomic inequities, including unequal access to prenatal and postpartum services.[4]

It is easy to become numb to these figures, to repeat them without really knowing what they mean. Studies of patients' experiences offer only piecemeal insight into a system that doles out care and neglect along familiar lines. We know, for example, that one in five women report mistreatment while receiving maternity care, and that Black, Hispanic, and uninsured patients are more likely to experience threats of withholding treatment from providers.[5,6] However, these studies do not account for what comes after—the grief, solitude, and, in some cases, recovery that follows maternal morbidity, miscarriage, or infant loss. The limited available research describes this process as one of intense isolation, where feelings of inadequacy and stigma shadow recovering patients.[7] Support groups, including the one I attended, provide a rare space for this grief to find voice and witness. In fact, one reason I continued returning to the group was to understand how people can forge hope and community amid such profound pain.

Through those meetings, I learned that numbers alone can obscure the firsthand experiences that make public health problems—and their potential solutions—concrete. Only when I moved beyond the data did I truly hear the stories of people like Alice, a Black woman who said her nurses dismissed her cries of stabbing spasms during labor. Another Black woman recalled how her physician insisted she repeatedly rate her pain on a scale of 1 to 10, as if he "didn't believe me the first time." I discovered that some group participants dislike being labeled as "patients" and prefer to be called "parents." ("I still feel like a mother, even if my son was only with me for a few hours," one woman told me.) Many had not dismantled their babies' cribs. These stories opened my eyes but also left me, as a young student unable to relate to these experiences, feeling like an imposter. This sense of inadequacy only grew as I tried to update the resource pamphlets I had brought to the group. My attempts to incorporate what I had learned felt shallow. For all my research and advocacy, I could not restore what these parents had lost.

Then, a few weeks later, I met the founder of the support group: a White, male ob-gyn without children, who had

AJPH June 2025, Vol. 115, No. 6

connected several former patients after they shared how isolated they felt in their sadness. "It's easy to feel helpless when the problem seems so overwhelming, especially if you haven't personally experienced it," he told me. "I couldn't begin to comprehend those parents' grief, let alone offer a straightforward solution. But I found that listening to people's stories is a good start."

I realized that I was clinging to the same mindset I had when I first joined the support group, trying to fit existing answers into the problem instead of truly considering what the parents had shared with me over many meetings: their beliefs, hopes, and visions for the future.

In public health interventions, health care facilitators are seen as the "knowledge holders" because of their professional status, and, by extension, are believed to hold the greatest power. Yet, as Ogunwole and Starks write,[8] the most meaningful connections form when we, as public health advocates, step back from this title and trust others as the true "knowers" of their own experiences. Ultimately, forging a community depends less on what we know and more on our willingness to learn—to recognize what we do not, and perhaps can never, fully understand, and to act with that humility.

Adopting this framework, I set aside my pamphlets and worked with the support group to organize a maternity clothes drive, offering the parents an opportunity to donate tangible reminders of their bereavement while connecting them with local families in need. "It's a way to give purpose to our pain," one group member said. As we packed up the remaining items at the end of the drive, Alice announced that she and her husband planned to apply for adoption next year. The group responded with hugs and cheers of genuine celebration, the kind grounded in a shared understanding of loss and belief in the possibility of healing. Moments like those embody the true work of public health: not just delivering resources or care, but walking alongside people in their darkest times and helping them find light again. In these spaces, we build community. AJPH

CORRESPONDENCE

Correspondence should be sent to Lucy Tu, The Faculty of Law, University of Oxford, St Cross Building, St Cross Road, Oxford OX1 3UL, United Kingdom (e-mail: lucy.tu@law.ox.ac.uk). Reprints can be ordered at https://www.ajph.org by clicking the "Reprints" link.

PUBLICATION INFORMATION

Full Citation: Tu L. Lessons in grief: public health and healing in community. *Am J Public Health*. 2025;115(6):856–857.

Acceptance Date: November 20, 2024.

DOI: https://doi.org/10.2105/AJPH.2024.307955

ORCID iD:

Lucy Tu https://orcid.org/0000-0002-7649-6634

ACKNOWLEDGMENTS

I am deeply grateful to the support group attendees for their compassion, vulnerability, and willingness to share their experiences with me. I also extend my heartfelt thanks to the anonymous *AJPH* reviewers for their invaluable feedback on earlier drafts.

CONFLICTS OF INTEREST

The author declares no conflicts of interest.

REFERENCES

1. Fleszar LG, Bryant AS, Johnson CO, et al. Trends in state-level maternal mortality by racial and ethnic group in the United States. *JAMA*. 2023;330(1):52–61. https://doi.org/10.1001/jama.2023.9043
2. Hill L, Rao A, Artiga S, Ranji U. Racial disparities in maternal and infant health: current status and efforts to address them. KFF. October 25, 2024. Available at: https://www.kff.org/racial-equity-and-health-policy/issue-brief/racial-disparities-in-maternal-and-infant-health-current-status-and-efforts-to-address-them. Accessed December 3, 2024.
3. Trost SL, Beauregard J, Njie F, et al. *Pregnancy-Related Deaths: Data From Maternal Mortality Review Committees in 36 US States, 2017-2019*. Atlanta, GA: Centers for Disease Control and Prevention, US Dept of Health and Human Services; 2022.
4. Tu L. Why maternal mortality rates are getting worse across the US. *Scientific American*. July 25, 2023. Available at: https://www.scientificamerican.com/article/why-maternal-mortality-rates-are-getting-worse-across-the-u-s. Accessed August 21, 2024.
5. Centers for Disease Control and Prevention. One in 5 women reported mistreatment while receiving maternity care. January 1, 2016. Available at: https://www.cdc.gov/media/releases/2023/s0822-vs-maternity-mistreatment.html. Accessed August 21, 2024.
6. Nguyen TT, Criss S, Kim M, et al. Racism during pregnancy and birthing: experiences from Asian and Pacific Islander, Black, Latina, and Middle Eastern women. *J Racial Ethn Health Disparities*. 2023;10(6):3007–3017. https://doi.org/10.1007/s40615-022-01475-4
7. Burden C, Bradley S, Storey C, et al. From grief, guilt, pain, and stigma to hope and pride—a systematic review and meta-analysis of mixed-method research of the psychosocial impact of stillbirth. *BMC Pregnancy Childbirth*. 2016;16(1):9. https://doi.org/10.1186/s12884-016-0800-8
8. Ogunwole SM, Starks FD. Cultivating critical love to improve black maternal health outcomes. *AMA J Ethics*. 2024;26(1):E72–E83. https://doi.org/10.1001/amajethics.2024.72

Notes From the Field: An Article Format Appropriate for the Current Times

Robert J. Kim-Farley, MD, MPH

ABOUT THE AUTHOR

The author is with the Departments of Epidemiology and Community Health Sciences, Fielding School of Public Health, University of California, Los Angeles, and is an associate editor of the American Journal of Public Health.

See also Ferguson, p. 814, Erwin, p. 859, and Brown, p. 862.

I wish to express my gratitude to the many authors of Notes From the Field (NFTF) who have contributed to this dynamic section of *AJPH* and for the vital role these NFTF articles play in sharing innovative public health programs and interventions. I warmly welcome more NFTF submissions as we move into the next 115 years of the journal.

In 2021, the *AJPH* editor-in-chief introduced the NFTF article format,[1] and in 2024 he wrote about the importance of NFTF's contribution to public health practice.[2] The new article format is conducive to reporting on current public health practices that are sustainable and potentially replicable in other localities and communities.

Over the past four years, the NFTF section has documented a wide range of public health challenges and responses highlighting its value in meeting a critical need in the public health community. In 2024 alone, *AJPH* published 15 NFTF articles in regular issues and 22 in four supplements. These articles have covered wide-ranging topics such as the health workforce, local health equity action teams, pediatric vaccination reporting, opt-out hepatitis C testing, and legalization of fentanyl test strips. The diverse institutional and geographical origins of NFTF articles demonstrate their relevance and appeal to a broad audience across the country.

NFTF articles provide valuable insights into the practical implementation and evaluation of public health interventions, offering "lessons learned" that can be applied in other settings. One of the key strengths of these articles is their ability to document fully implemented and evaluated interventions, ensuring that the information shared is based on real-world experiences and outcomes, making it more reliable and useful for public health practitioners.

From my viewpoint, I am always seeking NFTF articles that share successful and impactful field experiences, especially at the local level. The format ensures that key information is presented clearly, enabling replication in other contexts. Unlike research articles, NFTF focuses on describing processes and providing practical, actionable insights for public health practitioners. Importantly, the format allows for rapid dissemination through timely publication and social media sharing.

NFTF articles are structured to ensure comprehensive coverage of the intervention being described; specify the geographic location, implementation period, and targeted population; provide evidence on effectiveness and discussion of any adverse consequences; discuss factors supporting the ongoing continuation of the practice; and indicate the importance of the program for public health locally and more broadly.[2]

In conclusion, through timely publication in the NFTF section, we can ensure that it remains an essential resource for documenting and disseminating best practices and successful interventions. AJPH

CORRESPONDENCE

Correspondence should be sent to Robert J. Kim-Farley, MD, MPH, UCLA Department of Epidemiology, Room 71-279A CHS, 650 Charles E. Young Dr S, Los Angeles, CA 90095 (e-mail: robert@kimfarley.org). Reprints can be ordered at https://www.ajph.org by clicking the "Reprints" link.

PUBLICATION INFORMATION

Full Citation: Kim-Farley RJ. Notes From the Field: an article format appropriate for the current times. *Am J Public Health*. 2025;115(6):858–858.

Acceptance Date: March 17, 2025.

DOI: https://doi.org/10.2105/AJPH.2025.308121

ORCID iD:

Robert J. Kim-Farley https://orcid.org/0000-0003-3022-6548

ACKNOWLEDGMENTS

I acknowledge and appreciate having the opportunity to serve as an *AJPH* associate editor along with the dedicated team of the editor-in-chief, my editor colleagues, and the staff of *AJPH* for so many years. I wish to congratulate *AJPH* for its 115 years of serving the public's health and all of the professionals seeking to achieve social justice.

CONFLICTS OF INTEREST

The author reports no conflicts of interest.

REFERENCES

1. Morabia A. Notes from the field: a repository of best practices. *Am J Public Health*. 2022;112(8):1079. https://doi.org/10.2105/AJPH.2022.306957
2. Morabia A. Notes from the field: why they are important. *Am J Public Health*. 2024;114(11):1134–1135. https://doi.org/10.2105/AJPH.2024.307852

Whose Democracy, and Whose Public Health?

Paul Erwin, MD, DrPH

ABOUT THE AUTHOR

Paul C. Erwin serves as an associate editor of AJPH.

See also Ferguson, p. 814, Kim-Farley, p. 858, and Brown, p. 862.

The framed document on the otherwise bare wall lists the "Keys to Trust in Science and Public Health" as the following:

- Political will: health and education are rights
- An educated population
- Science as a pillar of education
- Accessible health services and information
- Media/social media explain science and health
- Health professionals trained in health messaging
- General public engaged in health

These would appear to be fundamental tenets of a public health system built within a thriving democracy; instead, this was a document in a health clinic, reflecting deeply held and commonly spoken beliefs of the one country in the Western hemisphere with a truly integrated public health and health care system—Cuba. And the biggest threat to Cuba? The United States government, the largest democracy in the same hemisphere.

As described in the 2012 *AJPH* article by Keck and Reed, "The Curious Case of Cuba," health outcomes in Cuba had—at least until the time of that article—been far ahead of what would otherwise be predicted by its economic output—for example, infant mortality and life expectancy equal to or better than in the United States, at an order of magnitude less in health expenditures per capita.[1] And what Cuba was able to implement during the COVID-19 pandemic—creating multiple new vaccines and conducting phased clinical trials through its health system to test those vaccines—resulted in far less COVID-19 morbidity and mortality compared with the US experience.[2] The credit for these achievements is the Cuban health system, a multitiered system with a strong foundation of primary care, free to all at every level, rooted in the concepts of "care according to need," well-integrated with the biotech and pharma sectors, with health care as a fundamental, constitutionally guaranteed right of every citizen.

During his first administration, President Trump added 243 more restrictions on Cuba, at a time when it was already suffering the longest and most comprehensive unilateral sanctions in modern history.[3] And the new constraints include the death blow of relisting Cuba on the State Department's state sponsors of terrorism (SSOT) list, joining Iran, Syria, and North Korea (an action opposed by many former Bush and Obama governmental officals[4]). As a result of that measure alone, Cuba has virtually no access to international banking, making normal trade in essential goods impossible. Although many had hoped that the Biden administration would take a different approach with Cuba, the Trump-imposed restrictions, including the SSOT listing, were left in place until the very end of the Biden administration. The SSOT was lifted on January 14, 2025, only to have it reinstated by the new president on January 20, 2025.[5,6] What does the United States have so much to fear about Cuba in 2025 that it continues an embargo in effect for over 60 years and layers on even more punitive measures? There is such inconsistency in US foreign policy. We somehow found a way to restore diplomatic relations with communist-led Vietnam, which has now become a vitally important trading partner in Southeast Asia. And see what we have built over more than 50 years through diplomatic relations with the largest communist-led presence in the world: China. Yet, we are so worried about Cuba and its 11 million people?

For more than 30 years—especially since Clinton signed the Helms–Burton Act, codifying the US embargo on Cuba into law—the hyperpartisanship surrounding *any* US action on Cuba appears to be driven solely to either appease or at least not anger the powerful slice of the Cuban-American community that remains steadfastly against the Cuban government. I'll put it out there: the previous administrations were—and the new administration remains—politically opportunistic with respect to these voters' opposition to Cuba. As if the Cuban-American vote could singlehandedly tilt the overall US electorate toward the Republicans—which it doesn't—or as if the Democrats could continue to hold out hope that appeasing such Cuban-Americans in Florida will somehow win back the state—which it won't. I think it comes down, mostly, to this: the United States just can't bear the lingering images

AJPH June 2025, Vol. 115, No. 6

of Fidel Castro thumbing his nose at the United States for so long. Perhaps the embarrassment started all the way back with José Martí, considered a national hero in Cuba for leading the revolution to liberate the country from Spain in the late 1800s, who believed in a free Cuba that could stand in the way of 19th-century US expansionism and forge an egalitarian society that would serve as a counter to the racist legacies of post-Reconstruction America. A small Caribbean island lighting the way to democracy, freedom, and equality? No way, José, as the saying goes.

I recently returned from my 10th visit to Cuba in as many years, and even during my short time there, I was able to witness the destructive impact of US policies. Following the brief return of full diplomatic relations under President Obama and the benefits this brought—especially through increased tourism and the promise of investment in both the private and public sectors—the nation has been on a slow downward slide. The additional US restrictions on Cuba, especially the SSOT listing, combined with the pandemic's impact on tourism and trade along with subsequent numerous hurricanes in rapid succession, have left the island cash poor.

The weight of the US insistence on allowing support only to the private sector (e.g., in the rare circumstances under which we can legally travel to Cuba, US citizens cannot stay in any of over 400 state-owned or managed hotels) has slowly created distinct economic layers in a society that previously was much more egalitarian. What policy changes the Biden administration did make only further promoted the private sector.[7] Cubans refer to the years following the Soviet collapse and subsequent withdrawal of support in the 1990s as the "Special Period," when, as a result of a loss of 85% of its trade and foreign aid, scarcity resulted in documented nutritional deficiencies and the outmigration of many Cubans. But even in those difficult years, the resilience of Cubans and their commitment to an egalitarian society were paramount. Cubans consider this current era to be a new Special Period, worse than the first, but with a clear distinction. As Gail Reed, a US journalist who has reported from Cuba for over 40 years, describes it, "In the Special Period, at least if I had only 6 eggs, you also had 6 eggs. Now I may have 10 eggs, and you may have 2." (Personal communication, January 10, 2025. Reed currently chairs the board of directors of Medical Education Cooperation with Cuba [MEDICC], a US nonprofit organization that fosters US–Cuba health collaboration aimed at extending the right to healthy lives for all, and under whose auspices I have traveled to Cuba.)

My overall impression following this most recent visit: Cuba is dying. It is Gaza in slow motion. The extent of outmigration, especially among younger Cubans (the 11 million population figure given earlier is likely much closer to 10 million or even less, particularly because of recent outmigration[8]), paired with a birth rate already below replacement levels, is fundamentally changing the landscape for what is possible for a healthy and thriving Cuba. This has a direct impact on the health system and the health care–public health workforce that is key to its success; lose that workforce and the system will not survive.

My point in this editorial? Although we are questioning whether a threat to democracy in the United States is a threat to *our* public health, perhaps we might, even for a moment, consider how our own much-touted democracy and democratic institutions are crushing a public health system that has worked *for its people*. In another twist of irony, recent polling data show that a majority of Americans favor expanding diplomatic ties with Cuba and lifting travel and economic restrictions.[9] Whose democratic voice is being heard? Saving democracy alone, without putting the core beliefs of what it means to be a democracy into practice both here and abroad, will not sustain us. Nor should it represent us. AJPH

CORRESPONDENCE

Correspondence should be sent to Paul C. Erwin, MD, DrPH, 3993 8th Court South, Birmingham, AL 35222 (e-mail: perwin57@gmail.com). Reprints can be ordered at https://www.ajph.org by clicking the "Reprints" link.

PUBLICATION INFORMATION

Full Citation: Erwin P. Whose democracy, and whose public health? *Am J Public Health*. 2025; 115(6):859–861.

Acceptance Date: March 15, 2025.

DOI: https://doi.org/10.2105/AJPH.2025.308127

ORCID iD:
Paul Erwin https://orcid.org/0000-0002-0580-4855

CONFLICTS OF INTEREST

The author serves on the Board of Directors for the Medical Education Cooperation with Cuba and receives no compensation for this voluntary service.

ACKNOWLEDGMENTS

I acknowledge Gail Reed for her assistance in clarifying and validating the Biden and Trump administrations' actions vis-à-vis Cuba and Sonia Kikeri for her review and comments on an earlier draft of the manuscript.

REFERENCES

1. Keck CW, Reed GA. The curious case of Cuba. *Am J Public Health*. 2012;102(8):e13–e22. https://doi.org/10.2105/AJPH.2012.300822
2. Powell MA, Erwin PC, Bermejo PM. Comparing the COVID-19 responses in Cuba and the United States. *Am J Public Health*. 2021;111(12):2186–2193. https://doi.org/10.2105/AJPH.2021.306526
3. Lippmann W. Compendium of Trump's measures against Cuba. *CubaNews*. January 15, 2022. Available at: https://walterlippmann.com/trumps-243-measures-against-cuba. Accessed January 11, 2025.
4. Bernal R. Bush, Obama alumni ask Biden administration to ease up on Cuba before Trump takes office. *The Hill*. December 17, 2024. Available at:

https://thehill.com/latino/5045016-bush-obama-biden-harris-trump-cuba-rules. Accessed January 10, 2025.

5. Hunnicutt T, Sherwood D. Biden looks to relax Cuba sanctions in final days before Trump. *Reuters.* January 15, 2025. Available at: https://www.reuters.com/world/americas/us-lift-designation-cuba-state-sponsor-terrorism-ap-reports-2025-01-14. Accessed January 28, 2025.
6. Spetalnick M. Trump revokes Biden removal of Cuba from US state sponsors of terrorism list. *Reuters.* January 20, 2025. Available at: https://www.reuters.com/world/americas/trump-revokes-biden-removal-cuba-us-state-sponsors-terrorism-list-2025-01-21. Accessed January 28, 2025.
7. DeYoung K. Biden administration eases some economic restrictions on Cuba. *Washington Post.* May 28, 2024. Available at: https://www.washingtonpost.com/national-security/2024/05/28/us-cuba-sanctions-biden-trump. Accessed January 11, 2025.
8. Augustin E. Biden's Cuba policy leaves the island in wreckage. *Drop Site.* October 1, 2024. Available at: https://www.dropsitenews.com/p/where-to-watch-the-debateand-a-dispatch. Accessed January 10, 2025.
9. Dandekar A, Fairclough T. Voters want Biden to continue advancing diplomatic ties with Cuba during his lame-duck session. *Data for Progress.* December 11, 2024. Available at: https://www.dataforprogress.org/blog/2024/12/11/voters-want-biden-to-continue-advancing-diplomatic-ties-with-cuba-during-his-lame-duck-session. Accessed January 11, 2025.

An American Health Dilemma 25 Years Later

Theodore M. Brown, PhD

ABOUT THE AUTHOR

Theodore M. Brown is professor emeritus of history and public health sciences, University of Rochester, Rochester, NY, and an AJPH associate editor.

See also Ferguson, p. 814, Kim-Farley, p. 858, and Erwin, p. 859.

When W. Michael Byrd and Lynda A. Clayton published their massive two-volume *An American Health Dilemma* (New York, NY: Routledge) in 2000 and 2002, the volumes were reviewed in major journals, such as the *Journal of the American Medical Association*, the *New England Journal of Medicine*, the *Journal of Health Politics, Policy, and Law*, and *Social Science and Medicine* and generally given accolades. One reviewer commended the two volumes as filling a void in "the way we think about the issues of health and health policy."[1(p875)] Another praised volume 1 (*A Medical History of African Americans and the Problem of Race: Beginnings to 1900*) for doing

> a masterful job of collecting information from disparate sources about the roles of illness and inequity. The strengths of the work . . . are the thoroughness of the research and comprehensive scope of coverage.[2(p458)]

A third praised the same volume as "staggeringly ambitious . . . compellingly written and meticulously documented" and added:

> *An American Health Dilemma* is not the first attempt to document race-based biomedical inequities, but it surely represents the most comprehensive effort to place black health in its full sociohistorical context.[3(p1219)]

The same reviewer applauded volume 2 (*Race, Medicine, and Health Care in the United States: 1900–2000*) as

> a detailed history of the rise of modern medicine and a devastatingly incriminating account of the complex ways in which prevailing conceptions of race and class in every era have informed medical education and training, medical and political discourse, relations between white and black practitioners, and, of course, clinical interactions with African-American and other poor patients.[4(p3009)]

The reviewer added:

> Practitioners who claim to treat all patients as individuals may find unsettling the authors' implication that bias so pervades the very marrow of health care that color-blind diagnosis and treatment are impossible.[4(p3009)]

Given its subject matter and scope, *An American Health Dilemma* would normally have been reviewed in *AJPH*. But it was not because, at the time it was published, the *Journal* was passing through a period when it reviewed no books at all, however significant for public health and US health policy they may have been. *AJPH* has since decided to review major books again, but its policies restrict reviews to newly or very recently published books. However, in the spirit of the *New York Times*' "Overlooked No More" obituaries begun in March 2018 to pay respect to individuals who were inappropriately overlooked when they passed away,[5] *AJPH* will include a set of reflective essays in this 115th anniversary volume under the rubric "An American Health Dilemma 25 Years Later."

These solicited and peer-reviewed essays by prominent historical scholars and policy analysts will assess the major contributions of Byrd and Clayton in ways that evaluate what those authors claimed about key issues and what those claims look like in light of modern scholarship and contemporary data. Topics will include long-standing ideas about racial differences in North America, slave health and medical treatment, childbearing and reproductive health under slavery, Black hospitals and professional organizations, disputed origins of 20th-century African American health disparities, Black medical professional leadership in the 20th century, Black patients in 20th-century urban and rural hospitals, Black struggles for medical education and postgraduate training, racial discrimination in federal policies and programs, and the cause and consequence of Black health disparities in the United States of the 20th-century. Leading scholars have accepted invitations to contribute reviews on these topics with a look both at what Byrd and Clayton wrote on those topics and at what contemporary data and analysis reveal. We will publish one or two of these retrospective essays per month beginning in July 2025. AJPH

CORRESPONDENCE

Correspondence should be sent to Theodore M. Brown, Department of History, University of Rochester, 362B Rush Rhees Library, P.O. Box 270070, Rochester, NY 14627 (e-mail: theodore_brown@urmc.rochester.edu) Reprints can be ordered at https://www.ajph.org by clicking the "Reprints" link.

PUBLICATION INFORMATION

Full Citation: Brown TM. *An American Health Dilemma* 25 years later. *Am J Public Health*. 2025; 115(6):862–863.

Acceptance Date: March 17, 2025.

DOI: https://doi.org/10.2105/AJPH.2025.308132

CONFLICTS OF INTEREST

The author has no conflicts of interest to disclose.

REFERENCES

1. Smith DB. *An American Health Dilemma: Race, Medicine, and Health Care in the United States, 1900–2000*. *J Health Polit Policy Law*. 2002;27(5): 873–876. https://doi.org/10.1215/03616878-27-5-873
2. Washington HA. *An American Health Dilemma. Vol. 1. A Medical History of African Americans and the Problem of Race: Beginnings to 1900*. *N Engl J Med*. 2002; 346(6):458. https://doi.org/10.1056/NEJM200202073460621
3. Race and Health: *An American Health Dilemma: A Medical History of African Americans and the Problem of Race—Beginnings to 1900*. *JAMA*. 2001;285(9):1219. https://doi.org/10.1001/jama.285.9.1219
4. Race and Health Care: *An American Health Dilemma: Race, Medicine, and Health Care in the United States 1900–2000, vol 2*. *JAMA*. 2002;287(22):3009. https://doi.org/10.1001/jama.287.22.3009-JBK0612-3-1
5. *The New York Times*. Overlooked. March 8, 2018. Available at: https://www.nytimes.com/spotlight/overlooked. Accessed March 15, 2025.

Passing Policies That Promote Urban Health: Lessons From the CityHealth Project

David H. Jernigan, PhD, Katrina Forrest, JD, Catherine Patterson, MPP, and Brian Castrucci, DrPH

Cities are important laboratories for cross-sectoral collaboration and advancing equity. CityHealth, a project of the de Beaumont Foundation and Kaiser Permanente, used legal epidemiology to identify, score, and promote nine city-level policies important to population health in the 40 largest US cities from 2017 to 2021. The project supported 86 policy changes over five years. These results demonstrate possibilities for encouraging passage of city-level health-enhancing policies and the need to move beyond scoring and ranking to direct policy advocacy. (*Am J Public Health*. 2025;115(6):864–867. https://doi.org/10.2105/AJPH.2025.308036)

AJPH June 2025, Vol. 115, No. 6

CityHealth, a project of the de Beaumont Foundation and Kaiser Permanente, used methods from legal epidemiology, the scientific study and deployment of law as a factor in the cause, distribution, and prevention of disease and injury,[1] to track, score, and promote nine city-level policies important to population health.[2]

INTERVENTION AND IMPLEMENTATION

Building on evidence that addressing social determinants of health through policy changes can improve population health,[3] over five years of published assessments, CityHealth supported 86 policy changes in the nation's 40 largest cities. This article describes what CityHealth did that led to these policy changes and lessons this may provide for the public health field.

PLACE, TIME, AND PERSONS

From 2017 to 2021, CityHealth engaged and worked with subject matter experts and technical assistance partners to identify or validate best practices in each policy domain. The project partnered with Legal Science LLC, now at Temple University, which searched city codes to find statutes embodying these best practices, their prevalence across the 40 cities, and the degree to which cities in various states were limited or "preempted" by state law from action on the policy. This research guided CityHealth's collaborations with city leadership and civil society partners to support policy change.

PURPOSE

Cities are significant population centers: 39% of the nation's population clusters in the roughly 800 cities with populations greater than 50 000, 19.3% live in the 100 largest, and 13.7% live in the 40 largest cities.[4] From parks to pollution, cities have the potential to influence health in both positive and negative ways.[5] Cities are often the first to face and test strategies for dealing with emerging health problems,[6] such as housing, transportation, food and economic security, mental health and substance use, and air quality. With persistent gridlock and partisanship at federal and state levels, cities may have more room for policy innovation[7]; one observer called local governments "an increasingly positive force, innovating and solving problems that would have been beyond them a decade ago."[8] Health departments in large cities are more likely than other local health departments to engage with local, state, and federal policy beyond the confines of the health department.[9]

EVALUATION AND ADVERSE EFFECTS

Details of the development of CityHealth's initial nine-policy package have been provided elsewhere[2] and are summarized briefly here. The project had four essential elements: (1) a curated, evidence-based, and informed policy package; (2) legal epidemiology tracking those policies across the nation's 40 largest cities; (3) annual reports awarding medals for cities that passed them; and (4) a focused government relations effort communicating the policy package and what cities would need to do to improve their medal standing.

Existing public health research provided evidence of health impact of policies and what policy elements were most important to that impact; these informed the project's definition of "best practices."[2,10] Further details about each policy, including public health evidence for their effectiveness and specific policy elements required for each medal level, may be found in the Appendix (available as a supplement to the online version of this article at https://ajph.org).

The project vetted its initial nine-policy package through consultation with a range of civil society partners, as well as a policy advisory committee composed of elected officials and leaders from academic public health, consumer health product retailers, hospital and health care systems, national membership organizations, and local chambers of commerce. CityHealth initially sought to address nine categories of city-level social determinants of health, many of which lie outside the strict purview of health departments: education, housing, employment and income, food and nutrition, active living and transportation, mental health and substance use, public health and emergency preparedness, public safety, and environment and air quality. In addition to likely impact on health, selection criteria for candidate policies included evidence of return on investment, bipartisan support, political feasibility demonstrated by successful implementation in at least one US city, being within city jurisdictional authority, ease of implementation, and potential for ameliorating health disparities. No formal weights were assigned to these criteria; the development process was deliberative and consultative, benefiting from input from the policy advisory committee, subject matter experts from academia and civil society organizations, and preliminary legal surveillance demonstrating feasibility through existing city ordinances that met or came close to meeting scoring criteria.

This research informed a scoring structure in which cities with best practice versions of the policies would receive a gold medal for that policy area, and cities with some elements of good policy could receive silver or bronze medals. CityHealth staff and consultants analyzed each city based on criteria for each policy and through the lens of how far cities were from achieving overall medals, as defined by an algorithm awarding overall gold for at least five gold medals, overall silver for five gold or silver medals but falling short of five golds, and bronze for four gold, silver, or bronze medals.

The project's initial primary focus was on the scoring itself. Expectations were that this and the positive media coverage accompanying it would be sufficient motivation for city leaders. However, key informant interviews with elected city leaders and focus groups with registered voters in four cities at the project's outset revealed that health policy advocates had a steep hill to climb: neither group viewed health as a priority, stressing instead economic development, public safety and crime, and housing affordability. Two possible communications strategies produced greater resonance: (1) emphasizing how health policies could affect the issues that most concerned city leaders and residents and (2) crafting messages about those policies that were uplifting, aspirational, and positive.[2]

Recognizing it was not inventing policy wheels but, rather, promoting and encouraging changes already underway in at least some cities, CityHealth collaborated with and provided financial support to existing organizations working in the policy spaces it selected, including the National Institute for Early Education Research, the Campaign for Tobacco-Free Kids, Smart Growth America, the American Heart Association, Family Values @ Work, A Better Balance, and the National Environmental Health Association. However, findings from the public opinion research as well as conversations early on with city leadership led the project to pivot from primary reliance on public communication and media advocacy as motors of change to an intensive government relations effort, enhancing both internal and external direct advocacy capacity to do "grasstops" organizing.[11] Resources from Kaiser Permanente permitted hiring consultants to deepen this approach in cities within its integrated health care services footprint. Because of the concentration of large cities in Texas, the project also added a part-time government relations consultant focused on cities there.

CityHealth staff and consultants used fora such as the US Conference of Mayors and the National League of

TABLE 1— Medals Awarded in the 40 Largest US Cities by Population for Nine Policies Addressing Social Determinants of Health: 2017 and 2021

	2017, No.			2021, No.		
Policy	**Gold**	**Silver**	**Bronze**	**Gold**	**Silver**	**Bronze**
Affordable housing	2	6	4	3	7	3
Earned sick leave	2	4	11	4	6	12
Complete streets	16	14	1	30	7	1
Food safety/restaurant rating	9	3	0	12	3	0
Healthy food procurement	8	2	5	9	7	3
Smoke-free indoor air	18	14	4	21	14	2
High-quality, accessible pre-K	8	6	17	15	3	15
Tobacco 21	13	0	0	40	0	0
Safer alcohol sales	8	6	0	8	8	0

Cities meetings to promote the policy package and recognize mayors of cities earning medals. At every step, City-Health collaborated closely with local health officials. The de Beaumont Foundation's close affiliation with the Big Cities Health Coalition, bringing together leading health officers of the nation's largest cities, facilitated consultation and communication with them.

Table 1 shows the changes by policy area, from 2017 to 2021. Figure 1 shows the progress in overall medals, using the algorithm described previously: 47.5% of cities received an overall medal in 2017, while 92.5% merited this recognition in 2021.

SUSTAINABILITY

By requiring that medal-earning policies be written into and findable through legal epidemiology in city codes (except the pre-K medals), the CityHealth approach ensured the sustainability of the policies it promoted. On the basis of its successes in the first five years, CityHealth received further funding from the two funders to develop and promote a revised and enlarged policy package in the nation's 75 largest cities from 2022 to 2026.

PUBLIC HEALTH SIGNIFICANCE

CityHealth's focus on policy passage rather than measurement of impact is a limitation. However, the project's experience has at least two key implications for the public health field. The first is that, even in partisan times, it is possible to make progress on policies that promote population health and safety. CityHealth, from its inception,

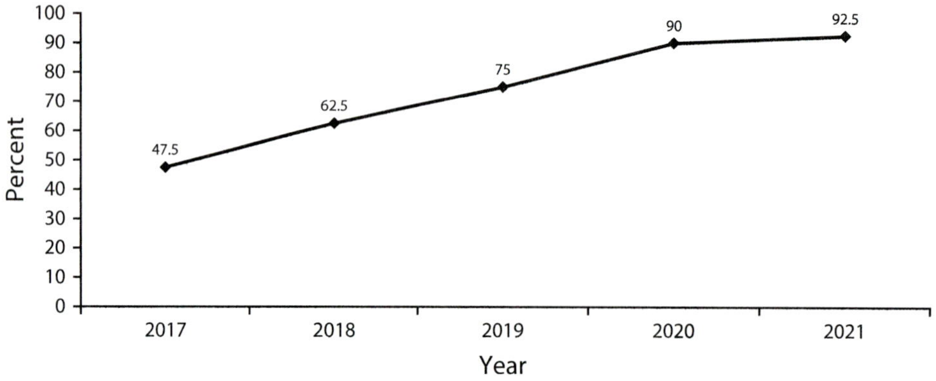

FIGURE 1— Percentage of 40 Largest US Cities Earning an Overall CityHealth Medal: 2017–2021

Note. Cities received an overall gold medal for passing policies meeting gold medal criteria in at least five of the nine policy areas, an overall silver for at least five gold or silver medals but falling short of five golds, and an overall bronze for four gold, silver, or bronze medals.

worked for and recognized individual policy achievements in all 40 cities, regardless of party of leadership; by 2021, overall medalist cities included Fort Worth, Texas; Houston, Texas; and Oklahoma City, Oklahoma (Republican leadership), as well as Las Vegas, Nevada, and San Antonio, Texas (led by independents).

The second is the need to move beyond ranking and scoring to coordinated advocacy to achieve changes beneficial to population health. Scoring systems usefully point to key health indicators and risk factors. But policies matter for health, and there is a need for greater implementation of the Institute of Medicine's 2011 recommendation for initiating and testing policy surveillance systems that track and report on specific health-enhancing policies.[12] For instance, the Center for Public Health Law and Research at Temple University operates LawAtlas, tracking public health–relevant policies across 20 topic areas.[13] However, tracking and reporting on health-enhancing policies is but the crucial first step in promoting evidence-based approaches to social determinants of health. Using these findings to stimulate policy change requires government relations and advocacy expertise and skills.[14] CityHealth's experience adds to the body of evidence showing how critical these skills are, both within and without public health departments,[15] for creating the environments that will support millions of people to live longer, better lives in vibrant, prosperous communities. AJPH

ABOUT THE AUTHORS

David H. Jernigan is with the Boston University School of Public Health, Boston, MA. Katrina Forrest, Catherine Patterson, and Brian Castrucci are with the de Beaumont Foundation, Bethesda, MD.

CORRESPONDENCE

Correspondence should be sent to David H. Jernigan, 715 Albany St, Talbot 349W, Boston, MA 02118 (e-mail: dhjern@bu.edu). Reprints can be ordered at https://www.ajph.org by clicking the "Reprints" link.

PUBLICATION INFORMATION

Full Citation: Jernigan DH, Forrest K, Patterson C, Castrucci B. Passing policies that promote urban health: lessons from the CityHealth project. *Am J Public Health*. 2025;115(6):864–867.

Acceptance Date: January 17, 2025.

DOI: https://doi.org/10.2105/AJPH.2025.308036

ORCID iD:
David H. Jernigan https://orcid.org/0000-0002-0789-6917

CONTRIBUTORS

All authors contributed to the conceptualization of the article. D. H. Jernigan drafted and all other authors contributed revisions to the article, and all authors gave final approval to the version to be published.

ACKNOWLEDGMENTS

All authors received support from the de Beaumont Foundation and Kaiser Permanente for the development of this article.

CONFLICTS OF INTEREST

The funders were involved in the decision to publish and with the preparation of the article. There are no other conflicts to disclose.

HUMAN PARTICIPANT PROTECTION

There were no human participants involved in the work described in this article.

REFERENCES

1. Ramanathan T, Hulkower R, Holbrook J, Penn M. Legal epidemiology: the science of law. *J Law Med Ethics*. 2017;45(1 suppl):69–72. https://doi.org/10.1177/1073110517703329
2. Castrucci BC, Corcoran EA, Hearne SL, Keith K, Voyles E, Patterson C. CityHealth: policies for today's urban health challenges. In: Galea S, Ettman CK, Vlahov D, eds. *Urban Health*. New York, NY: Oxford University Press; 2019:298–308. https://doi.org/10.1093/oso/9780190915858.003.0032
3. Thornton RLJ, Glover CM, Cené CW, Glik DC, Henderson JA, Williams DR. Evaluating strategies for reducing health disparities by addressing the social determinants of health. *Health Aff (Millwood)*. 2016;35(8):1416–1423. https://doi.org/10.1377/hlthaff.2015.1357
4. Toukabri A, Medina L. Latest city and town population estimates of the decade show three-fourths of the nation's incorporated places have fewer than 5,000 people. United States Census Bureau. October 8, 2021. Available at: https://www.census.gov/library/stories/2020/05/america-a-nation-of-small-towns.html. Accessed January 25, 2023.
5. Galea S, Freudenberg N, Vlahov D. Cities and population health. *Soc Sci Med*. 2005;60(5):1017–1033. https://doi.org/10.1016/j.socscimed.2004.06.036
6. Fielding JE. Public health in big cities: looking back, looking forward. *J Public Health Manag Pract*. 2015;21(suppl 1):S20–S23. https://doi.org/10.1097/PHH.0000000000000134
7. Institute of Medicine. *For the Public's Health. Revitalizing Law and Policy to Meet New Challenges*. Washington, DC: The National Academies Press; 2011.
8. Ehrenhalt A. How cities became the new laboratories of democracy. Available at: https://www.governing.com/archive/gov-urban-power.html. Accessed January 26, 2023.
9. Hearne S, Castrucci BC, Leider JP, Rhoades EK, Russo P, Bass V. The future of urban health: needs, barriers, opportunities, and policy advancement at large urban health departments. *J Public Health Manag Pract*. 2015;21(suppl 1):S4–S13. https://doi.org/10.1097/PHH.0000000000000166
10. Castrucci BC, Hearne S, Solomon L, Stoss JH. CityHealth: advancing strong policy to help cities thrive. *Natl Civ Rev*. 2019;108(2):34–40.
11. Joshi A, Heller RE, Acharya PT, Milla SS, Annam A. Pediatric radiology and advocacy: a professional responsibility. *Pediatr Radiol*. 2022;52(8):1412–1419. https://doi.org/10.1007/s00247-022-05369-9
12. Committee on Public Health Strategies to Improve Health; Institute of Medicine. Appendix G, For the Public's Health: Revitalizing Law and Policy to Meet New Challenges. In: *For the Public's Health: Investing in a Healthier Future*. Washington, DC: National Academies Press; 2012.
13. Center for Public Health Law and Research. LawAtlas. Temple University Beasley School of Law. Available at: https://lawatlas.org/topics. Accessed November 25, 2024.
14. Hearne S, Jernigan DH. Who will advocate to keep the public healthy? Establishing competency-based advocacy training for the public health field. *J Public Health Manag Pract*. 2024;30(1):3–7. https://doi.org/10.1097/PHH.0000000000001839
15. Hearne SA, Jernigan DH, Frey M, Matthews GW, Baker EL. Strengthening advocacy skills for public health leaders. *J Public Health Manag Pract*. 2023;29(6):950–952. https://doi.org/10.1097/PHH.0000000000001827

The Far Right, Authoritarian Power, and Public Health

Kenneth Rochel de Camargo, MD, PhD

ABOUT THE AUTHOR

Kenneth Rochel de Camargo is a full professor at the Instituto de Medicina Social, Universidade do Estado do Rio de Janeiro, Brazil, and an emeritus editor of AJPH.

See also Power, Politics, and Human Rights in Public Health, pp. 870–889.

The connection between public health and democratic policies has long been acknowledged. Two articles and an editorial in this issue add important themes to this discussion. On the one hand, they expand and make precise the threats that the resurgence of fascism or, more generally, far-right movements in various forms present to public health; on the other hand, they shed light on a frequently overlooked component of the social determinants approach: how power is held and wielded, how it affects inequality, and the differential risks it entails for various population groups. Taken together, these articles show how power imbalances are at the very heart of health inequities, and how such imbalances are a key feature of authoritarian, far-right politics, thus shedding more light on the inverse correlation between concentration of power and better health for all people.

In their analytic essay (p. 873)[1] the APLICA Cooperative points to the rise of far-right governments in various parts of the world, which have adopted a variety of antidemocratic policies that disrespect civil rights and consequently present a direct threat to public health. Despite variations in the character of those governments, they share a number of characteristics, described by the authors with regard to authoritarianism, injustice, racism, misogyny, LGBTQIA+phobia , divisive rhetoric, and a propensity for violence. For each of those aspects, the authors provide concrete examples of the threat they present to public health. Additionally, they show that the far right tends to adopt denialist positions with regard to scientific developments, which was plainly and painfully demonstrated before and during the COVID-19 pandemic by the response (or lack thereof) from governments aligned with that ideology, such as Brazil between 2019 and 2022 or the United States between 2016 and 2020.

Commenting on APLICA's article from a political science point of view, Greer (p. 870) adds important elements to their analysis. First, he stresses that rather than being an ideology of marginal parties, the far right is a form of political practice that unfortunately has permeated mainstream political parties in traditionally democratic countries. He also highlights the role played by institutions, such as political parties, that allow such practices to become part of the ruling body of government. Although some scholars might not share Greer's emphasis on presidentialism as an inherent contributor to political instability and a possible takeover of democracies by fascism, his analysis of recent political upheavals, particularly in the United States, is acute and pertinent.

Finally, Reynolds and Galea (p. 883) propose a thorough discussion of power and how it relates to public health issues. They invoke both the 19th-century physician, scientist, and social reformer Rudolph Virchow (1821–1902) and former Chilean president (and physician) Salvador Allende (1908–1973), who was assassinated by the September 1973 military coup that enthroned a military dictatorship in that country, as examples of authors who made the connection between power and health inequalities. Presenting distinct theoretical frameworks, they point out how power imbalances—that is, subjugation of certain groups of people by others along fracture lines of race, ethnicity, gender, and class—are directly related to the inequalities that translate into health risks as studied by the social determinants of health approach. Compared with authoritarian governments, a democratic government is more conducive to proper public health policies. Reynolds and Galea additionally articulate the growing literature on commercial determinants of health as also reflecting power relationship issues, to the extent that when commercial interests hold more weight and influence in governments, democracy tends to fade. Conversely, civil resistance can counteract some of the effects of the concentration of power in fewer hands. Options for furthering the research on power relations and public health are also presented.

The concrete consequences for public health of far-right governments have been in clear display recently in the Americas. The governments of the

United States (between 2016 and 2020) and Brazil (between 2019 and 2022) offered prime examples of far-right politicians. Faced with the challenge of the COVID-19 pandemic, both governments failed to rise to the occasion. Both displayed an antiscience streak, sowed fear, doubt, and uncertainty about vaccines, blamed China for the pandemic, and touted unproven therapeutics as a response to the crisis, simultaneously downplaying nonpharmacological interventions such as social distancing and using masks in public.[1,2] The current US administration is adopting even worse stances, cutting jobs and funding in essential areas of public service and research; a particularly troubling development from the point of view of public health is the nomination of a notorious antivaccine activist as secretary of the Department of Health and Human Services, despite strong protestation from several health organizations, including the APHA.[3] In Argentina, deep cuts in the public budget threw more than half the population under the poverty line, and compromised public health care and research.[4]

Modern far-right governments share one important characteristic with their early 20th-century precursors: they used the tools and institutions of democracy against itself, with varying degrees of success. Once they were elected or obtained a parliamentary majority, they dedicated themselves to promoting an authoritarian, unpopular agenda, especially with regard to the economy. And here lies an important interpretive key that was not brought to the fore in the articles analyzed here.

Decades of neoliberal, "trickle-down," structural adjustment policies produced a degree of wealth concentration unseen since the end of the 19th century. The concentration of wealth, as demonstrated by the French economist Thomas Piketty,[5] brought with it not only a corresponding concentration of power, with the rise of oligarchies that support the far-right movement, but also a high degree of instability, both political and economic. The many financial crises that took place beginning in the mid-1970s further deepened the gap between rich and poor, creating a sense of helplessness and disillusionment that proved to be a fertile ground for the propagation of far-right ideologies. By saving banks and leaving everyone else in the rain in 2008, governments all over the world contributed to an increasing distrust in democracy itself.

In 1848, Virchow wrote in his "Report on the Typhus Epidemic in Upper Silesia" that "[t]he interests of the human race are not served when, by an absurd concentration of capital and landed property in the hands of single individuals, production is directed into channels that always guide back the flow of the profits into the same hands. . . . Therefore, I abide by the doctrine which I have placed at the head of this discussion: Free and unlimited democracy."[6(p2104)]

Public health is inherently political, albeit not partisan. With the ascent of the far right, however, the political dispute is no longer between left and right in its various versions, but between democracy and authoritarianism, whose divisive and polarizing ideology is incompatible with public health.[7] AJPH

CORRESPONDENCE

Correspondence should be sent to Kenneth Rochel de Camargo, Instituto de Medicina Social, Universidade do Estado do Rio de Janeiro, R. S. Francisco Xavier, 524 7° Andar Bloco D, Rio de Janeiro, RJ 25.559-900, Brazil (e-mail: kencamargo@gmail.com). Reprints can be ordered at https://www.ajph.org by clicking the "Reprints" link.

PUBLICATION INFORMATION

Full Citation: Rochel de Camargo K. The far right, authoritarian power, and public health. *Am J Public Health*. 2025;115(6):868–869.

Acceptance Date: March 16, 2025.

DOI: https://doi.org/10.2105/AJPH.2025.308123

ORCID iD:
Kenneth Rochel de Camargo https://orcid.org/0000-0003-3606-5853

CONFLICTS OF INTEREST

The author declares no conflicts of interest.

REFERENCES

1. Yamey G, Gonsalves G. Donald Trump: a political determinant of covid-19. *BMJ*. 2020;369:m1643. https://doi.org/10.1136/bmj.m1643
2. Ortega F, Orsini M. Governing COVID-19 without government in Brazil: ignorance, neoliberal authoritarianism, and the collapse of public health leadership. *Glob Public Health*. 2020;15(9):1257–1277. https://doi.org/10.1080/17441692.2020.1795223
3. Benjamin GC. America deserves better than RFK Jr. American Public Health Association. Available at: https://www.apha.org/news-and-media/news-releases/apha-news-releases/2024/rfk-jr-hhs-nomination. Accessed February 13, 2025.
4. Santoro E. Están condenando a morir a la gente con cáncer y hay personas sufriendo por dolor porque Milei les sacó los medicamentos. Pagina12. Available at: https://www.pagina12.com.ar/810488-estan-condenando-a-morir-a-la-gente-con-cancer-y-hay-persona. Accessed March 14, 2025.
5. Piketty T. *Capital in the Twenty-First Century*. Cambridge, MA: Belknap Press; 2014. https://doi.org/10.4159/9780674369542
6. Virchow RC. Report on the typhus epidemic in Upper Silesia. *Am J Public Health*. 2006;96(12):2102–2105. https://doi.org/10.2105/AJPH.96.12.2102
7. Morabia A. The fascist threat. *Am J Public Health*. 2021;111(4):538–539. https://doi.org/10.2105/AJPH.2021.306169

What Can Be Done About the Global Far Right's Threat to Health?

Scott L. Greer, PhD

ABOUT THE AUTHOR

Scott L. Greer is professor of health management and policy, global public health, and political science (by courtesy) at the University of Michigan-Ann Arbor and senior expert advisor on health governance to the European Observatory on Health Systems and Policies, Brussels, Belgium.

See also Power, Politics, and Human Rights in Public Health, pp. 868–889.

The far right is a global phenomenon, and a successful one lately. As the APLICA Cooperative writes in this issue of *AJPH* (p. 873), it is also bad news for public health. There is no definition of public health that can accept the far right's "authoritarianism, injustice, racism, misogyny, LGBTQIA+phobia, divisive rhetoric, and . . . propensity for violence." Fortunately, political science research can help us address the rise of the global far right—and show us how adhering to the ethical commitments of public health is also a wise political strategy. This editorial highlights some especially relevant consensus findings from political science research on the topic.

WHAT EMPOWERS THE FAR RIGHT?

The APLICA Cooperative defines the far right as not just far-right parties but also "ultra-conservative moments, fascist groups, regimes with totalitarian tendencies, and all the discourses that are coming with them." This definition is awkwardly broad, but it does capture something important: the far right is a form of political practice, not the identity of marginal parties.

Mainstream parties are often the reason that far-right policies are adopted.[1] It was the United Kingdom's Conservatives that delivered Brexit. It is US Republicans who held signs reading "MASS DEPORTATION NOW" at 2024 campaign rallies and embarked on a campaign against birthright citizenship in 2025. Big established parties, trying to preempt rising far-right challenges, can implement policies that the radical right parties would never be strong enough to enact.

Political institutions decide what votes mean. For example, electoral rules that create two-party systems limit voter choice. There is no evidence that either Germany or the United States has a far-right majority, but electoral rules gave the United States a far-right government in 2024. The divergence emerged in two steps. First, the US far right was able to take over the Republicans in low-turnout primary elections. Second, in the general election, US voters discontented with Democrats were offered only one real alternative, and that alternative was Donald Trump. German electoral rules, by contrast, allowed voters in 2025 to express discontent with the incumbent government without voting for the far right, and then gave the far right a share of legislative seats proportionate to its actual support.

There are many institutional factors that affect democratic sustainability in ways that can be hard to tease out, but at the moment a particularly perilous one to highlight is presidentialism, the phenomenon of a directly elected president with a fixed term such as we see in the United States or France.[2] The problem with presidential systems is that they combine dual legitimacy (both the president and the legislature can claim a personal mandate from the people) with rigidity (the president is hard to remove outside elections). They create overmighty executives with weak democratic accountability who are hard to remove. Presidentialism is by no means the only cause of authoritarianism, but it creates the problem that an authoritarian president can be left in charge of the state after they have lost support, a combustible situation that the United States might soon face. Prime Minister Liz Truss in the United Kingdom lost public support and was famously removed by her political party in less time than it took a lettuce to go bad. In a presidentialist system, she would have had years more in office with no clear way to remove or even check her.

WHAT CAN PUBLIC HEALTH ADVOCATES DO?

For people motivated by public health, which in the 21st century includes a clear commitment to equity and human rights, political scientists' analysis offers some lessons.

Better Health Is a Political Intervention

Pay attention to directly exploring and combatting health-related roots of radical right politics. A variety of studies show that people in poor health are less likely to participate in politics and more likely to vote for the far right; more usefully still, they pinpoint the mechanism, which is reduced trust.[3] People failed by health care providers lose trust in society and either disengage or become open to extremist appeals. Rural American voters whose hospitals close shift toward Republicans, even if it was Republican policies that led to the closure.[4] Ill health can lead to distrust, which benefits the far right. Appeals to patient-centered, trustworthy, responsive health care take on a new edge if we can tell policymakers that the alternative is an increasing far-right vote in their constituency.

Political Reform Can Be a Public Health Policy

Political institutions can empower or disempower the far right and are therefore a fit object of advocacy. Consider the state of Michigan, a relatively poorly educated, aging state long stuck on a weak economic trajectory. Since 2020, its voters have liberalized regulations on unions, drawn state and federal legislative districts to maximize political competitiveness, and facilitated ballot access, producing one of the country's highest rates of registration of eligible voters. All of these political reforms are associated with better health and social outcomes.[5–7] If the political science is correct, Michigan's trajectory should change. Political determinants of public health matter.

Change the Subject

To a skittish mainstream political party, it can seem wise to adopt policies popularized by the far right. In particular, adopting far-right proposals on immigration, citizenship, and gender and reproductive issues can look like a way to win back socially conservative voters and redirect the conversation to other topics.

In practice, the strategy is very risky. Selling out members of your coalition creates friction and demobilizes them.[8] Meanwhile, adopting versions of far-right proposals increases the salience of those issues, normalizes far-right ideas and politicians, and does not win over far-right voters.[9] Echoing far-right views of immigration, in particular, contributes to far-right parties' success.[10]

Nor does letting the far right dictate the agenda affect the most persuadable, marginally decisive voters. Marginal voters generally decide on the basis of household income growth shortly before the election.[11] Xenophobia and transphobia do not improve average household incomes. The solution to a far-right challenge is not to embrace it; it is to change the topic.

Policy Is the Far Right's Weakness

Research on the populist radical right is disproportionately focused on what they say, not what they do in office. That bias in research veils their major weakness: the gap between rhetoric and reality. The rhetoric of populist radical right parties is frequently that of "welfare chauvinism," which promises a lavish welfare state for insider populations and exclusion for others. But decades of research have found that in office, these parties are rather conventionally right wing. They deliver stingier and more exclusive welfare states, reducing access to "outsiders" without making them more generous, while deregulating businesses and corrupting public administration.[12]

DOING GOOD IS DOING GOOD POLITICS

Broadly, the global far right that the APLICA Cooperative identifies reiterates a basic model that combines aggressive redistribution to the rich and protection for higher-income people with xenophobic rhetoric and policies. Pointing this out, rather than conceding their ideas, is wise before the election.

Once they are in office, what these parties do is frequently unpopular, and their signature issues can lose salience quickly. That is their weakness. The voters who support the far right because they like its ideology are a limited share of any electorate. The same marginal voters who vote their wallets, uninterested in appeals to democracy, continue to vote their wallets, uninterested in appeals to bigotry.

Opposing the far right requires renewed commitment to advocacy for equity, science, and human rights. It also requires collaboration with political science researchers and practitioners who understand the subtle ways that political institutions and public opinion work to empower or defeat the radical right, and the reforms that might change our direction. That is not just the foundation of 21st-century public health ethics; it is also the political practice that can defeat the far right. AJPH

CORRESPONDENCE

Correspondence should be sent to Scott L. Greer, Department of Health Management and Policy, University of Michigan School of Public Health, 1415 Washington Heights, Ann Arbor, MI 48109-2029 (e-mail: slgreer@umich.edu). Reprints can be ordered at https://www.ajph.org by clicking the "Reprints" link.

PUBLICATION INFORMATION

Full Citation: Greer SL. What can be done about the global far right's threat to health? *Am J Public Health*. 2025;115(6):870–872.

Acceptance Date: March 15, 2025.

DOI: https://doi.org/10.2105/AJPH.2025.308128

ORCID iD:
Scott L. Greer https://orcid.org/0000-0002-5288-0471

ACKNOWLEDGMENTS

I thank Holly Jarman for her comments.

CONFLICTS OF INTEREST

The author has no conflicts of interest to declare.

REFERENCES

1. Bale T, Kaltwasser CR, eds. *Riding the Populist Wave: Europe's Mainstream Right in Crisis.* Cambridge, UK: Cambridge University Press; 2021. https://doi.org/10.1017/9781009006866
2. Linz JJ. The perils of presidentialism. *J Democracy.* 1990;1(1):51–69. https://doi.org/10.1353/jod.2005.0026
3. Kavanagh NM, Menon A. *Health as a Driver of Political Participation and Preferences: Implications for Policy-Makers and Political Actors.* Brussels, Belgium: European Observatory on Health Systems and Policies; 2024.
4. Shepherd ME. The politics of rural hospital closures. *Polit Behav.* 2025. https://doi.org/10.1007/s11109-024-10000-8
5. Gamm G, Kousser T. Life, literacy, and the pursuit of prosperity: party competition and policy outcomes in 50 states. *Am Polit Sci Rev.* 2021;115(4):1442–1463. https://doi.org/10.1017/S0003055421000617
6. Montez JK, Beckfield J, Cooney JK, et al. US state policies, politics, and life expectancy. *Milbank Q.* 2020;98(3):668–699. https://doi.org/10.1111/1468-0009.12469
7. Bedekovics G, Maciolek A. *How Michigan Became a Blueprint for Strengthening Democracy.* Washington, DC: Center for American Progress; 2023.
8. Nicolaisen MH. Normalizing and absorbing the radical right: The Danish People's Party. In: Bourne AK, ed. *Democratic Defence as Normal Politics: Everyday Opposition to Populist Parties in Multilevel Europe.* Cham, Switzerland: Springer Nature; 2024:271–293. https://doi.org/10.1007/978-3-031-60483-6_11
9. Krause W, Cohen D, Abou-Chadi T. Does accommodation work? Mainstream party strategies and the success of radical right parties. *Political Sci Res Methods.* 2023;11(1):172–179. https://doi.org/10.1017/psrm.2022.8
10. Valentim V. *The Normalization of the Radical Right: A Norms Theory of Political Supply and Demand.* Oxford, UK: Oxford University Press; 2024. https://doi.org/10.1093/9780198926740.001.0001
11. Bartels LM. *Unequal Democracy: The Political Economy of the New Gilded Age.* Princeton, NJ: Princeton University Press; 2008.
12. Falkenbach M, Greer SL, eds. *The Populist Radical Right and Health: National Policies and Global Trends.* New York, NY: Springer; 2021.

Potential Global Effects of the Rise of the Far Right on Public Health

Sebastià March, José Miguel Carrasco, Álvaro Flores-Balado, Aitana Muñoz-Haba, Ana Pereira-Iglesias, and Gustavo Andrés Zaragoza on behalf of the APLICA Cooperative

See also Power, Politics, and Human Rights in Public Health, pp. 868–889.

The influence of the far right is growing globally. This calls for a critical examination of its potential public health implications.

Characterized by authoritarianism, injustice, racism, misogyny, homophobia, transphobia, divisive rhetoric, and a propensity for violence, the far right often employs denialist arguments against scientific evidence, including opposition to environmental protection policies. We conducted a narrative review of existing evidence to assess the impact of these elements on public health.

The findings suggest that the rise of the far right could have significant negative effects on population health. As a consequence, we advocate that the public health field and society at large must take a deliberate stance in response to this emerging reality. (*Am J Public Health*. 2025;115(6):873–882. https://doi.org/10.2105/AJPH.2025.308016)

AJPH June 2025, Vol. 115, No. 6

In recent years, the far right has gained presence and power in different regions of the world. In Europe, they are currently represented in the governments of countries such as Poland, Hungary, Switzerland, Finland, Turkey, Italy, and the Netherlands, and in the administration of regional governments in France, Germany, and Spain. In the Americas, the governments of Bolsonaro in Brazil (2019–2022), Milei in Argentina (2023), or Trump in the United States (2017–2021 and recently again in 2024) came to power under the same wake. Authoritarian forms of government and perspectives continue to exist in other parts of the world as well, such as in Israel, and their ideas and discourses are increasingly present in the media and social networks around the globe.[1–3] In this article, we examine how the rise of these far-right tendencies may affect the health of the global population.

For the purposes of this reflection, the concept of far right is not limited only to those parties that call themselves such but also includes ultraconservative movements, fascist groups, regimes with totalitarian tendencies, and all the discourses that come with them and that are permeating the rest of society.[1,4] These actors may take different forms in each region, although they share a common identity and ideological elements.[1,4] A fundamental one is that they understand that inequalities are intrinsic to human beings and, therefore, should not be corrected. In practice, this means upholding the power privileges of certain elites (e.g., racial, economic, gender) over the rest of society.[1] Among the common elements of the spreading far-right tendencies discussed in this article, the following stand out:

- the tendency toward authoritarianism,
- the defense of policies that increase social injustice and inequality related to economic neoliberalism,
- the discriminatory component of its ideas (racist, misogynist, homophobic, transphobic),
- the use of polarizing discourses that fragment social cohesion and generate a sense of fear and rupture,
- the self-interested denial of scientific evidence for political gain, and
- the antienvironment agenda, which defends private profit over the protection of the planet's habitability conditions.

Although these characteristics are not exclusive to the far right and can be found in other ideological spectrums, they do form substantial elements of its identity.

The approach of this article is that public health science, which is by definition a promoter and protector of health and well-being, has a responsibility to position itself and denounce those actions that are negative for the health of the population. These actions include the maintenance of inequalities, the promotion of discrimination, or the maintenance of patriarchy, all of which are related to and promoted by the far right. Furthermore, it is understood that public health must be aligned with the protection and defense of human rights, and it has been argued that the rise of the far right poses a serious risk of regression of these rights.[5]

Therefore, this context of the far-right escalation demands a reflection on its potential impacts on health,[6] especially following the experience of the COVID-19 pandemic, which provided several examples of where far-right health policies might be heading.[7,8] With this essay, we aim to deepen this reflection from a public health perspective, carrying out a narrative review of the scientific literature to point out the impacts that the advance of the far right already has or could have on population health.

THE FAR RIGHT IS AUTHORITARIAN

The discourses of the far right are associated with authoritarian ideas and values that undermine plurality and democratic freedoms.[1] There is evidence that authoritarian governments, compared with democratic ones, have worse population health indicators: a study, using longitudinal data from 168 countries collected between 1960 and 2010, found that, adjusted for gross domestic product, countries with democratic elections have, on average, 11 years longer life expectancy and 62.5% lower infant mortality than those without.[9] One explanation for this phenomenon is that democratic regimes tend to protect their citizens better, more effectively, and more equitably, as could be seen during the COVID-19 pandemic.[8]

But authoritarianism is not just about the type of government regime but also about the values that underpin it. The far right is associated with authoritarian ideas that can also be defended within democratic regimes, such as the claim of the leader or of "strong" governments, or the valorization and use of law enforcement and "repressive" actions to uphold the law.[1] Moreover, actors with authoritarian ideas are also more likely to support antidemocratic measures to defend their positions.[10] These authoritarian values affect the development and quality of democracy, which is also related to population health indicators. For example, having more representative and pluralistic governments and having more political competition and party alternation in power are factors associated with higher life expectancy at birth and lower infant mortality.[11,12]

A recent example of the health risks of authoritarianism is the Hungarian government under Viktor Orbán. His government has been accused of undermining democratic institutions, restricting press freedom, and repressing political opposition.[13] These authoritarian tendencies may have hampered the ability of health experts and institutions to provide transparent and evidence-based guidance during crises such as the COVID-19 pandemic. In addition, the erosion of democratic norms may lead to reduced accountability in health systems, which could result in decisions that prioritize political considerations over public health needs and unequal access to health resources, thereby reinforcing inequities.[13]

THE FAR RIGHT IS UNFAIR

The evidence that epidemiology has provided on health inequities is so compelling that it is now difficult to justify any public health action that does not incorporate an equity perspective.[14] It is recognized that structural social inequalities in the distribution of power, whether by income, race, gender, or any other determinant, create unjust and avoidable health inequities.[14] Far-right parties and movements often ignore this aspect, taking an incomplete scientific view of population health, which can lead them to develop discourses and promote policies that can generate harm to society.[15]

Structural factors that determine these inequalities could be governance and policies.[14] In recent decades, the far right has adapted the neoliberal positions supporting free markets, financial deregulation, and the reduction of the capacities of welfare states to provide social protection to their citizens.[4,15] The implementation of these neoliberal policies points to an increase in socioeconomic inequalities.[15,16] In turn, rising income inequalities are associated with poorer outcomes on diverse indicators ranging from general and infant mortality to violent crime, adolescent pregnancy, obesity, social distrust, and depression.[17] There is evidence that indicates that in countries with more right-wing governments, less egalitarian traditions, or less developed welfare states, there is an increase in inequalities, and, consequently, this has a negative impact on population health indicators such as life expectancy, infant mortality, or general health.[16]

A circular relationship between the far right and inequalities should be noted[18]: its policy proposals promote inequality, and, in turn, the increase in social inequality is associated with an increase in the far-right vote. Therefore, it is in the interests of these actors not only to defend privilege but also to increase disparity, even though this may harm the health of the most privileged.[17]

Another strand of neoliberal policies embraced by the far right is cuts in public services. There is evidence that these cuts are harmful to population health, impacting such substantial and robust indicators as overall mortality.[19] In general, these cuts, whether in health or not, affect marginalized groups more, widening the health gap. Bolsonaro's far-right government in Brazil implemented specific cuts for the indigenous population.[20] Trump's government in the United States has also made specific cuts, targeting those with fewer economic resources, mostly Black people.[21] Therefore, inequality is promoted in these countries through cuts to the welfare system.

THE FAR RIGHT IS RACIST

A common feature of the far right's public approach is the xenophobic discourse that dehumanizes and criminalizes foreigners.[1,2] These approaches are also related to the defense of a hierarchical structure of power and privilege based on a supposed race.[1,22] Race is a construct of social classification, determined by perceived physical or ancestral appearance, and has an important effect on health that operates at both the individual and the structural or community level.[22,23] Racism can lead to forms of cultural, ethnic, religious, or place-of-origin discrimination, which also have an impact on health.[23]

The effects of racism on health may vary depending on the context and the population affected, although there are common factors in the impacts studied.[22] It can act indirectly, affecting other social determinants, such as socioeconomic status, but also directly, as an independent factor.[22] At the individual level, experiencing racism can generate negative behavioral, psychological, and physiological responses.[22] The experience of racism is associated with poorer health habits, less physical activity, poorer diet, and abuse of tobacco and other toxic substances.[22] Racism is a stressor that is also associated with poorer mental health outcomes, with a higher prevalence of depression, anxiety, low self-esteem, relationship difficulties, and suicide attempts.[22,23] This also affects the biological level, with poorer physical health outcomes and chronic diseases.[22,23] The cumulative effects of racism can lead to metabolic changes, which would explain impacts such as low birth weight, higher infant mortality, cognitive impairment, dementia, and risk of premature death.[22]

Racism also operates on population health at the community and structural levels.[22] For example, it promotes spatial segregation that leads to inequalities in access to resources and services and exposure to health risks.[22] At the collective level, we speak of institutional racism when there are policies or administrative actions that are prejudicial based on the conception of race.[24] This is the case with far-right policy proposals, which tend to disadvantage minoritized groups. One example, as mentioned earlier, is the application of cuts in social benefits within the framework of neoliberal policies, which mostly affects populations of certain races or origins. This is a particular form of necropolitics, where it is decided who has the right to live and who does not.[22,25] Another example is border, migration, and asylum policies, which have their most dramatic effect on border deaths but also affect the health and lives of asylum seekers in host countries.[25] Far-right groups have an identity element in pushing for the tightening of these policies, insensitive to the impact they have on the future of entire generations.

THE FAR RIGHT IS MISOGYNISTIC

The far right is conservative and traditional in its understanding of the world.[1] Their discourses and attitudes are clearly related to ideas that promote patriarchy (i.e., the maintenance of a hierarchical social structure where men prevail over women) through the preservation of differentiated gender roles.[26] In general, the far right spreads messages that deny the scientific and social advances related to gender that feminist theories have contributed, downplaying their value.[26] All of this leads them to promote a transnational agenda that denies gender and feminism and, therefore, discriminates against a large part of the population.[26]

In public health, it has long been well-known that gender inequalities have an impact on health.[14,27] Countries with worse indicators of gender equality (greater wage or care gaps) also have worse health indicators for women than for men.[27] Because of gender roles or social norms associated with gender in a patriarchal society, inequities are created in exposure to risks, behavioral differences, and other factors, which determine health inequities between men and women.[14]

These inequalities are reproduced in health institutions in the form of implicit biases of professionals, who may provide different care depending on gender because of their own stereotypes, independent of biological factors.[28]

One of the most serious forms of inequality produced by patriarchy is gender-based violence, as has been recognized by multiple international entities such as the United Nations and the World Health Organization. Worldwide, 27% of the female population aged 15 to 49 years have experienced physical or sexual violence by an intimate partner or another man.[29] Violence against women has known long-term effects on their health, such as worsening menopausal symptoms and increasing the risk of contracting infectious diseases or developing diabetes, substance abuse, chronic diseases, and pain.[30] To deny existing knowledge about the effects of patriarchy is to deny the structural causes of the gender gap in health and to downplay the importance of the global public health problem of gender-based violence.

Another of the issues where the action against gender equality and public health of the far right is exemplified is in their antiabortion policies.[31,32] The public health evidence on the suitability of safe abortion is compelling[31,32]: lower maternal and infant mortality, lower cost to the system and families, and lower socioeconomic and community impact on society. In contrast, in countries that have practiced antiabortion policies, the opposite effects have occurred, without reducing the prevalence of abortion.[31,32] According to a 2016 systematic review,[33] the stigma caused by antiabortion discourse on women receiving this benefit also has a negative impact on their health, with increased self-judgment, fear of social judgment, and the need to hide their experience, leading to increased symptoms of psychological distress and social isolation. This stigma is promoted by conservative and ultra–right-wing discourses that single out women who have abortions.

THE FAR RIGHT IS HOMOPHOBIC AND TRANSPHOBIC

In their gender-denialist stance, the far right also discriminates against those who step outside the traditional, patriarchal framework of gender roles.[1] They defend heteronormative masculinity and femininity, as well as a vision of the traditional family that leads them to wield homophobic and transphobic narratives.[1] These forms of discrimination on the basis of gender identity or sexual orientation also have important health impacts on the population and individuals.[34]

Societies with policies that discriminate on the basis of sexual orientation and gender identity are known to have poorer physical and mental health indicators and lower life expectancy in men.[34] Because of this discrimination, gay and lesbian youths suffer greater bullying, lower self-esteem and social support, poorer school performance, higher rates of sexually transmitted infections, and higher prevalence of suicide, anxiety, and depression than heteronormative youth.[35] Queer people also have higher barriers to accessing the health care system and, therefore, are more likely to self-medicate, with detrimental consequences for their health.[36]

Furthermore, in countries where discrimination is more prevalent, queer people are more likely to experience an effect known as internalized homophobia and transphobia, which leads them not to accept their sexuality or gender identity.[37] This phenomenon is associated with increased mental health problems (e.g., anxiety, depression) and higher rates of suicide, drug use, and eating disorders and has a negative impact on social relationships.[37] The homophobic and transphobic loudspeaker that is the discriminatory voices of the far right can increase negative health impacts for these populations.

THE FAR RIGHT IS DIVISIVE

The maintenance of social inequalities defended by the far right is closely related to a detriment to social cohesion, which is, in turn, a fundamental determinant of population health.[38] Different conceptualizations of social cohesion converge around the ideas of trust in others or identification with the same common good.[38] Those are the elements that the far right tends to break with their discourses. They frequently use confrontational narratives, whose central axis is the logic of "us versus them," creating social polarization and promoting social discrimination.[1,2,39] They also use fear-based discourses and policies and alarmist rhetoric (e.g., "the country is breaking up"; "there is a cultural invasion"; "decay of institutions"; "increase in crime") to facilitate support for the discriminatory and authoritarian measures commonly found in their programs.[1,39] These discourses cause a constant sense of fear and tension in the population and severely erode social cohesion, directly affecting population health. The effects described in the literature range from increased stress, depression, anxiety, fatigue, and anger to loss of sleep, temper, or control over certain actions.[40] These rupturing discourses also serve as a justification and a call for discrimination and violence.[39,41]

To disseminate these narratives, far-right groups use digital media and social networks.[39,41] In particular, they relate to the use of fake news, conspiracy theories, and, in general, disinformation, with the intention of boosting their discourse. Conspiracy theories, even if false, can have consequences on real people, such as negative impacts on interpersonal relationships, perceptions of security, or social distancing that can promote violent tendencies.[42]

An example of this strategy of fragmentation and fear was experienced in many countries during the COVID-19 pandemic, where far-right-wing groups launched messages that questioned the preventive actions promoted by health institutions. The consequence was to promote resistance to these measures, increasing fear, depression, and fatigue.[43] At a time when there was an important need for social cohesion, for everyone to walk together, various sectors of the far right throughout the world promoted disagreement and conflict, calling for division, which in some cases could lead to violence.[7]

THE FAR RIGHT IS VIOLENT

The discriminatory discourses of the far right not only fragment society but also promote hatred and fear of what is different with hyperbolic and radical rhetoric that points to violence as a solution.[39,41] Their more or less veiled calls for violence and their amplification in the media and social networks seem to be related to the increase in aggressions.[2,3,39]

Violence spiraling is a public health problem, affecting not only those who suffer from it but also the perpetrators and the whole community.[44] Apart from the impact of aggression, violence can cause long-term impacts on the brain, the immune response, and the neuroendocrine system, which can lead to increased incidence of depression, anxiety, posttraumatic stress disorder, and suicide, or increased cardiovascular risk and premature death.[44] Interpersonal violence can also affect the community as a whole: witnesses of violence or members of the same community as those who receive violence are more at risk for depression or intergenerational trauma.[44]

Particularly relevant because of their relation to right-wing extremist discourses are hate crimes—attacks on people for being different in terms of religion, nationality, sexual orientation, gender identity, etc.[3] These are a worrying and growing reality that is also a public health problem. Examples of this violence on minoritized populations include the assaults on people of Asian origin during the COVID-19 pandemic[7] and those received by transgender people.[45] In the latter group, having suffered violence is related to suicide attempts and the consumption of toxic substances.[45] The far right, with its inflammatory speeches, promotes and even perpetrates these crimes and violent actions,[2] including terrorist actions associated with these ideas.[46]

THE FAR RIGHT IS ANTISCIENCE

Another common feature of the far right in modern times is the dissemination of an antiscience discourse that triggers resistance and reinterpretations of societal research advancements. This has already been pointed out in the denial of the impact of inequalities on health. However, when it aligns with their interests in political agitation and social division, it can also encompass other equally important health-related issues. For instance, the use of denialist discourses can lead people to alter healthy behaviors or reject advice provided by institutions to improve their health, avoiding evidence-based therapeutic or preventive interventions (such as contraceptives or vaccines).[47,48]

Moreover, there was resistance to preventive public health measures during the COVID-19 pandemic. There was already evidence linking far-right ideologies to vaccine resistance before the pandemic,[47] but it became particularly relevant during this time.[49] There was also resistance toward other preventive measures, such as the use of masks.[50] Therefore, the far right can not only harm the health of populations but also undermine actions designed to improve it by spreading and legitimizing messages that go against these actions.[48]

THE FAR RIGHT IS ANTIENVIRONMENTAL

In the line of denying advances in scientific knowledge, the far right also promotes skeptical discourses regarding climate change or the acknowledgment of human responsibility for it.[51] There is solid evidence on the causes and consequences of climate change and its negative health effects,[52] to the extent that it has been identified as the main challenge for public health in the 21st century. Again, these effects are unevenly distributed, exacerbating health inequities.[52] The far right

BOX 1— Synthesis of Results of Far-Right Impacts on Population Health

Far-Right Is	What They Do	Known Health Impacts
Authoritarian	They hold more authoritarian and less pluralistic and democratic regimes and values.	Authoritarian regimes have worse life expectancy and maternal and infant mortality, adjusted for income. Less pluralistic governments are associated with lower life expectancy and higher maternal and infant mortality.
Unfair	They do not recognize an equity perspective, favor privilege, and promote neoliberal policies that foster inequalities, welfare state cuts, and the disempowerment of marginalized groups.	Neoliberal policies increase health inequalities between and within countries. Greater income inequalities are associated with higher rates of overall and infant mortality, obesity, depression, violent crime, adolescent pregnancy, and social distrust. Governments with less egalitarian traditions are associated with poorer life expectancy, infant mortality, and general health indicators. Cuts in public services are associated with increased overall mortality and have a greater impact on marginalized and minoritized groups.
Racist	They maintain xenophobic and racist discourses and promote the resurgence of necropolitics against migrant and minoritised populations.	The experience of racism is associated with poorer health habits such as less physical activity, poorer diet, and consumption of toxic substances. It is also associated with poorer mental health, depression, anxiety, and self-esteem, and increased suicide attempts. Suffering from racism is associated with poorer physical health indicators, more chronic diseases, lower birth weight, and higher premature mortality, cognitive impairment, and dementia. Racism promotes spatial discrimination that leads to inequities in access to resources and services and exposure to health risks. Necropolitics, such as those related to migration, have a substantial impact on people's health.
Misogynist	They maintain an antigender and antifeminist agenda that denies the contributions of gender theory, including equality policies. They uphold the privileges of men over women in the distribution of roles. They maintain an antiabortion stance and a denial of gender-based violence.	Gender roles create inequities in health, starting in childhood and continuing into adulthood. Countries with worse equity rates have worse health indicators for women. Structural gender inequalities underpin gender-based violence. Abortions continue to occur, even with antiabortion laws, albeit with poorer safety conditions. Unsafe abortions increase maternal and infant mortality, the cost to the system and families, and the resulting harm from stigma to the women who have them.
LGBTQIA+phobic	They uphold the privileges of normative gender roles and traditional family structures and discriminate against people with diverse gender identities or sexual orientations.	In the most homophobic societies, there are poorer physical and mental health indicators, and men have lower life expectancy. Young gay men suffer higher rates of bullying, poorer self-esteem and academic performance, and higher prevalence of suicide, anxiety, and depression. Queer people have more difficulty accessing the health care system. Where there is discrimination, there is greater internalized homophobia, which is associated with higher rates of depression, anxiety, and suicide, and increased drug use and eating disorders. Discrimination has a negative impact on social support and difficulties in relating to others.
Divisive	They sustain polarizing discourses, alarmist narratives, and the politics of fear, which fragment social cohesion.	Social cohesion is an important component of population health. Discourses of fear and polarization are associated with increased stress, depression, anxiety, loss of sleep, and worsening physical health. Conspiracy theories can have negative impacts on interpersonal relationships, perceptions of safety, or social distancing. Fake news can alter people's behavior, creating resistance to public health recommendations.
Violent	They wield inflammatory and dehumanizing narratives that justify and promote certain forms of violence, including terrorism.	Violence is a public health problem that affects those on the receiving end, the perpetrators, and the community. Increased assaults are associated with the spread of far-right discourses. Violence can cause long-term health effects, such as increased depression, anxiety, posttraumatic stress disorder, or suicide, and increased risk of cardiovascular disease or premature death. Suffering more violence is collectively associated with a higher prevalence of depression, lower social cohesion, and higher rates of premature births and intergenerational trauma.
Antiscience	They deny scientific knowledge when it goes against their interests.	Denialist discourses can erode the impact of public health interventions and the prestige of the institutions that promote them.

Continued

BOX 1— Continued

Far-Right Is	What They Do	Known Health Impacts
Antienvironmental	They deny climate change, promoting deregulation and delegitimization of environmental protection policies.	Climate change has serious effects on the health of populations and their inequities. Increased air pollution is closely linked to the rise in respiratory and cardiovascular diseases, resulting in millions of deaths per year. The scientific consensus is that pollution and human impact on global warming and the planet's other biophysical and ecological limits must be regulated.

Note. LGBTQIA+ = lesbian, gay, bisexual, transgender, queer or questioning, intersexual, or asexual plus.

engages in a transnational climate change denial agenda.[51] This agenda often presents neoliberal approaches, advocates for deregulation, and defends the interests of private entities and large multinational corporations.[51]

In addition to the false debate on climate change, other well-known and undeniable phenomena related to the environment and caused by human action have a negative impact on health. An example is air pollution. Its impact on health, especially respiratory and cardiovascular diseases, is well-documented, and it is estimated that more than 4 million premature deaths annually can be attributed to outdoor air pollution.[53] Improving air safety would prevent deaths and illnesses, leading to economic savings and increased social productivity.[54] However, the antienvironmentalist policies promoted by the far right go in the opposite direction: less control of pollutant emissions, discrediting environmental protection institutions, reducing sanctions, and withdrawing from international commitments to reduce air pollution, among others.[55] These obstructionist actions can, in the most authoritarian regimes where they hold power, lead to persecution and even violence against environmental activists,[51] often linked to indigenous populations, introducing a racial and discriminatory component once again.

Beyond all these actions, the mere legacy of discredit and erosion that the far right wields against environmental protection actions and institutions has a significant and difficult-to-erase impact on society. The messages of the previous Trump administration denying human pollution's responsibility for climate change (calling it a racist "Chinese hoax") or claiming that protective measures would cost jobs resonated with the American population, resulting in less support for environmental policies and institutions.[56] Therefore, it can be concluded that the far right has its own agenda that it defends despite the interests of the planet and the global population.

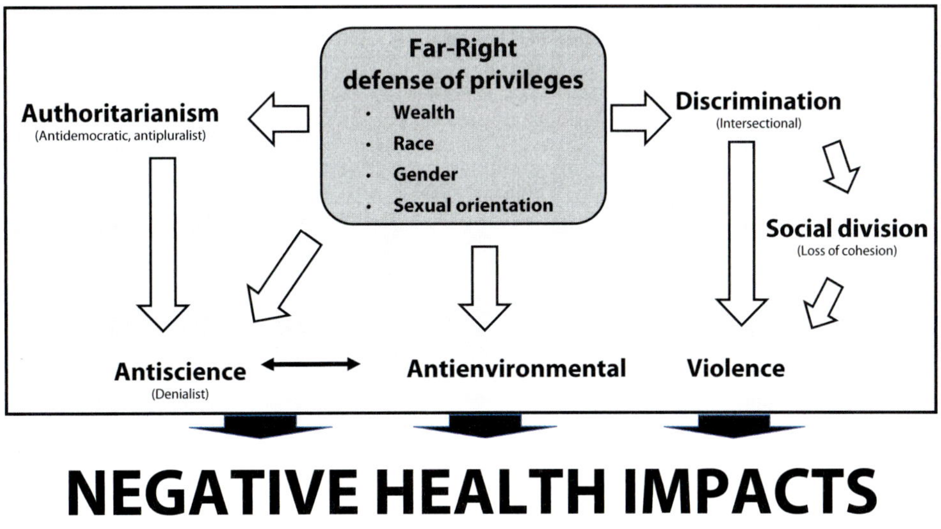

FIGURE 1— Explanatory Framework of the Relation Between the Far Right and Negative Health Impacts

Note. Some examples of negative health impacts related to the far right are represented in Box 1.

CONCLUSION AND CALL TO ACTION

The far right, in its many forms and guises, is gaining power in various parts of the world. Its discourses are permeating society and promoting or reinforcing policies that have a negative impact on population health and worsen inequities (Box 1). These impacts are broad, affecting mental, physical, and social health, and are reflected in robust indicators such as mortality. Because of the defense of their privileges in power axes (e.g., wealth, race, gender, sexual orientation), the far right maintains denialist positions against science, environmental issues, and discriminatory practices, ultimately fueling social division and violence (Figure 1). Far-right ideas, movements, parties, and policies represent, therefore, a threat to health. Public health as a discipline and its professionals as a community cannot remain on the sidelines in the face of this reality and must take a clear, critical stance.[57] The existence of public health based on scientific evidence is necessary to highlight these impacts and advocate actions to neutralize and prevent them.

There are public health interventions designed to reduce some of the effects that far-right policies can have, such as actions to promote equality,[27] reduce discrimination[58] and social inequalities,[59] and mitigate the impact of climate change.[60] This palliative approach to impacts is necessary but proves insufficient. There is also a need to identify the root of the problem that generates changes in discourse. The far right must be denounced, not engaged in a sterile dialectical battle of differing opinions. It must be confronted as an infection that spreads. We need health promotion interventions, vaccines, protective networks, monitoring, and treatment of the infected. But the goal, let us not forget, is to eradicate it.

We are not alone in this task. Various sectors and social movements are organizing to confront the values promoted by the far right, a task for the entire society. Public health can add another dimension to this struggle. We have the responsibility to contribute our knowledge and experience to expose policies that will harm the health of the population. These are not times to hide behind a supposed neutrality of science. Scientific knowledge has supported positions in favor of equity, health, social cohesion, the promotion of freedoms, and human rights for years without fear of taking a stand to defend the health of the population.[5] It is, then, appropriate to denounce those approaches that go against these principles.

If you work for a better public health, be critical against far-right policies; do not whitewash their ideas, movements, and parties; and be proud to be antifascist. AJPH

ABOUT THE AUTHORS

The authors are members of APLICA Cooperative, Madrid, Spain.

CORRESPONDENCE

Correspondence should be sent to Sebastià March, APLICA Cooperative, 22 Alameda St, 28014, Madrid, Spain (e-mail: sebastia.march@gmail.com). Reprints can be ordered at https://www.ajph.org by clicking the "Reprints" link.

PUBLICATION INFORMATION

Full Citation: March S, Carrasco JM, Flores-Balado Á, Muñoz-Haba A, Pereira-Iglesias A, Zaragoza GA. Potential global effects of the rise of the far right on public health. *Am J Public Health*. 2025;115(6):873–882.

Acceptance Date: January 2, 2025.

DOI: https://doi.org/10.2105/AJPH.2025.308016

ORCID iD:
Sebastià March https://orcid.org/0000-0001-7238-9519

CONTRIBUTORS

S. March had the idea and prepared the first draft. S. March and A. Pereira-Iglesias carried out the review. The structure of the work was discussed collectively by the entire APLICA team, and all authors reviewed and made contributions to the document.

ACKNOWLEDGMENTS

The APLICA cooperative is dedicated to and specialized in public health research. We are part of a social economy network, and our mission is to develop research that impacts the well-being of the community. Therefore, we are antifascists, and we position ourselves against far-right ideas, movements, parties, and policies. We appreciate the collaboration of Elisa García-Mingo, Maite Cruz, and Elena de la Vega in revising the first drafts of the article.

Note. This review does not make these collaborators responsible for the opinions expressed, nor for any errors we may have made in writing.

CONFLICTS OF INTEREST

This work has been self-financed by APLICA Cooperative.

HUMAN PARTICIPANT PROTECTION

This study did not conduct direct research with humans.

REFERENCES

1. Jupskås AR, Leidig E. *Knowing What's (Far) Right. A Compendium.* C-REX. University of Oslo. 2020:100. Available at: https://www.sv.uio.no/c-rex/english/groups/compendium/c-rex-compendium-print-version.pdf. Accessed November 13, 2023.
2. Wahlström M, Törnberg A, Ekbrand H. Dynamics of violent and dehumanizing rhetoric in far-right social media. *New Media Soc.* 2021;23(11):3290–3311. https://doi.org/10.1177/1461444820952795
3. Müller K, Schwarz C. Fanning the flames of hate: social media and hate crime. *J Eur Econ Assoc.* 2021;4(19):2131–2167. https://doi.org/10.1093/jeea/jvaa045
4. Saull R. Capitalism, crisis and the far-right in the neoliberal era. *J Int Relat Dev.* 2015;18(1):25–51. https://doi.org/10.1057/jird.2013.14
5. Meier BM, Evans DP, Kavanagh MM, Keralis JM, Armas-Cardona G. Human rights in public health: deepening engagement at a critical time. *Health Hum Rights.* 2018;20(2):85–91.
6. Morabia A. The fascist threat. *Am J Public Health.* 2021;111(4):538–539. https://doi.org/10.2105/AJPH.2021.306169
7. Liu M, Anastasio N, LeFreniere H, Perliger A. Public health crisis and hate crimes: deciphering the proliferation of anti-Asian violence in the US before and during Covid-19. *Terror Count-Terror Stud.* 2023;17(1). https://doi.org/10.19165/YWMK7593
8. Karabulut G, Zimmermann KF, Bilgin MH, Doker AC. Democracy and COVID-19 outcomes. *Econ*

Lett. 2021;203:109840. https://doi.org/10.1016/j.econlet.2021.109840

9. Patterson AC, Veenstra G. Politics and population health: testing the impact of electoral democracy. *Health Place*. 2016;40:66–75. https://doi.org/:10.1016/j.healthplace.2016.04.011
10. Pasek MH, Ankori-Karlinsky LO, Levy-Vene A, Moore-Berg SL. Misperceptions about out-partisans' democratic values may erode democracy. *Sci Rep*. 2022;12(1):16284. https://doi.org/10.1038/s41598-022-19616-4
11. Wigley S, Akkoyunlu-Wigley A. Do electoral institutions have an impact on population health? *Public Choice*. 2011;148(3-4):595–610. https://doi.org/10.1007/s11127-010-9686-6
12. Wang Y, Mechkova V, Andersson F. Does democracy enhance health? New empirical evidence 1900–2012. *Polit Res Q*. 2019;72(3):554–569. https://doi.org/10.1177/1065912918798506
13. Ádám Z, Csaba I. Populism unrestrained: Policy responses of the Orbán regime to the pandemic in 2020–2021. *Eur Policy Anal*. 2022;8(3):277–296. https://doi.org/10.1002/epa2.1157
14. Commission on Social Determinants of Health. Closing the gap in a generation: health equity through action on the social determinants of health: final report of the Commission on Social Determinants of Health. 2008. Available at: https://iris.who.int/bitstream/handle/10665/69832/WHO_IER_CSDH_08.1_eng.pdf?sequence=1. Accessed March 25, 2025.
15. Rinaldi C, Bekker MPM. A scoping review of populist radical right parties' influence on welfare policy and its implications for population health in Europe. *Int J Health Policy Manag*. 2021;10(3):141–151. https://doi.org/10.34172/ijhpm.2020.48
16. McCartney G, Hearty W, Arnot J, Popham F, Cumbers A, McMaster R. Impact of political economy on population health: a systematic review of reviews. *Am J Public Health*. 2019;109(6):e1–e12. https://doi.org/10.2105/AJPH.2019.305001
17. Pickett KE, Wilkinson RG. Income inequality and health: a causal review. *Soc Sci Med*. 2015;128:316–326. https://doi.org/10.1016/j.socscimed.2014.12.031
18. Jay S, Batruch A, Jetten J, McGarty C, Muldoon OT. Economic inequality and the rise of far-right populism: a social psychological analysis. *J Community Appl Soc Psychol*. 2019;29(5):418–428. https://doi.org/10.1002/casp.2409
19. Budhdeo S, Watkins J, Atun R, Williams C, Zeltner T, Maruthappu M. Changes in government spending on healthcare and population mortality in the European Union, 1995–2010: a cross-sectional ecological study. *J R Soc Med*. 2015;108(12):490–498. https://doi.org/10.1177/0141076815600907
20. Massuda A, Dall'Alba R, Chioro A, Temporão JG, Castro MC. After a far-right government: challenges for Brazil's Unified Health System. *Lancet*. 2023;401(10380):886–888. https://doi.org/10.1016/S0140-6736(23)00352-5
21. Woolhandler S, Himmelstein DU, Ahmed S, et al. Public policy and health in the Trump era. *Lancet*. 2021;397(10275):705–753. https://doi.org/10.1016/S0140-6736(20)32545-9
22. Selvarajah S, Corona Maioli S, Deivanayagam TA, et al. Racism, xenophobia, and discrimination: mapping pathways to health outcomes. *Lancet*. 2022;400(10368):2109–2124. https://doi.org/10.1016/S0140-6736(22)02484-9
23. Paradies Y, Ben J, Denson N, et al. Racism as a determinant of health: a systematic review and meta-analysis. *PLoS One*. 2015;10(9):e0138511. https://doi.org/10.1371/journal.pone.0138511
24. Needham BL, Ali T, Allgood KL, Ro A, Hirschtick JL, Fleischer NL. Institutional racism and health: a framework for conceptualization, measurement, and analysis. *J Racial Ethn Health Disparities*. 2023;10(4):1997–2019. https://doi.org/10.1007/s40615-022-01381-9
25. Mayblin L, Wake M, Kazemi M. Necropolitics and the slow violence of the everyday: asylum seeker welfare in the postcolonial present. *Sociology*. 2020;54(1):107–123. https://doi.org/10.1177/0038038519862124
26. Graff A, Kapur R, Walters SD. Introduction: gender and the rise of the global right. *Signs J Women Cult Soc*. 2019;44(3):541–560. https://doi.org/10.1086/701152
27. Borrell C, Palencia L, Muntaner C, Urquia M, Malmusi D, O'Campo P. Influence of macrosocial policies on women's health and gender inequalities in health. *Epidemiol Rev*. 2014;36(1):31–48. https://doi.org/10.1093/epirev/mxt002
28. FitzGerald C, Hurst S. Implicit bias in healthcare professionals: a systematic review. *BMC Med Ethics*. 2017;18(1):19. https://doi.org/10.1186/s12910-017-0179-8
29. Sardinha L, Maheu-Giroux M, Stöckl H, Meyer SR, García-Moreno C. Global, regional, and national prevalence estimates of physical or sexual, or both, intimate partner violence against women in 2018. *Lancet*. 2022;399(10327):803–813. https://doi.org/10.1016/S0140-6736(21)02664-7
30. Stubbs A, Szoeke C. The effect of intimate partner violence on the physical health and health-related behaviors of women: a systematic review of the literature. *Trauma Violence Abuse*. 2022;23(4):1157–1172. https://doi.org/10.1177/1524838020985541
31. Fathalla MF. Safe abortion: the public health rationale. *Best Pract Res Clin Obstet Gynaecol*. 2020;63:2–12. https://doi.org/10.1016/j.bpobgyn.2019.03.010
32. Singh S. Global consequences of unsafe abortion. *Womens Health*. 2010;6(6):849–860. https://doi.org/10.2217/WHE.10.70
33. Hanschmidt F, Linde K, Hilbert A, Riedel-Heller SG, Kersting A. Abortion stigma: a systematic review. *Perspect Sex Reprod Health*. 2016;48(4):169–177. https://doi.org/10.1363/48e8516
34. Lamontagne E, d'Elbée M, Ross MW, Carroll A, Plessis AD, Loures L. A socioecological measurement of homophobia for all countries and its public health impact. *Eur J Public Health*. 2018;28(5):967–972. https://doi.org/10.1093/eurpub/cky023
35. Douglas Scott S, Pringle A, Lumsdaine C. *Sexual Exclusion: Homophobia and Health Inequalities: A Review of Health Inequalities and Social Exclusion Experienced by Lesbian, Gay and Bisexual People*. UK Gay Men's Health Network. 2004:374. Available at: https://citeseerx.ist.psu.edu/document?repid=rep1&type=pdf&doi=53b8b565a5819edf62bc953ad081ecee46d4ea73. Accessed November 13, 2023.
36. Alencar Albuquerque G, De Lima Garcia C, Da Silva Quirino G, et al. Access to health services by lesbian, gay, bisexual, and transgender persons: systematic literature review. *BMC Int Health Hum Rights*. 2016;16(1):2. https://doi.org/10.1186/s12914-015-0072-9
37. Williamson IR. Internalized homophobia and health issues affecting lesbians and gay men. *Health Educ Res*. 2000;15(1):97–107. https://doi.org/10.1093/her/15.1.97
38. Miller HN, Thornton CP, Rodney T, Thorpe RJ, Allen J. Social cohesion in health: a concept analysis. *Adv Nurs Sci*. 2020;43(4):375–390. https://doi.org/10.1097/ANS.0000000000000327
39. Marcks H, Pawelz J. From myths of victimhood to fantasies of violence: how far-right narratives of imperilment work. *Terror Polit Violence*. 2022;34(7):1415–1432. https://doi.org/10.1080/09546553.2020.1788544
40. Smith KB. Politics is making us sick: the negative impact of political engagement on public health during the Trump administration. *PLoS One*. 2022;17(1):e0262022. https://doi.org/10.1371/journal.pone.0262022
41. Lewis J, Lewis B, Cameron R, Pond P, Ghumkhor S, Mohamud H. *Mediating Extremist Violence: A Report on the Role of Media, Far-Right Politics and Gender in Extremist Violence and Social Cohesion in Victoria*. Central for Global Research. RMIT University; 2017:137. Available at: https://www.rmit.edu.au/content/dam/rmit/documents/research/centres/centre-for-global-research/mediating-extremist-violence.pdf. Accessed March 25, 2025.
42. van Prooijen JW, Douglas KM. Belief in conspiracy theories: basic principles of an emerging research domain. *Eur J Soc Psychol*. 2018;48(7):897–908. https://doi.org/10.1002/ejsp.2530
43. Rocha YM, De Moura GA, Desidério GA, De Oliveira CH, Lourenço FD, De Figueiredo Nicolete LD. The impact of fake news on social media and its influence on health during the COVID-19 pandemic: a systematic review. *J Public Health*. 2023;31(7):1007–1016. https://doi.org/10.1007/s10389-021-01658-z
44. Rivara F, Adhia A, Lyons V, et al. The effects of violence on health. *Health Aff (Millwood)*. 2019;38(10):1622–1629. https://doi.org/10.1377/hlthaff.2019.00480
45. Testa RJ, Sciacca LM, Wang F, et al. Effects of violence on transgender people. *Prof Psychol Res Pract*. 2012;43(5):452–459. https://doi.org/10.1037/a0029604
46. Koehler D. Violence and terrorism from the far-right: policy options to counter an elusive threat. International Centre for Counter-Terrorism – The Hague. February 2019. Available at: https://icct.nl/sites/default/files/import/publication/Koehler-Violence-and-Terrorism-from-the-Far-Right-February-2019.pdf. Accessed March 25, 2025.
47. Baumgaertner B, Carlisle JE, Justwan F. The influence of political ideology and trust on willingness to vaccinate. *PLoS One*. 2018;13(1):e0191728. https://doi.org/10.1371/journal.pone.0191728
48. Hotez PJ. Antiscience extremism in America: escalating and globalizing. *Microbes Infect*. 2020;22(10):505–507. https://doi.org/10.1016/j.micinf.2020.09.005
49. Serrano-Alarcón M, Wang Y, Kentikelenis A, Mckee M, Stuckler D. The far-right and antivaccine attitudes: lessons from Spain's mass COVID-19 vaccine roll-out. *Eur J Public Health*. 2023;33(2):215–221. https://doi.org/10.1093/eurpub/ckac173
50. Gonzalez KE, James R, Bjorklund ET, Hill TD. Conservatism and infrequent mask usage: a study of US counties during the novel coronavirus (COVID-19) pandemic. *Soc Sci Q*. 2021;102(5):2368–2382. https://doi.org/10.1111/ssqu.13025

51. McCarthy J. Authoritarianism, populism, and the environment: comparative experiences, insights, and perspectives. *Ann Am Assoc Geogr.* 2019; 109(2):301–313. https://doi.org/10.1080/24694452.2018.1554393
52. Romanello M, Napoli CD, Green C, et al. The 2023 report of the Lancet Countdown on Health and Climate Change: the imperative for a health-centered response in a world facing irreversible harms. *Lancet.* 2023;402(10419):2346–2394. https://doi.org/10.1016/S0140-6736(23)01859-7
53. Forouzanfar MH, Afshin A, Alexander LT, et al. Global, regional, and national comparative risk assessment of 79 behavioral, environmental and occupational, and metabolic risks or clusters of risks, 1990–2015: a systematic analysis for the Global Burden of Disease Study 2015. *Lancet.* 2016;388(10053):1659–1724. https://doi.org/10.1016/S0140-6736(16)31679-8
54. Pascal M, Corso M, Chanel O, et al. Assessing the public health impacts of urban air pollution in 25 European cities: results of the Aphekom project. *Sci Total Environ.* 2013;449:390–400. https://doi.org/10.1016/j.scitotenv.2013.01.077
55. Vale MM, Berenguer E, Argollo De Menezes M, Viveiros De Castro EB, Pugliese De Siqueira L, Portela RDCQ. The COVID-19 pandemic as an opportunity to weaken environmental protection in Brazil. *Biol Conserv.* 2021;255:108994. https://doi.org/10.1016/j.biocon.2021.108994
56. Bomberg E. The environmental legacy of President Trump. *Policy Stud.* 2021;42(5-6):628–645. https://doi.org/10.1080/01442872.2021.1922660
57. Smith R. How "both-sideism" harms health. *BMJ.* 2022;378:o2136. https://doi.org/10.1136/bmj.o2136
58. Abubakar I, Gram L, Lasoye S, et al. Confronting the consequences of racism, xenophobia, and discrimination on health and health-care systems. *Lancet.* 2022;400(10368):2137–2146. https://doi.org/10.1016/S0140-6736(22)01989-4
59. Pons-Vigués M, Diez È, Morrison J, et al. Social and health policies or interventions to tackle health inequalities in European cities: a scoping review. *BMC Public Health.* 2014;14(1):198. https://doi.org/10.1186/1471-2458-14-198
60. Whitmee S, Green R, Belesova K, et al. Pathways to a healthy net-zero future: report of the Lancet Pathfinder Commission. *Lancet.* 2024;403(10421):67–110. https://doi.org/10.1016/S0140-6736(23)02466-2

Advancing the Study of Power: Opportunities and Priorities for Understanding Population Health Inequities

Megan M. Reynolds, PhD, and Sandro Galea, MD, DrPH, MPH

See also Power, Politics, and Human Rights in Public Health, pp. 868–882.

In this essay, we provide an overview of how power has been conceptualized in public health and allied fields and describe recent advances connecting power to the topic of health inequities.

To aid researchers in capitalizing on these historical and contemporary insights, we offer 6 concrete suggestions for empirical work.

Systematic analyses involving these recommendations can help return public health scholars to foundational principles of the field and test the limits of power as an explanatory factor in population health inequities. (*Am J Public Health*. 2025;115(6):883–889. https://doi.org/10.2105/AJPH.2025.308015)

AJPH June 2025, Vol. 115, No. 6

Recent years have seen innovation in our thinking and in empirical work about the role that power plays in shaping the health of populations.[1–9] Although this emergent work is new, the insights motivating such efforts are not. To mention 2 seminal thinkers in the area, Rudolf Virchow, the father of modern pathology, conducted a study of Prussian typhus in the mid-1800s and concluded that improved employment opportunities, higher taxation, and better wages were the most effective remedies to the typhus epidemic. According to Virchow:

> If we get free and well-educated people then we shall undoubtedly have healthy ones as well. I do want to stress that such measures, combined with a just and direct system of taxation and the abolition of all privileges and feudal duties, would enable the poorer classes to make good use of their wages and, at the same time, to get pleasure out of their work.[10(p208)]

Here Virchow emphasized not only the importance of education and economic redistribution but the abolition of feudalism. As a system in which landed aristocracy held power over peasants who worked the land in exchange for protection, feudalism prohibited the translation of socioeconomic resources into a better life. The importance of empowering the working classes with education ran throughout Virchow's subsequent work and helped contribute to the emergence of the field of social medicine, a discipline that heavily informed the social determinants of health literature.

At the end of the 1930s, as a young physician and minister of health, Salvador Allende wrote *La Realidad Médico-Social Chilena* (*Chile's Medical-Social Reality*).[11] In this text, he outlined how mortality, communicable diseases, emotional disturbances, and occupational illness were byproducts of the poor living conditions of Chile's working class. Central to Allende's agenda was the expansion of government and the empowerment of workers. Allende believed that shifting economic power from domestic elites and foreign corporations to the state and the working class would be more effective than medical interventions in ameliorating the problem of poor population health.

CONCEPTUALIZING POWER

In its simplest terms, power is the ability to act or to make others act in a particular way. More sophisticated definitions of power have been offered by scholars across the ages. Among the most influential have been those of Emile Durkheim, Max Weber, and Karl Marx. Durkheim originated power as emanating from the ability of society to create a "collective consciousness" that binds people together through shared norms, values, and beliefs. Weber defined power as the probability that one actor within a social relationship will be able to carry out his or her own will despite resistance, regardless of the basis on which this probability rests. According to Marx, power is a resource that the ruling class employs to dominate the working class in the economic sphere to amass wealth.

Theories on power have centered on the various forms that power takes. Notions of "power over," the predominant view of power, center on dynamics of domination and cast power in a repressive (i.e., negative) light. They presume an asymmetrical relationship in which one party (the dominant party) exercises control over a subordinate party. Typically, the dominant party occupies a higher position in some institutional hierarchy. In power-over scenarios, the controlling party's gain is the subordinate party's loss. Notions of "power to" center on dynamics of empowerment and cast power in an emancipatory (i.e., positive) light. They presume an asymmetrical relationship in which one party resists being controlled by another party. Typically, the subordinate party occupies a lower position in an organizational hierarchy. In power-to scenarios, the subordinate party's gain is the controlling party's loss.

Although these 2 notions differ in their normative assumptions about power, they are not mutually exclusive. As noted by McCartney et al.,

> Campaigns for social justice can be seen as mobilising "power to" and "power with" in order to exert "power over" dominant interests. Conversely, "power over" in a context of domination entails "power to" and "power with" for those actors in control.[3(p24)]

Moreover, both notions assume antagonistic relationships between groups competing for social and economic resources. Unlike notions of power over and power to that focus on domination of one group over another, power with emphasizes collaboration and shared power among groups. Here power need not be a zero-sum game in which one party's gain is necessarily the other party's loss.

Theories of power concern themselves not only with forms of power but the processes through which they function, especially in the case of power over. Steven Lukes[12] provides what is arguably the most widely used framework for understanding these processes. Lukes's "three faces of power" framework examines how power manifests as the ability to resolve, address, and define societal priorities. The first face, commonly referred to as "overt power," is the power to influence whether issues are resolved (i.e., decision-making power). Decision-making power typically operates within formal political institutions (e.g., government, law) through the implementation of rules and regulations that determine the behavior of others. It responds contemporaneously to readily observable issues to settle conflicts.

The second face is the power to influence the issues that are addressed (i.e., agenda-setting power). This has been described elsewhere as "covert power." Agenda-setting power operates within and outside of formal political institutions by promoting norms and values that determine the considerations of others. It responds early to less observable issues to suppress conflict.

The third face (invisible power) is the power to influence how issues are defined. Invisible power primarily operates outside of formal political institutions by shaping perceptions that determine the wishes of others. Unlike the first 2 faces of power, invisible power does not presume a conflict of interest; rather, it responds preemptively to anticipated issues to avoid conflict. Integrating this third face into previous understandings of both overt and covert power provides a holistic view of how power permeates all aspects of how society is structured.

POWER AS A SOCIAL DETERMINANT OF HEALTH

The role of power in shaping health has been brought back to the fore as part of a growing global focus on the social determinants of health. The World Health Organization's 2008 report titled *Closing the Gap in a Generation*[13] spurred a paradigm shift that encouraged health scientists to think about health inequities not as the result of individual risk factors but as the result of "circumstances in which people grow, live, work, and age, and the systems put in place to deal with illness. . .. These circumstances are shaped by the distribution of money, power, and resources at global, national, and local levels."

The report's discussion of power did not, by some standards, go far enough. Some critiqued the final version as not providing sufficiently strong foundational policy recommendations to ameliorate well-documented health inequities.[14] Others issued more full-throated commentaries on areas of improvement:

> The Commission's studious avoidance of the category of power (class power, as well as gender, race, and national power) and how power is produced and reproduced in political institutions is the greatest weakness of the report.[15(p440)]

In the years that followed, the "Barcelona group" (as it came to be known by some) and a small group of American scholars[7] advanced efforts to emphasize how power and power relations shaped health inequities within and across nations.[9] They argued that cross-national health inequities observed in the welfare state literature were reflective of inequities in the distribution of power.[5] This was even more true of the stark and often-overlooked health inequities between the Global North and Global South[14] in which dominant classes of developed and developing countries united to consolidate their power and shape neoliberalism in directions that benefited them.[15] Scholars of public and population health echoed these sentiments in major reports[16] and integrative frameworks that placed power squarely at the center of research on global health inequities.[17]

Around the same time, the shrinking health advantage of the United States relative to peer nations became an object of interest. In 2013, the National Research Council and the Institute of Medicine[18] released *US Health in International Perspective: Shorter Lives, Poorer Health*, which documented in stark terms health disparities between the United States and other rich countries. The report generated a body of work in which scholars imported comparative emphases of welfare state effects on health to the domestic sphere,[8] producing a wealth of empirical research on social policy as health policy.[19] A parallel body of literature reinforced the notion of US states as entities that "vary in policies, resources, and opportunity structures in ways that affect population health."[20(p624)] This research on the political economy of health presented institutions as the context in which risk factors for health are engendered,[21] underpinned by a definition of institutions as a combination of schemas and resources that organize power.

THEORIES OF POWER IN HEALTH RESEARCH

More recently, there have been unified theoretical frameworks articulated that attempt to explain how power might operate across institutions to influence health.[1] McCartney et al.[3] provided a wealth of information on the forms, sources, and positions of power as well as where power resides. Heller et al. discussed the relationship between structural determinants of health and power, describing power as representing "a continual struggle and negotiation in which actors draw on social, political, and economic resources to maintain or alter social constraints (i.e., structures)."[2(p6)] In their framework, structures take shape, maintain, and change because of the power that distinct groups have to shape decision making, agendas, and worldviews.

Health power resources (HPR) theory[6] provides a framework for understanding how power dynamics within society, particularly rich modern democracies, affect the distribution of health across populations. Unlike prevailing approaches that depict empowerment as an individual trait arising from social conditions, HPR theory underscores how the consolidation of power in major societal domains (e.g., health care, labor markets) acts as a collective resource harnessed in ways that influence social conditions and, therefore, health disparities across major social axes such as race, class, and gender.

The theory suggests that although many social determinants of health imply power imbalances between groups, the effects of these imbalances have seldom been explicitly theorized or tested. HPR theory contends that regardless of the quantity of socioeconomic and health-relevant resources one has, their impact on health is determined by how necessary, valuable, and useful they are. Therefore, whereas many theories focus chiefly on the distribution of resources, HPR theory delineates 3 power-related processes (commodification, discrimination, and devitalization) that shape the meaning of resources in ways that matter for health.

HPR theory offers several advantages to public health researchers interested in social determinants of health. First, by focusing on power distributions across groups, one shifts from individual traits to the underlying social factors that make these traits significant. As reflected in the burgeoning research on structural determinants of health, health advantages and disadvantages associated with these traits reflect complex dynamics originating "upstream" rather than arising because of "downstream" risk factors.

Second, HPR theory can help understand why differences in traditional social determinants do not always correlate as expected with differences in health. For example, research has shown that despite their higher income and education, supervisors often exhibit worse mental health than their supervisees. Because it contradicts established patterns, this association might be regarded as a health paradox of sorts. It is less paradoxical, however, when we account for the contradictory class location[22] of supervisors who are in conflict with workers as well as upper management.[23] As such, supervisors may possess the lowest levels of workplace power as they are simultaneously responsible to leadership and excluded from many workplace protections.

Third, HPR theory extends research on institutions and health by explaining how an institution's effects on health are influenced by the power dynamics within the institution. For example, power resources determine the benefits or costs that an institution aims to deliver to specific groups.

Fourth, HPR theory provides a new interpretation of individuals' adoption of unhealthy behaviors even when healthier options are readily available. According to its concept of devitalization, lifestyle choices are a logical response to chronic deprivation and repeated opportunity blockages.

PRIORITIES TO ADVANCE UNDERSTANDING OF HEALTH INEQUITIES

Empirical public health work on macrolevel sources of health inequity has yet to fully capitalize on the conceptual and theoretical advances that have unfolded over the past couple of decades. Two groups of literature have proven to be exceptions. The rapidly growing literature on structural determinants of health examines hierarchical power wielded by the few and affecting many. Although the role of power in this literature is varied and sometimes murky, it is assumed to be both a cause and an effect of the "rules of the game" that determine who gets what.[24]

A separate but related group of literature focuses not on axes of inequity (e.g., race, sex, nativity) but on institutional sources of inequity. Two of the institutions that have gained increased attention in recent years are government[25] and commerce.[26] Research suggests that population health tends to fare better when democracies and good governance thrive.[27] Given the links between government and business, especially in an era of multinationalism (or supranationalism), the literature on the "corporate" and "commercial" determinants of health has grown over the past decade.[28] This research suggests that the distribution of power between corporations and governments is at the heart of the distribution of health between people and places.[29]

To guide efforts toward translating conceptual and theoretical advances into empirical ones, we provide 6 concrete suggestions as to what a capacious version of this research might include. We offer these specific suggestions because we believe that they constitute significant departures from current approaches, are well suited to the strengths of public health scholars, and would most substantially advance research on upstream drivers of health and health inequities. These suggestions also each treat power not only as something that an individual or even a group has but in terms of relations between at least 2 groups with opposing goals. As Muntaner et al.[4] point out, inequity is an inherently relational phenomenon and, as such, relational approaches should be used to understand it. We concur and prioritize suggestions that reflect this sentiment.

First, we encourage this body of research to explore power as a force that emerges from the coalescence of individuals into groups. Collective action enables groups to wield power that is more potent than that possessed by the sum of their members. Embarking on a wider and more intensive exploration of such group-level power will enable researchers to address a dissonance in the literature wherein potential remedies to inequities are prioritized over investigation into their cause. In much of the literature on power and health, this dissonance manifests as a preoccupation with individual empowerment in which people (or patients) are encouraged to believe that they are capable of autonomous decision making and action.[30] Such personal empowerment is highly relevant to improving individual health but has limited ability to address far-reaching inequities.[31]

We suggest that there is a need for research acknowledging that the circumstances from which individual health status emerges are shaped by powerful entities and therefore cannot be addressed without paying attention to how those entities function. For example, "empowerment-type therapies" in which (predominantly low-income) patients acquire knowledge to encourage healthier choices offer the potential for enhanced decision making among those with diabetes; the public health benefit of such therapies, however, will necessarily be circumscribed in the context of the limited power held by consumers (relative to industry) to influence the food environments in which metabolic disorders arise. As Hannah Arendt famously stated,

> Power corresponds to the human ability not just to act but to act in concert. Power is never the property

AJPH June 2025, Vol. 115, No. 6

> of an individual; it belongs to a group and remains in existence only so long as the group keeps together.[32(p24)]

Second, we posit an important role for Lukes's power framework described earlier. Researchers interested in investigating the impact of power on population health inequities are faced with a broad array of definitions of power from which to choose. Many of these definitions are motivated by a desire to understand political dynamics, particularly in relation to how power shapes democracy and democratic processes. But these definitions often lack the necessary insight to fully understand the complex machinations of how power affects health. Lukes described power as the ability to set and resolve societal objectives, to influence the way people feel and think about those objectives, and to help or hinder the accumulation and deployment of resources in the pursuit of those objectives. By emphasizing control across the goal-setting life cycle, Lukes's formulation lends itself nicely to the study of health inequities. Later in the article we interpret public health scholarship on incarceration and health through the lens of Luke's framework.

Third, there is a critical need for studies of power in broad-based institutions. There has been some work investigating how power is distributed between certain groups within specific organizations or environments and how that is associated with health inequities between groups. This scholarship is a vital first step toward understanding how group-based power can ameliorate health inequities. We contend that this focus should be extended to major societal institutions (e.g., government, labor markets, law) that transcend the boundaries of a single organization or environment. Unlike organizations—which are defined by specific purposes, people, places, and times (e.g., churches)—institutions are defined by broad purposes, constant population replacement, diffuse geographical reach, and reproduction over time. Therefore, the effects of institutions on people's lives and health can be more far-reaching than those of organizations.

By way of illustration, we point to the work of Michener,[33] who examined the potential for tenant organizations to force policy changes that improve the housing circumstances of low-income Black Americans. Expanding this analysis to examine the distribution of power in real estate markets offers the opportunity to advance our understanding of racial health inequities that are linked to housing conditions, such as why Black Americans are at significantly greater risk of asthma and other respiratory diseases.

Fourth, although it is important to also understand the potential of informal social institutions (e.g., grassroots or community-based social movements, including those related specifically to health), we submit that adding an examination within formal institutions such as legislatures, industries, and science systems is crucial. Because these institutions are structured according to binding rules and regulations, they offer opportunities to

> solve the coordination problems of groups, multiply the power of otherwise disconnected individuals, have the necessary resources to make a difference, and carry greater legitimacy in the national political arena where welfare policy gets decided.[34(p11)]

Research on corrections and health serves as an example of what this work might look like. Well before the proliferation of research on structural oppression and health, public health scholars were examining the relationship between incarceration and racial health disparities such as higher rates of infectious diseases (e.g., tuberculosis and HIV) among Black men.[35] Much of this research framed hyper-incarceration among Black Americans as a result of a largely White federal administration exerting overt power (Lukes's first face of power) through a war on drugs that was ostensibly about crime but, in truth, was a backlash against the gains made in the civil rights movement.[36]

In the institution of science, there have been campaigns to include incarceration in public health systems and training.[37] This highlights how public health stakeholders (e.g., federal health agencies, state and local health departments, professional associations) hold unique agenda-setting power (Lukes's second face of power) to define the province of public health and invisible power (Lukes's third face of power) to reify the existence of factors such as institutional racism that fall within it. Complementary scholarship on both social movements and formal institutions can offer a richer understanding of how the study of all faces of power can be leveraged and unified in the future.

Fifth, research would benefit from studying groups that occupy similar social locations. We propose that there is even greater potential for theoretical and public health advancement in studying the consolidation of power among groups defined by status-related (e.g., race, class, gender) rather than health-related (e.g., tobacco control) goals. Such groups are larger in size than those with a singular health-related focus and are therefore able to concentrate higher degrees of power.

Moreover, focusing on social status groups complicates the notion of "interests" in a way that can bring nuance to our understanding of power dynamics. Social science research on power often invokes the concept of interests because it helps to explain why individuals desire a specific outcome. Individuals attempt to unite with others who share a common interest because they believe that it will more effectively convey their desires and pressure decision makers to satisfy them. In the case of social status groups, the more diverse mix of desires presents unique challenges and opportunities for research. For instance, the increasing power of working women (relative to men) has the potential to influence workplace customs and laws, such as flexible scheduling and paid family leave, that do not aim to address the comparatively high maternal mortality rates in the United States but nonetheless have significant potential to do so.

Sixth, we suggest that public health research expand its scope beyond those who are the worst off in terms of health status. We recognize that public health research is driven in large part by the desire to improve health among those who are least healthy, and accordingly voluminous research has been dedicated to investigation and intervention among these populations. Remedying the starkest health disparities allows public health to alleviate the deepest suffering in the United States. However, we urge that scholarly attention be widened to social groups that constitute a larger—even if slightly healthier—percentage of the populace.

For example, many of the two thirds of Americans who constitute the working class have lower rates of cardiovascular disease than those classified as poor but still have significantly higher rates than those with high incomes. By expanding the focus of research from the deeply affected but smaller group to the moderately affected but larger group, we may be able to identify factors that can be modified to reduce diseases with high mortality and prevalence rates among large segments of the US population.

CONCLUSION

We suggest that the kind of work described here will bring us back to an often-overlooked foundation of the social determinants of health, one that underpinned public health's early incarnation as "social medicine." The conditions in which people live may be important social determinants of health, but those conditions are distributed nonrandomly on the basis of who has power. In a now 20-year-old publication, Hilary Graham[38(p104)] argued for the importance of distinguishing between social determinants of health and social determinants of health inequity:

> Using a single term to refer to both the social factors influencing health and the social processes shaping their social distribution would not be problematic if the main determinants of health—like living standards, environmental influences, and health behaviors—were equally distributed between socioeconomic groups. But the evidence points to marked socioeconomic differences in access to health-promoting resources.

She pointed even further back to the Diderichsen et al. model,[39] one of the first to visualize the social determinants of health; this model distinguished between the conditions in which we live (the social determinants of health) and the factors that shaped those conditions (the social determinants of health inequity) by generating and distributing "power, wealth, and risks." We suggest, along with others in the annals of *AJPH*,[40] that a systematic approach to the study of power is within the ken of population health scholars and stands to be a critical part of advancing social determinants of health research in coming decades. AJPH

ABOUT THE AUTHORS

Megan M. Reynolds is with the Department of Sociology, University of Utah, Salt Lake City. Sandro Galea is with the School of Public Health, Washington University in St. Louis, St. Louis, MO.

CORRESPONDENCE

Correspondence should be sent to Megan M. Reynolds, PhD, University of Utah, Department of Sociology, 1530 E 380 S, Salt Lake City, UT 84121 (e-mail: megan.reynolds@soc.utah). Reprints can be ordered at https://www.ajph.org by clicking the "Reprints" link.

PUBLICATION INFORMATION

Full Citation: Reynolds MM, Galea S. Advancing the study of power: opportunities and priorities for understanding population health inequities. *Am J Public Health*. 2025;115(6):883–889.

Acceptance Date: January 2, 2025.

DOI: https://doi.org/10.2105/AJPH.2025.308015

ORCID iD:

Megan M. Reynolds https://orcid.org/0000-0002-8864-0613

CONTRIBUTORS

M. M. Reynolds was responsible for the conceptualization and drafting of the article. S. Galea contributed to the design and critical revision of the essay.

ACKNOWLEDGMENTS

Megan M. Reynolds thanks Rita Hamad for inspiring the idea of an essay piece and Ashley Fox for improving it with her expert feedback.

CONFLICTS OF INTEREST

The authors declare no conflicts of interest.

HUMAN PARTICIPANT PROTECTION

No protocol approval was needed for this research because no human participants were involved.

REFERENCES

1. Beckfield J, Bambra C, Eikemo TA, Huijts T, McNamara C, Wendt C. An institutional theory of welfare state effects on the distribution of population health. *Soc Theory Health*. 2015;13(3–4): 227–244. https://doi.org/10.1057/sth.2015.19
2. Heller JC, Givens ML, Johnson SP, Kindig DA. Keeping it political and powerful: defining the structural determinants of health. *Milbank Q*. 2024;102(2):351–366. https://doi.org/10.1111/1468-0009.12695
3. McCartney G, Dickie E, Escobar O, Collins C. Health inequalities, fundamental causes and power: towards the practice of good theory. *Sociol Health Illn*. 2021;43(1):20–39. https://doi.org/10.1111/1467-9566.13181
4. Muntaner C, Ng E, Chung H, Prins SJ. Two decades of neo-Marxist class analysis and health inequalities: a critical reconstruction. *Soc Theory Health*. 2015;13(3–4):267–287. https://doi.org/10.1057/sth.2015.17
5. Raphael D, Bryant T. Power, intersectionality and the life-course: identifying the political and economic structures of welfare states that support or threaten health. *Soc Theory Health*. 2015;13(3–4):245–266. https://doi.org/10.1057/sth.2015.18
6. Reynolds MM. Health power resources theory: a relational approach to the study of health inequalities. *J Health Soc Behav*. 2021;62(4): 493–511. https://doi.org/10.1177/00221465211025963
7. Beckfield J, Krieger N. Epi + demos + cracy: linking political systems and priorities to the magnitude of health inequities—evidence, gaps, and a research agenda. *Epidemiol Rev*. 2009;31(1):152–177. https://doi.org/10.1093/epirev/mxp002
8. Bambra C. *Health Divides: Where You Live Can Kill You*. Policy Press and Bristol University Press; 2017.
9. Muntaner C, Borrell C, Ng E, et al. Politics, welfare regimes, and population health: controversies and evidence. *Sociol Health Illn*. 2011;33(6):946–964. https://doi.org/10.1111/j.1467-9566.2011.01339.x
10. Taylor R, Rieger A. Medicine as social science: Rudolf Virchow on the typhus epidemic in Upper Silesia. *Int J Health Serv*. 1985;15(4):547–559. https://doi.org/10.2190/XX9V-ACD4-KUXD-C0E5
11. Allende S. *La Realidad Médico-Social Chilena*. Ministerio de Salubridad; 1939.
12. Lukes S. *Power: A Radical View*. Palgrave Macmillan; 1974.
13. Marmot M, Friel S, Bell R, Houweling TAJ, Taylor S. Closing the gap in a generation: health equity through action on the social determinants of health. Available at: https://iris.who.int/bitstream/handle/10665/43943/9789241563703_eng.pdf. Accessed December 20, 2024.
14. Muntaner C, Sridharan S, Solar O, Benach J. Against unjust global distribution of power and money: the report of the WHO Commission on the Social Determinants of Health: global inequality and the future of public health policy. *J Public Health Policy*. 2009;30(2):163–175. https://doi.org/10.1057/jphp.2009.15
15. Navarro V. What we mean by social determinants of health. *Int J Health Serv*. 2009;39(3):423–441. https://doi.org/10.2190/HS.39.3.a
16. Ottersen OP, Dasgupta J, Blouin C, et al. The political origins of health inequity: prospects for change. *Lancet*. 2014;383(9917):630–667. https://doi.org/10.1016/S0140-6736(13)62407-1
17. Kentikelenis A, Rochford C. Power asymmetries in global governance for health: a conceptual framework for analyzing the political-economic determinants of health inequities. *Global Health*. 2019;15(suppl 1):70. https://doi.org/10.1186/s12992-019-0516-4
18. *US Health in International Perspective: Shorter Lives, Poorer Health*. National Research Council and Institute of Medicine; 2013.
19. Woolf SH. Social policy as health policy. *JAMA*. 2009;301(11):1166–1169. https://doi.org/10.1001/jama.2009.320
20. Montez JK, Zajacova A, Hayward MD, Woolf SH, Chapman D, Beckfield J. Educational disparities in adult mortality across US states: how do they differ, and have they changed since the mid-1980s? *Demography*. 2019;56(2):621–644. https://doi.org/10.1007/s13524-018-0750-z
21. Gkiouleka A, Huijts T, Beckfield J, Bambra C. Understanding the micro and macro politics of health: inequalities, intersectionality & institutions - a research agenda. *Soc Sci Med*. 2018;200:92–98. https://doi.org/10.1016/j.socscimed.2018.01.025
22. Wright EO. *Classes*. Verso; 1997.
23. Muntaner C, Borell C, Benach J, Pasarin MI, Fernandez E. The associations of social class and social stratification with patterns of general and mental health in a Spanish population. *Int J Epidemiol*. 2003;32(6):950–958. https://doi.org/10.1093/ije/dyg170
24. Krieger N. Measures of racism, sexism, heterosexism, and gender binarism for health equity research: from structural injustice to embodied harm-an ecosocial analysis. *Annu Rev Public Health*. 2020;41:37–62. https://doi.org/10.1146/annurev-publhealth-040119-094017
25. Dawes D, Gonzalez J. The politics of population health. *Milbank Q*. 2023;101(suppl 1):224–241. https://doi.org/10.1111/1468-0009.12603
26. Maani N, Petticrew M, Galea S, eds. *The Commercial Determinants of Health*. Oxford University Press; 2022.
27. Wang Y-t, Mechkova V, Andersson F. Does democracy enhance health? New empirical evidence 1900–2012. *Polit Res Q*. 2018;72(3): 554–569. https://doi.org/10.1177/1065912918798506
28. Lee K, Freudenberg N. Public health roles in addressing commercial determinants of health. *Annu Rev Public Health*. 2022;43:375–395. https://doi.org/10.1146/annurev-publhealth-052220-020447
29. McKee M, Stuckler D. Revisiting the corporate and commercial determinants of health. *Am J Public Health*. 2018;108(9):1167–1170. https://doi.org/10.2105/AJPH.2018.304510
30. Friel S, Townsend B, Fisher M, Harris P, Freeman T, Baum F. Power and the people's health. *Soc Sci Med*. 2021;282:114173. https://doi.org/10.1016/j.socscimed.2021.114173
31. Zimmerman FJ. Habit, custom, and power: a multi-level theory of population health. *Soc Sci Med*. 2013;80:47–56. https://doi.org/10.1016/j.socscimed.2012.12.029
32. Arendt H. *Crises of the Republic: Lying in Politics, Civil Disobedience on Violence, Thoughts on Politics, and Revolution*. Harcourt Brace Jovanovich; 1972.
33. Michener J. Racism, power, and health equity: the case of tenant organizing. *Health Aff (Millwood)*. 2023;42(10):1318–1324. https://doi.org/10.1377/hlthaff.2023.00509
34. Brady D. *Rich Democracies, Poor People: How Politics Explain Poverty*. Oxford University Press; 2009.
35. Treadwell HM, Nottingham JH. Standing in the gap. *Am J Public Health*. 2005;95(10):1676. https://doi.org/10.2105/AJPH.95.10.1676
36. Dumont DM, Brockmann B, Dickman S, Alexander N, Rich JD. Public health and the epidemic of incarceration. *Annu Rev Public Health*. 2012;33: 325–339. https://doi.org/10.1146/annurev-publhealth-031811-124614
37. McCauley EJ, LeMasters K, Behne MF, Brinkley-Rubinstein L. A call to action to public health institutions and teaching to incorporate mass incarceration as a sociostructural determinant of health. *Public Health Rep*. 2023;138(5):711–714. https://doi.org/10.1177/00333549221120243
38. Graham H. Social determinants and their unequal distribution: clarifying policy understandings. *Milbank Q*. 2004;82(1):101–124. https://doi.org/10.1111/j.0887-378X.2004.00303.x
39. Diderichsen F, Evans T, Whitehead M. The social basis of disparities in health. In: Evans T, Whitehead M, Diderichsen F, Bhuiya A, Wirth M, eds. *Challenging Inequities in Health: From Ethics to Action*. Oxford University Press; 2001:12–23. https://doi.org/10.1093/acprof:oso/9780195137408.003.0002
40. Jahn JL, Hernandez SM. Mortality inequities: power, theory, and data considerations. *Am J Public Health*. 2023;113(7):726–728. https://doi.org/10.2105/AJPH.2023.307322

Medicaid Expansion and US Mortality Rates During the COVID-19 Pandemic, 2018–2022

Xuesong Han, PhD, Kewei Sylvia Shi, MPH, Qinjin Fan, PhD, Parichoy Pal Choudhury, PhD, Xin Hu, PhD, and K. Robin Yabroff, PhD

See also Allen, p. 833.

Objectives. To examine the association of state Medicaid expansion status with mortality changes during the COVID-19 pandemic in the United States.

Methods. Deaths among individuals 20 to 64 years of age in 3142 counties were identified from 2018 to 2022 mortality surveillance data. Age-adjusted mortality rates were calculated for each county and by cause of death. Changes in mortality rates before and after the onset of the COVID-19 pandemic (2018–2019 vs 2021–2022) in Medicaid expansion states relative to nonexpansion states were calculated after adjustment for county sociodemographic factors and state COVID-19 vaccination rates.

Results. All-cause mortality rates increased in 2020–2021 nationwide and decreased slightly in 2022. Overall, the increase was slower in Medicaid expansion states, leading to a net decrease of 31.8 (95% confidence interval [CI] = 20.9, 42.8) deaths per 100 000 person-years associated with Medicaid expansion from 2018–2019 to 2021–2022. The decrease was largest for deaths from heart disease and liver disease and was observed across subpopulations stratified by sex, age, and race.

Conclusions. Increases in mortality rates were slower in Medicaid expansion states than in nonexpansion states during the COVID-19 public health emergency, suggesting a protective effect of Medicaid expansion on population health during the pandemic. (*Am J Public Health*. 2025;115(6): 890–899. https://doi.org/10.2105/AJPH.2025.308045)

AJPH June 2025, Vol. 115, No. 6

The Affordable Care Act expanded Medicaid eligibility to adults with incomes up to 138% of the federal poverty level regardless of parental status in states that opted to expand coverage. A total of 24 states and the District of Columbia implemented Medicaid expansion in January 2014; 7 additional states implemented expansion in 2014 to 2016, 5 states did so in 2019–2020, and 4 states did so during 2021 to 2023. As of February 2025, 10 states had not adopted Medicaid expansion.[1] Substantial research has linked Medicaid expansion with increased insurance coverage and access to care as well as improvements in multiple health outcomes for low-income residents,[2,3] including a study showing significant reductions in mortality rates associated with Medicaid expansion before the COVID-19 pandemic.[4]

Between 2020 and 2023, the COVID-19 pandemic disrupted health care access and delivery and imposed potentially long-lasting effects on health outcomes, yielding a natural experiment of Medicaid expansion and resilience to the public health emergency. During the COVID-19 pandemic, the United States was among the high-income countries bearing the highest excess mortality.[5,6] A significant share of the excess mortality in the country was due to a fragmented health care system and a lack of universal health insurance coverage.[7]

Amid the health care disruption and economic instability caused by the pandemic, maintaining insurance coverage became especially crucial for low-income populations. The Families First Coronavirus Response Act of 2020 required state Medicaid programs to maintain continuous enrollment for beneficiaries through the end of the COVID-19 public health emergency in exchange for enhanced federal funding. Data from national surveys have shown that Medicaid expansion helped offset losses in coverage during pandemic economic downturns.[8,9] Through stabilizing health insurance coverage, Medicaid expansion might not only ensure timely access to care for COVID-19 related illnesses but also provide broader protections that could help shield against overall mortality.

Although previous studies showed positive associations of Medicaid expansion with improvements in self-reported health outcomes[10] and access to care[11] during the early onset of the pandemic, a comprehensive evaluation of whether state Medicaid expansion policies had long-lasting effects on overall and cause-specific deaths during the later phases of the pandemic is lacking. Moreover, the distinct COVID-19 outbreak patterns in Medicaid expansion states versus nonexpansion states in the first year of the pandemic limited earlier efforts to evaluate associations between Medicaid expansion and mortality.[12] In this study, we used recent surveillance data to examine changes in mortality rates during the pandemic in Medicaid expansion and nonexpansion states.

METHODS

We conducted a multiyear cross-sectional study with a quasi-experimental design.

Data

We identified deaths in 2018 to 2022 from the National Cancer Institute's Surveillance, Epidemiology, and End Results Program mortality database; underlying death certificate data for US residents were provided by the National Center for Health Statistics.[13] Deaths among individuals 20 to 64 years of age were included given that individuals 65 years or older are nearly universally covered by Medicare and thus are not the target population for Medicaid expansion. Medicaid expansion states included states that adopted Medicaid expansion by December 31, 2020; nonexpansion states included states that had not adopted Medicaid expansion by December 31, 2022. Oklahoma and Missouri, which expanded Medicaid eligibility on July 1, 2021, and October 1, 2021, respectively, were excluded from our main analysis.

Statistical Analysis

We assumed that death counts had a Poisson distribution and calculated age-adjusted mortality rates as a weighted average of crude age-specific mortality rates, with the weights being the proportions of individuals in the corresponding age groups of the 2000 US standard population.[14] We then generated maps to visualize yearly age-adjusted mortality rates for each county. Changes in age-adjusted mortality rates from 2018–2019 (before the COVID-19 pandemic) to 2021–2022 (after the pandemic onset) were also mapped for each county.

Furthermore, we calculated yearly age-adjusted mortality rate for Medicaid expansion states and nonexpansion states and graphed trends. Using county-level yearly age-adjusted mortality rate data, we applied a difference-in-differences approach and fit bivariate and multivariable linear mixed-effect models to estimate differences in changes in mortality rates before and after the onset of the pandemic between counties in Medicaid expansion and nonexpansion states. This modeling approach has been applied in previous studies evaluating changes in age-adjusted mortality rates in US counties after implementation of various policies.[4,15]

Our outcome variables included all-cause and cause-specific mortality rates from the 15 most common underlying causes of death, including COVID-19. Notably, because COVID-19 was added as a cause of death in 2020, we examined trends in COVID-19 deaths only for 2020 to 2022. Our primary independent variables were Medicaid expansion status, pre- or post-COVID-19 onset status, and the interaction of the 2 variables; all of these variables were included in the models as fixed effects.

Andersen and colleagues' behavioral model of health service utilization[16] was used to guide the selection of potential confounders, and our multivariable linear models were adjusted for (1) fixed effects of 2018 to 2022 estimates of county-level percentages of residents 65 years or older, non-Hispanic White residents, unemployed residents, and residents with incomes under 100% of the federal poverty level as measures of counties' socioeconomic status and (2) counties' metropolitan status according to the 2013 Rural-Urban Continuum Code.[17,18] We also adjusted for the fixed effect of state-level percentage of residents 18 years or older who had a COVID-19 vaccination by December 31, 2021, as a proxy for state public health policies and adherence to recommended practices.[19]

Moreover, state random intercepts were included in multivariable models to account for potential clustering effects at the state level. Stratified analyses were conducted by sex, age group, and race/ethnicity. We focused on changes in 2021–2022, the second and third years of the pandemic, to avoid confounding resulting from geographically unbalanced pandemic patterns in

2020 and to incorporate effects of COVID-19 vaccinations, which became widely available in 2021. We did not control for county-level insurance rate because it was part of the causal pathway of the hypothesized association between Medicaid expansion and changes in mortality rates. The parallel trends assumption of the difference-in-differences method was confirmed by null findings in models of pre-COVID-19 pandemic data comparing changes in 2019 versus 2018 mortality rates in Medicaid expansion and nonexpansion states (Table A, available as a supplement to the online version of this article at http://www.ajph.org).

We conducted several sensitivity analyses as robustness checks. First, we compared mortality rates in 2021 and 2022 separately (after the onset of the COVID-19 pandemic) with those in 2018 and 2019 (before the pandemic) in multivariable models to examine different patterns in the second and third years of the pandemic. Second, we restricted Medicaid expansion states to those that expanded before 2018 (i.e., excluding the 5 states that expanded Medicaid in 2018–2020: Virginia, Maine, Idaho, Utah, and Nebraska) given that Medicaid expansion may have a delayed effect.

Third, to further account for availability of health care resources, we included counties' hospital bed capacities and shortages of primary care physicians in 2018 in multivariable models. Finally, we conducted a propensity score matching analysis of Medicaid expansion counties and nonexpansion counties based on the following county-level characteristics: percentage of residents who were non-Hispanic White, percentage of residents with incomes under 100% of the federal poverty level, and metropolitan status. We then fit models using a subsample of 1944 counties.

We used SEER*STAT version 8.4.4 (NCI & IMS, Calverton, MD) to calculate mortality rates. Maps were generated through ArcGIS version 10.8.2 (ESRI, Redlands, CA). All other analyses were conducted with SAS version 9.4 (SAS Institute Inc, Cary, NC). All statistical tests were 2-sided with a significance level of .05.

RESULTS

A total of 3142 counties were included in our analysis (1834 in Medicaid expansion states and 1135 in nonexpansion states). The remaining 173 counties from Oklahoma and Missouri were used only in generating maps and producing state-level estimates. Relative to counties in expansion states, counties in nonexpansion states tended to have higher percentages of racial minority populations, higher poverty rates, and lower percentage of residents with COVID-19 vaccinations (Table 1).

As shown in Figure 1 and Figure A (available as a supplement to the online version of this article at http://www.ajph.org), spatially high mortality rates for residents 20 to 64 years of age were generally observed in Appalachia, Southeast areas, and areas with high concentrations of American Indian and Alaska Native (AIAN) residents (e.g., certain counties in South Dakota, Arizona, New Mexico, and Alaska). During the 5 years from 2018 to 2022, mortality rates were highest in 2020 and 2021, the first 2 years of the COVID-19 pandemic. A comparison of 2018–2019 and 2021–2022 showed that the mortality increase was highest in counties of Appalachia and the Southeast and areas with high percentages of AIAN residents.

Nationwide, all-cause mortality rates increased from 312.0 (per 100 000 person-years) in 2018 and 311.1 in 2019 to 373.7 in 2020, continued to increase to 419.2 in 2021, and then decreased to 366.8 in 2022. Changes in mortality rates, measured as differences between 2021–2022 and 2018–2019, varied by state. Medicaid expansion states New Mexico, West Virginia, Louisiana, and Alaska and nonexpansion states Mississippi, Tennessee, and Alabama exhibited the highest increases in mortality rates (Figure B, available as a supplement to the online version of this article at http://www.ajph.org). When examined according to Medicaid expansion status, all-cause mortality trends in Medicaid expansion and nonexpansion states were parallel during 2018–2020; increases slowed in expansion states but not in nonexpansion states in 2021, followed by a decrease in both expansion and nonexpansion states (Figure 2a).

With respect to COVID-19 mortality rates, expansion and nonexpansion states started similarly at around 30.0 (per 100 000 person-years) in 2020, after which rates increased to 49.0 in expansion states and 81.9 in nonexpansion states in 2021 and then fell to 16.3 in expansion states and 18.1 in nonexpansion states in 2022 (Figure 2b). Trends for other major causes of death are presented in Figure C (available as a supplement to the online version of this article at http://www.ajph.org).

Multivariable modeling at the county level showed that, on average, the all-cause mortality rate increased by 100.1 (95% confidence interval [CI] = 91.3, 108.9) deaths per 100 000 person-years in Medicaid expansion states and 132.7 (95% CI = 121.5, 143.9) in nonexpansion states from 2018–2019 to 2021–2022, leading to a net decrease

AJPH June 2025, Vol. 115, No. 6

TABLE 1— County Characteristics by Medicaid Expansion Status: United States, 2018–2022

	Total (3142 Counties), Mean ±SD or No. (%)	Expansion States (1834 Counties), Mean ±SD or No. (%)	Nonexpansion States (1135 Counties), Mean ±SD or No. (%)
Percentage of population			
Age ≥ 65 y	19.7 ±4.8	19.9 ±4.8	19.4 ±5.1
Non-Hispanic White	74.8 ±20.2	79.2 ±18.2	66.8 ±21.5
Income under 100% of federal poverty level	14.3 ±6.0	13.4 ±5.6	15.7 ±6.5
In labor force but unemployed	5.0 ±2.5	4.9 ±2.4	5.0 ±2.7
Age ≥ 18 y and had COVID-19 vaccination by December 31, 2021	70.2 ±6.7	72.6 ±7.0	67.3 ±4.7
Rural–urban continuum			
Metropolitan	1171 (37.0)	704 (38.4)	415 (36.6)
Urban	1333 (42.2)	758 (41.3)	481 (42.4)
Rural	649 (20.5)	364 (19.8)	239 (21.1)
Unknown	8 (0.3)	8 (0.4)	

Note. Counties from 50 states and the District of Columbia were included in the analysis. Medicaid expansion states included the following 36 states (in addition to the District of Columbia) that had implemented Medicaid expansion by December 31, 2020: Alaska, Arizona, Arkansas, California, Colorado, Connecticut, Delaware, Hawaii, Idaho, Illinois, Indiana, Iowa, Kentucky, Louisiana, Maine, Maryland, Massachusetts, Michigan, Minnesota, Montana, Nebraska, Nevada, New Hampshire, New Jersey, New Mexico, New York, North Dakota, Ohio, Oregon, Pennsylvania, Rhode Island, Utah, Vermont, Virginia, Washington, and West Virginia. The 12 nonexpansion states were Alabama, Florida, Georgia, Kansas, Mississippi, North Carolina, South Carolina, South Dakota, Tennessee, Texas, Wisconsin, and Wyoming. Oklahoma and Missouri, which adopted Medicaid expansion in 2021, were excluded from the models.

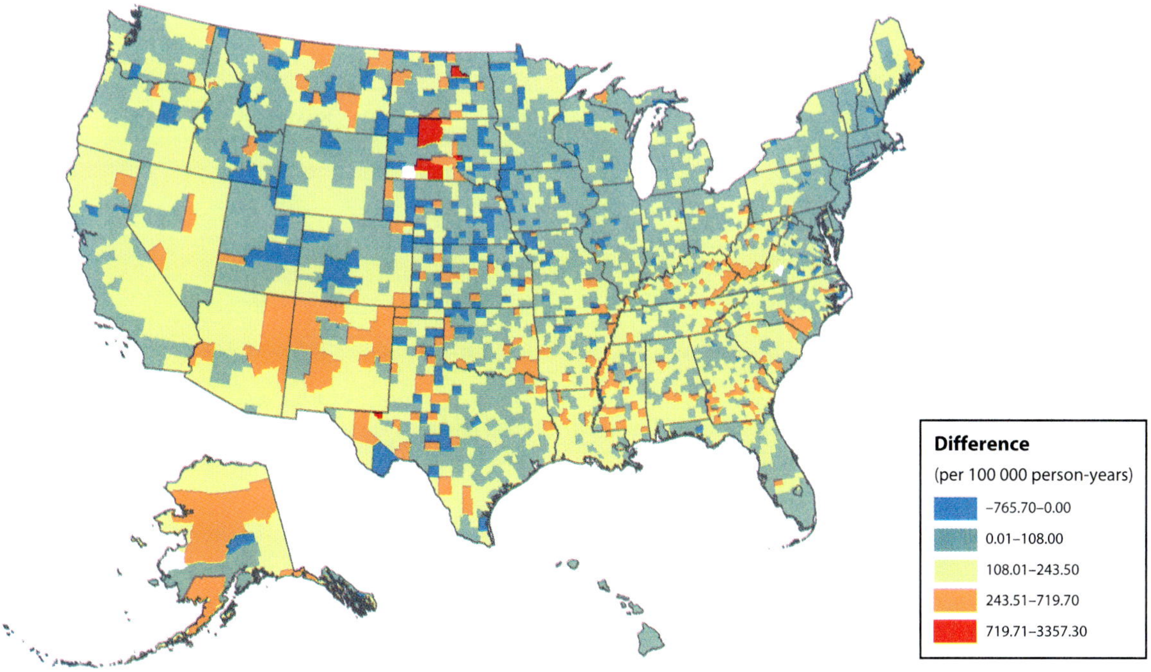

FIGURE 1— Mortality Differences Among Individuals 20–64 Years of Age Between 2021–2022 (Post-COVID-19 Pandemic Onset) and 2018–2019 (Pre-COVID-19 Pandemic) in US Counties

Note. Blue indicates lower mortality rates in 2021–2022 than in 2018–2019, and red indicates higher increases in rates in 2021–2022 than in 2018–2019.

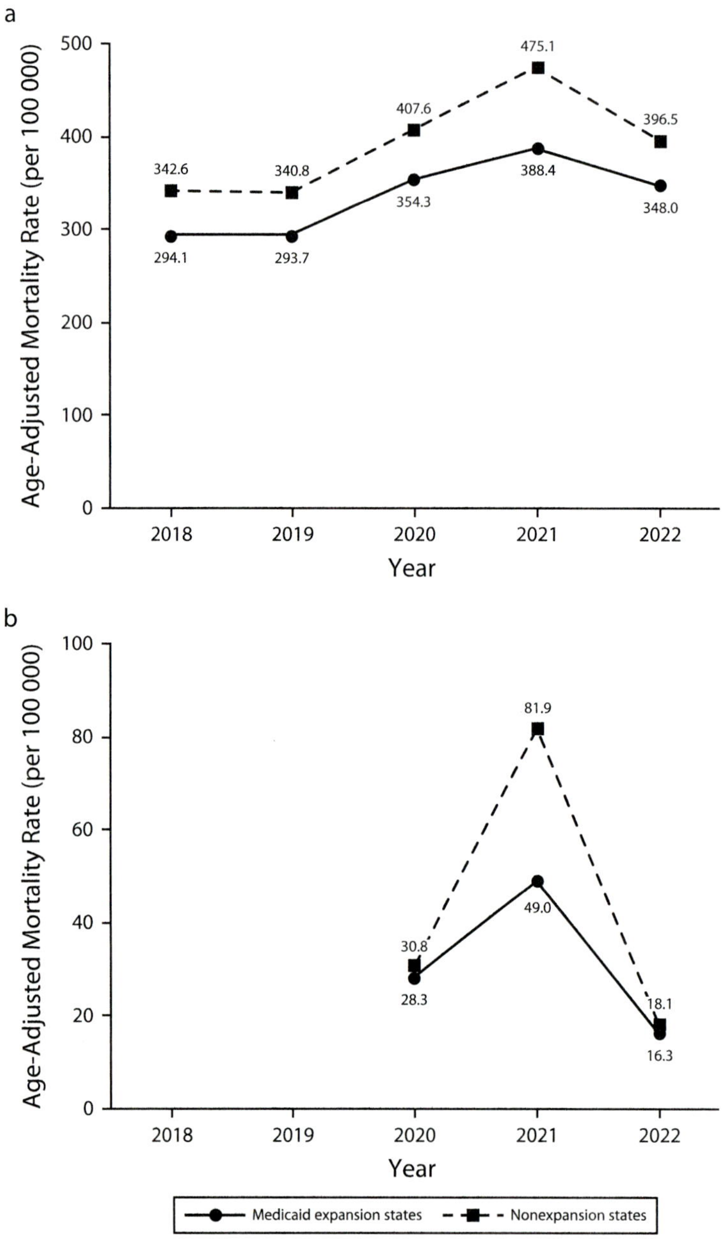

FIGURE 2— Trends in Age-Adjusted Mortality Rates (per 100 000 Person-Years) Among Individuals 20–64 Years of Age by State Medicaid Expansion Status During 2018–2022 for Deaths From (a) All Causes and (b) COVID-19: United States

of 31.8 (95% CI = 20.9, 42.8) deaths per 100 000 person-years associated with Medicaid expansion after the COVID-19 pandemic (Table 2). Net decreases in cause-specific mortality rates were observed for most major causes of death, with statistically significant decreases for heart disease and liver disease (Table 2). Of note, mortality rates from chronic lower respiratory disease, a major competing cause of death with COVID-19, decreased by 1.1 (95% CI = 0.3, 2.0) deaths per 100 000 person-years in nonexpansion states from 2018–2019 to 2021–2022 but remained nearly unchanged in expansion states, leading to a net increase of 1.2 (95% CI = 0.3, 2.2) chronic lower respiratory disease deaths per 100 000 person-years associated with Medicaid expansion.

When the data were stratified according to demographic variables, net decreases in all-cause mortality rates in expansion states were observed in almost all groups. The decreases were largest among males (34.9; 95%

TABLE 2— Associations Between Medicaid Expansion and Changes in Age-Adjusted Mortality Rates (per 100 000 Person-Years) Among Individuals 20–64 Years of Age Before and After the Onset of the COVID-19 Pandemic: United States, 2018–2019 vs 2021–2022

	Medicaid Expansion States			Nonexpansion States			Adjusted Difference in Changes (95% CI)[a]
	2018–2019	2021–2022	Difference (95% CI)	2018–2019	2021–2022	Difference (95% CI)	
All cause	353.1	453.2	100.1 (91.3, 108.9)	421.0	553.7	132.7 (121.5, 143.9)	−31.8 (−42.8, −20.9)
By disease[b]							
Cancer	74.1	72.9	−1.3 (−3.2, 0.7)	84.0	83.1	−0.9 (−3.4, 1.6)	−0.3 (−3.3, 2.7)
Heart disease	60.5	68.6	8.1 (5.8, 10.4)	79.3	91.1	11.8 (8.9, 14.7)	−3.7 (−6.9, −0.5)
Accident	62.7	85.1	22.4 (19.6, 25.2)	64.6	90.4	25.9 (22.4, 29.4)	−3.3 (−7.5, 0.9)
Suicide	25.2	26.1	0.9 (−0.8, 2.6)	25.8	25.1	−0.7 (−2.8, 1.5)	1.5 (−1.2, 4.2)
Liver disease	14.6	20.8	6.2 (4.7, 7.6)	16.8	25.5	8.7 (6.9, 10.6)	−2.7 (−4.8, −0.6)
Diabetes	12.7	15.6	2.9 (2.0, 3.8)	16.4	20.1	3.7 (2.6, 4.8)	−0.7 (−2.1, 0.6)
Chronic lower respiratory disease	12.3	12.4	0.1 (−0.6, 0.7)	15.0	13.9	−1.1 (−2.0, −0.3)	1.2 (0.3, 2.2)
Cerebrovascular disease	8.6	10.1	1.6 (0.9, 2.2)	12.8	14.9	2.1 (1.3, 2.9)	−0.6 (−1.6, 0.4)
Assault (homicide)	6.4	8.2	1.8 (1.1, 2.5)	10.6	13.1	2.6 (1.6, 3.5)	−0.8 (−1.9, 0.3)
Septicemia	4.4	5.2	0.7 (0.28, 1.12)	6.5	7.3	0.7 (0.2, 1.3)	−0.01 (−0.7, 0.6)
Kidney disease	3.9	4.8	0.9 (0.5, 1.3)	6.0	7.4	1.4 (0.9, 2.0)	−0.5 (−1.2, 0.2)
Influenza and pneumonia	4.7	4.6	−0.2 (−0.6, 0.2)	6.1	5.7	−0.4 (−0.9, 0.2)	0.2 (−0.5, 0.8)
Hypertension	2.4	3.6	1.1 (0.7, 1.5)	4.2	5.8	1.6 (1.1, 2.1)	−0.5 (−1.1, 0.1)
HIV	0.9	1.1	0.2 (−0.1, 0.4)	2.4	2.4	0.1 (−0.3, 0.4)	0.1 (−0.2, 0.5)
By gender							
Male	439.1	565.6	126.5 (115.2, 137.9)	522.3	684.9	162.5 (148.1, 177.0)	−34.9 (−49.4, −20.4)
Female	266.4	339.0	72.6 (64.9, 80.3)	321.0	417.5	96.5 (86.8, 106.3)	−23.6 (−33.6, −13.5)
By age, y[c]							
15–44	175.5	235.0	59.5 (52.8, 66.1)	199.5	275.9	76.5 (68.1, 84.9)	−17.5 (−27.1, −7.9)
45–54	455.4	583.5	128.0 (114.0, 142.0)	538.0	703.8	165.8 (148.0, 183.5)	−38.2 (−57.1, −19.2)
55–64	964.1	1202.6	238.5 (214.3, 262.7)	1158.2	1475.5	317.3 (286.7, 347.9)	−77.7 (−110.2, −45.3)
By race/ethnicity							
Hispanic	192.5	280.3	87.9 (69.3, 106.5)	221.6	340.8	119.2 (95.5, 142.9)	−30.4 (−60.4, −0.5)
Non-Hispanic AIAN	327.2	455.9	128.7 (81.4, 175.9)	296.4	431.9	135.5 (75.5, 195.5)	−5.4 (−80.5, 69.8)

Continued

TABLE 2— Continued

	Medicaid Expansion States			Nonexpansion States			Adjusted Difference in Changes (95% CI)[a]
	2018–2019	2021–2022	Difference (95% CI)	2018–2019	2021–2022	Difference (95% CI)	
Non-Hispanic API	142.4	210.8	68.5 (36.7, 100.2)	156.2	214.4	58.1 (17.8, 98.4)	11.5 (−40.3, 63.2)
Non-Hispanic Black	372.3	471.3	99.0 (54.3, 143.7)	487.0	630.0	142.9 (86.1, 199.8)	−45.4 (−117.4, 26.6)
Non-Hispanic White	349.6	439.5	89. 9 (79.6, 100.2)	421.9	540.0	118.1 (105.0, 131.1)	−27.4 (−42.0, −12.7)

Note. CI = confidence interval; AIAN = American Indian/Alaska Native; API = Asian and Pacific Islander. Medicaid expansion states included the following 36 states (in addition to the District of Columbia) that had implemented Medicaid expansion by December 31, 2020: Alaska, Arizona, Arkansas, California, Colorado, Connecticut, Delaware, Hawaii, Idaho, Illinois, Indiana, Iowa, Kentucky, Louisiana, Maine, Maryland, Massachusetts, Michigan, Minnesota, Montana, Nebraska, Nevada, New Hampshire, New Jersey, New Mexico, New York, North Dakota, Ohio, Oregon, Pennsylvania, Rhode Island, Utah, Vermont, Virginia, Washington, and West Virginia. The 12 nonexpansion states were Alabama, Florida, Georgia, Kansas, Mississippi, North Carolina, South Carolina, South Dakota, Tennessee, Texas, Wisconsin, and Wyoming. Oklahoma and Missouri, which adopted Medicaid expansion in 2021, were excluded from the models.

[a]Models were adjusted for county-level percentages of residents 65 years or older, non-Hispanic White residents, residents with incomes under 100% of the federal poverty line, and residents who are in the labor force but unemployed; counties' metropolitan status; and the percentage of adult residents who had COVID-19 vaccinations by December 31, 2021, after accounting for clustering at the state level.

[b]*International Classification of Diseases, 10th Revision* codes for causes of death can be found in Table A.

[c]Age-specific mortality rates are presented.

CI = 20.4, 49.4), individuals 55 to 64 years of age (77.7; 95% CI = 45.3, 110.2), and non-Hispanic Black individuals (45.4; 95% CI = −26.6, 117.4; Table 2).

Separate supplemental analyses of all-cause mortality for 2021 and 2022 showed that, in comparison with 2018–2019, Medicaid expansion was associated with net decreases of 49.8 (95% CI = 33.1, 66.6) in 2021 and 14.9 (95% CI = 3.1, 26.7) in 2022 (Tables B and C, available as supplements to the online version of this article at http://www.ajph.org).

Sensitivity analyses that excluded the 5 states that expanded Medicaid eligibility during 2018 to 2020 (Table D, available as a supplement to the online version of this article at http://www.ajph.org), further adjusted for hospital bed capacity and shortage of primary care physicians (Table E, available as a supplement to the online version of this article at http://www.ajph.org), or incorporated propensity score matching (Tables F and G, available as supplements to the online version of this article at http://www.ajph.org) showed similar results and did not lead to changes in our conclusions.

DISCUSSION

Using death surveillance data from more than 3000 US counties across 2018 to 2022, we found that Medicaid expansion was associated with lower mortality increases during the COVID-19 pandemic at the population level among individuals 20 to 64 years of age, a population that was susceptible to employment and health insurance coverage disruptions during the pandemic. This pattern was observed for 11 of 14 major causes of death and statistically significant for all-cause mortality and cause-specific mortality from heart disease and liver disease, suggesting a protective effect of Medicaid expansion policies among people in this age group. Our study, which incorporated the most recent data available from the second and third years of the pandemic, provides the first evidence to our knowledge of benefits from state Medicaid expansion policies with respect to mortality.

Although COVID-19 deaths contributed to the increase in mortality during 2020 to 2022 nationwide, our analysis by state Medicaid expansion status showed that COVID-19 mortality rates were higher in nonexpansion states than in expansion states, and the pattern was most striking in 2021 before the omicron variant, when death rates associated with the dominant COVID-19 variants were still high[20] and the first doses of vaccines were being delivered. Others have reported that Medicaid expansion was associated with increased health insurance coverage among low-income residents,[2] ensuring timely access to COVID-19 vaccination and treatment. In recognition of the correlation between state Medicaid expansion status and states' policies and norms regarding COVID-19 prevention and control,[21] we included state-level vaccination rates at the end of 2021 in our adjusted models along with other county-level demographic and socioeconomic characteristics; net decreases in all-cause mortality rates associated with Medicaid expansion remained statistically significant for both 2021 and 2022.

In addition to COVID-19 infections, inadequate access to care for other health conditions and exacerbated economic distress during the pandemic may have contributed to excess mortality, especially among historically disadvantaged and medically underserved populations.[22] Medicaid plays a crucial role in providing health insurance coverage for vulnerable populations, ensuring their access to COVID-19 vaccinations and care as well as necessary chronic disease management. In our analysis by cause of death, slower increases (or faster decreases) in Medicaid expansion states than nonexpansion states were observed for 11 of 14 major causes of death; the results for heart disease and liver disease, 2 common chronic conditions that require ongoing disease management, were statistically significant. Our findings reinforce prepandemic evidence showing associations between Medicaid expansion and reductions in mortality related to cardiovascular disease and liver disease.[23,24]

It is notable that chronic lower respiratory disease was an exception. Its mortality rate was nearly unchanged in expansion states but decreased in nonexpansion states after the COVID-19 outbreak, leading to a statistically significant net increase associated with Medicaid expansion. Chronic lower respiratory disease is closely related to COVID-19, with both affecting the respiratory system, and their co-occurrence can lead to severe complications and fatal outcomes. When COVID-19 is noted on death certificates, it is more likely to be selected as the underlying cause of death per rules set by the World Health Organization, leaving chronic lower respiratory diseases recorded as a contributing cause of death.[25,26]

Therefore, given the much higher COVID-19 mortality rate in nonexpansion states than in expansion states (81.9 vs 49.0 per 100 000 person-years in 2021), the decrease in chronic lower respiratory disease mortality in nonexpansion states is likely a larger offset of the increase in mortality from COVID-19 as a competing cause of death. The same mechanism may apply to influenza and pneumonia, for which statistically nonsignificant net increases associated with Medicaid expansion were observed.

Moreover, in addition to improving insurance coverage and access to care, recent studies showed positive spillover effects of Medicaid expansion on the financial performance of hospitals and providers, state economies, social determinants of health, and disparities in health care access and health outcomes that could indirectly but substantially contribute to improvements in population health among people of all ages.[27,28] For example, we found that, although the result was not statistically significant, Medicaid expansion was associated with slower increases in mortality rates from accidents and assaults, 2 causes not directly affected by insurance coverage or access to care; this suggests that Medicaid expansion may have been associated with improvements in broader social services that reduced social dysfunction during the pandemic.

When stratified by demographic characteristics, the net decrease in all-cause mortality associated with Medicaid expansion was seen in nearly all population subgroups, suggesting a broad protective effect of Medicaid expansion during the public health emergency. Meanwhile, the increase in all-cause mortality during the COVID-19 pandemic was greatest among AIAN and non-Hispanic Black individuals in both expansion and nonexpansion states. As a result of long-standing structural inequalities and systemic racism in the United States, AIAN and Black communities have experienced high poverty and limited access to health care, which exacerbated the death toll during the pandemic.[6]

Our findings reinforce the importance of investment in social determinants of health and targeted public health interventions addressing health-related social needs, especially among AIAN and Black communities. Achieving sustainable and meaningful change for these vulnerable populations requires multidisciplinary collaboration to dismantle institutionalized racism and inequities while providing relief and fostering long-term enhancement in broader socioeconomic infrastructures.[29,30]

Limitations

Our study has limitations. First, because county-level mortality rate data were available only for underlying causes of death, we examined underlying causes of death but not multiple causes of death. This approach could have led to underestimation of deaths from diseases other than COVID-19 because (as discussed) COVID-19 is more likely to be selected as the underlying cause of death.[26,31] There is no evidence that there was any differential misclassification by Medicaid expansion status, which could have biased some of our observed associations for non–COVID-19 causes of death toward the null. Second, we could not control for all variations in state policies and political ideologies, although we did account for potential clustering effects at the state level and believe that including COVID-19 vaccination rates in multivariable models served as a reasonable proxy for many state-level policy variations.

Third, we did not account for the staggered implementation of Medicaid expansion across expansion states during the study period; however, a sensitivity analysis excluding states that expanded Medicaid income eligibility during the study period showed robust findings. Finally, although our study provides evidence of the benefits of Medicaid expansion in terms of county-level population health outcomes, future studies at the individual level are warranted to confirm the protective association between Medicaid expansion and mortality during the COVID-19 pandemic.

Public Health Implications

In conclusion, using newly available death surveillance data during the COVID-19 public health emergency, we found that despite the increase in mortality rates nationwide, the increase was slower in Medicaid expansion states than in nonexpansion states even after we controlled for multiple county-level demographic and socioeconomic factors as well as COVID-19 vaccination rates, suggesting a protective effect of Medicaid expansion on population health during the pandemic. With 10 states having yet to expand Medicaid eligibility and with the 2024 US election featuring contrasting views on Medicaid's future and its outcome adding uncertainty,[32,33] our findings contribute to the growing body of evidence of the benefits of Medicaid expansion. Our findings also highlight the importance of monitoring lasting effects of the COVID-19 pandemic on access to care and population health, especially as millions of people have lost coverage during Medicaid unwinding after the pandemic.[34] AJPH

ABOUT THE AUTHORS

Xuesong Han, Kewei Sylvia Shi, Qinjin Fan, Parichoy Pal Choudhury, and K. Robin Yabroff are with Surveillance & Health Equity Science, American Cancer Society, Atlanta, GA. Kewei Sylvia Shi is also with the Department of Health Policy and Management, Gillings School of Global Public Health, University of North Carolina at Chapel Hill. Xin Hu is with the Department of Radiation Oncology, School of Medicine, Emory University, Atlanta, GA.

CORRESPONDENCE

Correspondence should be sent to Xuesong Han, PhD, American Cancer Society, 270 Peachtree St, Atlanta, GA 30303 (e-mail: xuesong.han@cancer.org). Reprints can be ordered at https://www.ajph.org by clicking the "Reprints" link.

PUBLICATION INFORMATION

Full Citation: Han X, Shi KS, Fan Q, Choudhury PP, Hu X, Yabroff KR. Medicaid expansion and US mortality rates during the COVID-19 pandemic, 2018–2022. *Am J Public Health*. 2025;115(6): 890–899.

Acceptance Date: January 26, 2025.

DOI: https://doi.org/10.2105/AJPH.2025.308045

ORCID iDs:

Xuesong Han https://orcid.org/0000-0001-7159-7949

Parichoy Pal Choudhury https://orcid.org/0000-0002-7072-0535

K. Robin Yabroff https://orcid.org/0000-0003-0644-5572

CONTRIBUTORS

All of the authors contributed to conceptualization, investigation, review, and editing. X. Han contributed to original writing and project administration. X. Han and K. S. Shi contributed to the analysis.

CONFLICTS OF INTEREST

Xin Hu received funding from the PhRMA Foundation, St. Jude Children's Hospital, Pfizer, and Johnson & Johnson outside of the submitted work. K. Robin Yabroff has received honoraria from the National Comprehensive Cancer Network for workgroup participation. The other authors have no conflicts of interest to disclose.

HUMAN PARTICIPANT PROTECTION

No protocol approval was needed for this study because all data were deidentified.

REFERENCES

1. Kaiser Family Foundation. Status of state action on the Medicaid expansion decisions: interactive map. Available at: https://www.kff.org/medicaid/issue-brief/status-of-state-medicaid-expansion-decisions-interactive-map. Accessed February 23, 2021.
2. Guth M, Garfield R, Rudowitz R. The effects of Medicaid expansion under the ACA: updated findings from a literature review. Available at: https://files.kff.org/attachment/Issue-Brief-The-Effects-of-Medicaid-Expansion-Under-the-ACA-Updated-Findings-from-a-Literature-Review. Accessed December 28, 2024.
3. Soni A, Wherry LR, Simon KI. How have ACA insurance expansions affected health outcomes? Findings from the literature. *Health Aff (Millwood)*. 2020;39(3):371–378. https://doi.org/10.1377/hlthaff.2019.01436

4. Lee BP, Dodge JL, Terrault NA. Medicaid expansion and variability in mortality in the USA: a national, observational cohort study. *Lancet Public Health*. 2022;7(1):e48–e55. https://doi.org/10.1016/S2468-2667(21)00252-8
5. COVID-19 Excess Mortality Collaborators. Estimating excess mortality due to the COVID-19 pandemic: a systematic analysis of COVID-19-related mortality, 2020–21. *Lancet*. 2022;399(10334): 1513–1536. https://doi.org/10.1016/S0140-6736(21)02796-3
6. Shiels MS, Haque AT, Haozous EA, et al. Racial and ethnic disparities in excess deaths during the COVID-19 pandemic, March to December 2020. *Ann Intern Med*. 2021;174(12):1693–1699. https://doi.org/10.7326/M21-2134
7. Campbell T, Galvani AP, Friedman G, Fitzpatrick MC. Exacerbation of COVID-19 mortality by the fragmented United States healthcare system: a retrospective observational study. *Lancet Reg Health Am*. 2022;12:100264. https://doi.org/10.1016/j.lana.2022.100264
8. Benitez J. Comparison of unemployment-related health insurance coverage changes in Medicaid expansion vs nonexpansion states during the COVID-19 pandemic. *JAMA Health Forum*. 2022; 3(6):e221632. https://doi.org/10.1001/jamahealthforum.2022.1632
9. Jacobs PD, Moriya AS. Changes in health coverage during the COVID-19 pandemic. *Health Aff (Millwood)*. 2023;42(5):721–726. https://doi.org/10.1377/hlthaff.2022.01469
10. Rakus A, Soni A. Association between state Medicaid expansion status and health outcomes during the COVID-19 pandemic. *Health Serv Res*. 2022;57(6):1332–1341. https://doi.org/10.1111/1475-6773.14044
11. Figueroa JF, Khorrami P, Bhanja A, Orav EJ, Epstein AM, Sommers BD. COVID-19-related insurance coverage changes and disparities in access to care among low-income US adults in 4 southern states. *JAMA Health Forum*. 2021;2(8): e212007. https://doi.org/10.1001/jamahealthforum.2021.2007
12. SharedGeo. US spread of COVID-19: maps and analytics. Available at: https://www.sharedgeo.org/COVID-19. Accessed December 28, 2024.
13. National Cancer Institute. Surveillance, Epidemiology, and End Results Program. Available at: https://seer.cancer.gov. Accessed December 28, 2024.
14. Surveillance, Epidemiology, and End Results Program. SEER*Stat Software. Available at: https://seer.cancer.gov/seerstat. Accessed December 28, 2024.
15. Bruch JD, Barin O, Venkataramani AS, Song Z. Mortality before and after border wall construction along the US-Mexico border, 1990–2017. *Am J Public Health*. 2021;111(9):1636–1644. https://doi.org/10.2105/AJPH.2021.306329
16. Andersen RM, Rice TH, Kominski GF. *Changing the US Health Care System: Key Issues in Health Services Policy and Management*. John Wiley & Sons; 2011.
17. Surveillance, Epidemiology, and End Results Program. SEER*Stat database: county attributes—total US, 1969–2022. Available at: www.seer.cancer.gov/seerstat/variables/countyattribs. Accessed December 28, 2024.
18. US Census Bureau. ACS demographic and housing estimates. Available at: https://data.census.gov/table/ACSDP5Y2022.DP05?q=DP05:%20ACS%20Demographic%20and%20Housing%20Estimates&g=010XX00US$0500000. Accessed May 22, 2024.
19. Centers for Disease Control and Prevention. COVID data tracker: COVID-19 vaccinations in the United States. Available at: https://covid.cdc.gov/covid-data-tracker/#vaccinations_vacc-people-booster-percent-pop5. Accessed February 15, 2024.
20. Tabatabai M, Juarez PD, Matthews-Juarez P, et al. An Analysis of COVID-19 mortality during the dominancy of alpha, delta, and omicron in the USA. *J Prim Care Community Health*. 2023;14: 21501319231170164. https://doi.org/10.1177/21501319231170164
21. Woolf SH, Sabo RT, Chapman DA, Lee JH. Association between partisan affiliation of state governments and state mortality rates before and during the COVID-19 pandemic. *Milbank Q*. 2023;101(4):1191–1222. https://doi.org/10.1111/1468-0009.12672
22. Paglino E, Lundberg DJ, Zhou Z, et al. Monthly excess mortality across counties in the United States during the COVID-19 pandemic, March 2020 to February 2022. *Sci Adv*. 2023;9(25): eadf9742. https://doi.org/10.1126/sciadv.adf9742
23. Kumar SR, Khatana SAM, Goldberg D. Impact of Medicaid expansion on liver-related mortality. *Clin Gastroenterol Hepatol*. 2022;20(2):419–426.e411. https://doi.org/10.1016/j.cgh.2020.11.042
24. Khan SS, Lloyd-Jones DM, Carnethon M, Pool LR. Medicaid expansion and state-level differences in premature cardiovascular mortality by subtype, 2010–2017. *Hypertension*. 2020;76(5):e37–e38. https://doi.org/10.1161/HYPERTENSIONAHA.120.15968
25. World Health Organization. International guidelines for certification and classification of COVID-19 as cause of death. Available at: https://www.who.int/publications/m/item/international-guidelines-for-certification-and-classification-(coding)-of-covid-19-as-cause-of-death. Accessed March 19, 2024.
26. Fedeli U, Schievano E, Avossa F, et al. Different approaches to the analysis of causes of death during the COVID-19 epidemic. *Eur Rev Med Pharmacol Sci*. 2021;25(9):3610–3613. https://doi.org/10.26355/eurrev_202105_25844
27. Guth M, Ammule M. Building on the evidence base: studies on the effects of Medicaid expansion, February 2020 to March 2021. Available at: https://www.kff.org/report-section/building-on-the-evidence-base-studies-on-the-effects-of-medicaid-expansion-february-2020-to-march-2021-report. Accessed March 18, 2024.
28. McInerney M, McCormack G, Mellor JM, Sabik LM. Association of Medicaid expansion with Medicaid enrollment and health care use among older adults with low income and chronic condition limitations. *JAMA Health Forum*. 2022;3(6): e221373. https://doi.org/10.1001/jamahealthforum.2022.1373
29. Erhunmwunsee L, Seewaldt VL, Rebbeck TR, Winn RA. From COVID-19 to cancer, watching social determinants decide life: when will we stop spectating? *J Natl Med Assoc*. 2021;113(4): 436–439. https://doi.org/10.1016/j.jnma.2021.02.003
30. Webb Hooper M, Marshall V, Perez-Stable EJ. COVID-19 health disparities and adverse social determinants of health. *Behav Med*. 2022;48(2): 133–140. https://doi.org/10.1080/08964289.2021.1990007
31. Zhao J, Han X, Miller KD, et al. Association of the COVID-19 pandemic and changes in patterns of cancer-related mortality in the United States. *JCO Oncol Pract*. 2023;19(7):501–508. https://doi.org/10.1200/OP.22.00522
32. Amba V, Cooper MSL, Sommers BD. History repeats—the election battle for Medicaid in 2024. *JAMA*. 2024;332(11):867. https://doi.org/10.1001/jama.2024.13100
33. Tolbert J, Bell C, Rudowitz R. *Medicaid Expansion Is a Red and Blue State Issue*. Kaiser Family Foundation; 2024.
34. Rosenbaum S, Collins SR, Musumeci M, Somodevilla A. Unwinding continuous Medicaid enrollment. *N Engl J Med*. 2023;388(12):1061–1063. https://doi.org/10.1056/NEJMp2301021

Medicaid Eligibility Expansion Regardless of Immigration Status and Insurance Coverage Among Latinos Seen in Community Health Centers, 2018–2023

Nathalie Huguet, PhD, Jorge Kaufmann, ND, MS, Heather Holderness, MPH, Jeremy Erroba, BS, Gretchen Mertes, MPH, Anna Steeves-Reece, PhD, MPH, Rachel Springer, MS, John Heintzman, MD, MPH, and Miguel Marino, PhD

See also Bustamante et al., p. 830.

AJPH June 2025, Vol. 115, No. 6

Objectives. To assess whether Latino patients receiving care in community-based health centers (CHCs) in US states that expanded Medicaid eligibility regardless of immigration status to adults 50 years and older had greater insurance coverage after the eligibility amendment compared with states that did not expand eligibility.

Methods. We performed a retrospective cohort study, using electronic health record data from 40 602 nonpregnant CHC patients aged 50 to 64 years living in states that expanded eligibility (OR, CA) or that did not (AK, CT, IN, MN, MT, NC, NJ, OH, WA) with a visit in both 2018–2019 (before policy change) and 2021–2023 (after policy change).

Results. Among Spanish-preferring Latinas, the overall Medicaid-insured difference-in-difference estimate across all 3 years after the amendment was positively moderate (average treatment effect on treated [ATT] = +7.04; 95% confidence interval [CI] = 0.10, 13.98); however, this effect was greatest in the third year after the amendment (ATT = +21.82; 95% CI = 14.04, 29.59), and this was accompanied by a substantial drop in third year uninsured visit rates (ATT = −15.45; 95% CI = −24.77, -6.13). We observed the same pattern for Spanish-preferring Latinos.

Conclusions. The findings suggest that expanding Medicaid eligibility regardless of immigration status improved access to health insurance for some Latino communities. (*Am J Public Health*. 2025;115(6): 900–909. https://doi.org/10.2105/AJPH.2025.308052)

The Latino community—the largest, youngest, and one of the most rapidly growing communities in the United States—persistently has the highest uninsured rate (4 times higher) of any racial or ethnic group, despite improvements in insurance coverage access after the Patient Protection and Affordable Care Act (ACA).[1] Latinos who are immigrants or part of a mixed-immigration-status household are especially at risk for being uninsured.[2–5] According to US Census data, in 2022, 20 million US residents were foreign-born Latinos.[6] A report from US Department of Homeland Security estimates that 30% of foreign-born Latinos are undocumented.[6,7] Half of likely undocumented immigrant adults report being uninsured compared with less than 1 in 10 naturalized citizen (6%) and US-born citizen (8%) adults.[8] Federal and state policies restricting or prohibiting coverage based on documentation status directly contribute to higher uninsured rates among undocumented populations.

Recognizing that immigration status is a critical factor in the willingness and ability of Latino community members to seek health insurance and access health care services,[9] several US states and the District of Columbia (DC) have expanded access to health insurance (via Medicaid eligibility, marketplace eligibility, specific local program) to provide coverage for children (12 states and DC) and adults (6 states and DC) regardless of immigration status.[10] Considering the importance of health insurance for prevention and disease management, these eligibility amendments could significantly mitigate care-access barriers and health disparities for many Latinos and their families in these states. For example, studies have shown that Latinos who gained insurance showed the greatest improvement in diabetes control, one of the most costly diseases.[11,12] Furthermore, health care utilization and total expenditures for low-income immigrants is less than one half of US-born adults.[13] Therefore, increasing access to health insurance for all Latinos could be cost-saving.

In 2021, California and Oregon both expanded Medicaid eligibility to adults aged 50 years and older, regardless of immigration status.[14,15] We evaluated the association of this eligibility expansion on insurance coverage among Latino patients receiving care in community-based health centers (CHCs). These clinics provide care regardless of insurance to a large proportion of socioeconomically disadvantaged patients. We compared changes in insured and uninsured visit rates before and after eligibility amendments in California and Oregon relative to states without this eligibility expansion. We did so by comparing changes in insured and uninsured visits among Latino patients by language preference (Spanish or English) and sex (male or female). We chose to disaggregate Latinos by language preference as preferred language has been shown to be a proxy for acculturation and cultural status and has been shown to be associated with differing health care utilization.[16,17] Lastly, evidence shows that Latino men are less likely to seek care than Latinas; therefore, we evaluated changes in Medicaid coverage separately for men and women.[18,19] We hypothesized that the rate of Medicaid-insured visits among Spanish-speaking Latino and Latina patients will have a greater increase than English-speaking Latino and Latina patients in states that expanded eligibility regardless of immigration status related to their peers in states that did not expand eligibility.

METHODS

This retrospective cohort study centers on California and Oregon because they are the only states to expand their Medicaid eligibility to adults aged 50 years and older regardless of immigration status in 2021. As a comparison, we included states that did not expand Medicaid eligibility regardless of immigration. These included states that expanded Medicaid to low-income adults in accordance with the ACA Medicaid expansion and that had clinics with more than 30 Latino patients on panel, did not have other insurance program (e.g., local program or marketplace) to assist undocumented immigrants, and participated in the OCHIN network in the pre- and postperiod. These states were Alaska, Connecticut, Indiana, Minnesota, Montana, North Carolina, New Jersey, Ohio, and Washington.

Data Source

We sourced patient-level data from the OCHIN Epic electronic health record (EHR) system. OCHIN provides a fully hosted and shared EHR platform across a nationwide network of health centers. OCHIN is part of the Accelerating Data Value Across a National Community Health Center Network (ADVANCE) Clinical Research Network of PCORnet.[20] ADVANCE clinical data are routinely assessed for completeness and quality following PCORnet's standard analytic queries and data quality check process and have low missingness on relevant variables. All study data, including patient self-reported ethnicity and preferred language, are collected in the routine course of clinical care in structured, preexisting fields in the OCHIN Epic EHR system. We use the label "Latino" because it is often preferred in our study population; however, the actual ethnicity information collected by the clinics is most often "Hispanic or non-Hispanic."

Population

The study population consisted of English- and Spanish-preferring Latino adults aged 50 to 64 years; we only used data from participants within this age range in analyses. Patients' age was restricted to align with the eligibility amendment in Oregon and California during the study period. We included all patients with at least 1 primary care visit (ambulatory visit) within the OCHIN network both before (2018–2019) and after (2021–2023) the eligibility amendment. Primary care visits were identified as those occurring with a physician (allopath, osteopath, or naturopath), physician assistant, or nurse practitioner in combination with encounters utilizing any the following Current Procedural Terminology codes 99201–99205, 99212–99215, 99241–99245,

99386–99387, and 99396–99397 (https://www.ama-assn.org/practice-management/cpt). We excluded patients seen in clinics located in both states that did and did not expand eligibility (n = 134), patients who were ever pregnant during the study (n = 360), and those who were dually eligible (n = 11 801; Medicaid plus Medicare), because pregnant individuals and those who are dually eligible have different eligibility criteria for Medicaid than other adults. We also excluded the year 2020 because of the pandemic and its impact on primary care delivery. The year 2020 had different visit trends with significant reductions in March to June.[21] The final study sample consisted of 40 602 Latino and Latina patients aged 50 to 64 years in Oregon, California, Alaska, Connecticut, Indiana, Minnesota, Montana, North Carolina, New Jersey, Ohio, and Washington.

Dependent Variables

Our 3 outcome measures included monthly clinic rates of (1) Medicaid-insured, (2) privately insured, and (3) uninsured visits for each ethnicity–language group. Rates were measured as the count of the insured-type visit over the total visits for each group in each month.

Independent Variables

Our primary exposure variable was a binary variable indicating location in states that expanded eligibility (California and Oregon) or states that did not expand eligibility (Alaska, Connecticut, Indiana, Minnesota, Montana, North Carolina, New Jersey, Ohio, and Washington). Our main independent variable differentiated patient's preferred language (Spanish or English preference), and we stratified analyses by sex (male or female).

Covariates

To describe the study groups, we extracted the following EHR-derived variables: year of first visit, distinct number of years with clinic visits, age at first study visit, total study visits over the time period, an indicator if the patient was a single clinic user (vs visiting multiple clinics), and last known income. In regression-based analyses that were clinic-level analyses, we included clinic's urban or rural status and percentage of clinic's patient population being at or below 138% of the US federal poverty level (FPL; as determined by the Department of Health and Human Services) as covariates.

Statistical Analysis

We first described characteristics of the full sample and by preferred language study groups. Next, we estimated and reported unadjusted sex- and language-stratified insured-type visit rates for Latinos before and after the amendment by eligibility expansion groups. We also produced profile plots that visually describe these rates over the study period. Then, to evaluate changes in insurance rates over time by eligibility expansion status, our primary analytic approach was done at the clinic level where insurance-type visit data and patient-level data were rolled up to the clinic–month level. We evaluated all 3 outcome measures (Medicaid, private, and uninsured visits) at the clinic–month level, where each insured-type visit was operationalized to reflect a percentage of the total visits within the clinic in the month of study by language preference. Specifically, all 3 outcome rates were estimated at the clinic–month level for Latinos who prefer English and Latinos who prefer Spanish.

To evaluate the association of this eligibility expansion on insurance coverage, we used a doubly robust covariate-adjusted difference-in-difference approach proposed by Sant'Anna and Zhao.[22] In short, this approach uses an outcome regression model and a propensity score model to address concerns about model misspecification, heterogeneity of treatment effects across patients, and lack of efficiency. Our outcome regression model was the standard difference-in-difference estimator that uses ordinary least squares with an indicator for expansion group start period, categorical time variable denoting month of study, and their interaction. The propensity score model was a logistic regression model that modeled the outcome of expansion group as a function of the pre-expansion clinic-level covariates listed previously (including the patient-level covariates that were rolled up to the clinic level). We used these propensity scores to produce stabilized inverse probability weighting with additional standard error adjustment for clustering of patients within clinics. This method combines the outcome and propensity score models by weighting the outcome regression with the propensity scores, ensuring that the treatment effect estimates remain consistent even if 1 of the models (either the outcome regression or propensity score) is misspecified.

Stratified by sex, we report the average treatment effect on the treated (ATT) with 95% confidence intervals (CIs) for each study group (English-preferring and Spanish-preferring Latinos) along with linear combinations of dynamic treatment effects showing separate effects for each of the 3 years (2021, 2022, and 2023) following initiation of the Medicaid eligibility expansion. The reported ATTs describe the difference-in-difference in insured-type visit rates before to after the amendment (difference 1) between states that did or did not expand eligibility (difference 2). The reported values reflect differences in percentage-point change of insured-type visit rates. We visually inspected parallel trends between the eligibility expansion groups using adjusted event study plots and interaction tests using preperiod data.

Sensitivity Analysis

Lastly, while our primary analysis used patients and clinics that were not exposed to this 2021 eligibility expansion as a comparison group, it is possible to conceptualize an alternative comparison group. Specifically, we could compare patients aged 50 to 64 years (who were eligible for the expansion) with those aged 30 to 49 years (who were not eligible) within California and Oregon. As such, we performed this sensitivity analysis by replacing our original comparison group to Latino patients in California or Oregon who were aged 30 to 49 years (n = 53 975). We then redid our difference-in-difference approach replacing our primary exposure to age group (50–64 vs 30–49 years). Of note, in July of 2023, Oregon expanded eligibility to all ages regardless of immigration status, and, thus, we further break out policy effects in the last year (2023) into January to June 2023 and July to December 2023.

We created the analytic data set using R version 4.3.0 (R Foundation for Statistical Computing, Vienna, Austria) and conducted analyses with the CSDID package in Stata version 15.1 (StataCorp LP, College Station, TX) using 2-sided testing and type I error set to 5%.

RESULTS

The full sample aged 50 to 64 years consisted of 40 602 Spanish-preferring Latino (81%) and English-preferring Latino (19%) adults with a median age of 55 years. A higher proportion of Spanish-preferring Latinos were female (62%), lived at or below 138% of the FPL (72%), and utilized eligibility expansion-state clinics (92%) than English-preferring Latinos (Table 1).

Average unadjusted insured-type visit rates for the pre- and postamendment periods are shown in Table 2 by eligibility expansion status. In general, eligibility expansion states had higher rates of Medicaid visits and lower rates of private and uninsured visits compared with states that did not expand eligibility. These patterns did not differ by language preference, and, overall, rates between Latinas and Latinos were comparable. The average preamendment rate of Medicaid visits for Latinas was 30.7% (SD = 36.7%) in states that did not expand and 43.0% (SD = 29.5%) in eligibility expansion states. The average preamendment rate of Medicaid visits for Latinos was 25.0% (SD = 33.6%) in states that did not expand and 36.4% (SD = 28.4%) in eligibility expansion states.

Figure 1, which depicts average monthly unadjusted Medicaid-insured rates, shows Medicaid rates for Spanish-preferring Latinas (Figure 1a) and Latinos (Figure 1b) in eligibility expansion states began rising in the second-year after the amendment and then leveled out in the third year. In contrast, rates appear steady throughout the study period for both English-preferring Latino groups in eligibility expansion states and for all Latino groups in states that did not expand eligibility.

Difference-in-difference analyses (Table 3) show a statistically significant association between eligibility expansion and insured rates exclusively for the Spanish-preferring Latino and Latina groups aged 50 to 64 years. Among Spanish-preferring Latinas, the overall Medicaid-insured difference-in-difference estimate across all 3 years after the amendment was moderate (ATT = +7.04; 95% CI = 0.10, 13.98); however, this effect was greatest in the third year after the amendment (ATT = +21.82; 95% CI = 14.04, 29.59), and this was accompanied by a substantial drop in third year uninsured visit rates (ATT = −15.45; 95% CI = −24.77, -6.13). The same pattern was observed for Spanish-preferring Latinos (Medicaid rate overall across the 3-year follow-up: ATT = 16.08 [95% CI = 7.32, 24.84]; Medicaid third year: ATT = 26.56 [95% CI = 16.75, 36.37]; uninsured third year: ATT = −11.44 [95% CI = −21.63, −1.26]).

In our evaluation of the parallel trends assumption (Appendices A and B, available as supplements to the online version of this article at https://ajph.org), we found that the parallel trends assumption holds for 10 of the 12 comparisons. For 2 groups (private female English-speaking and Medicaid male English-speaking), those *P* values were significant, suggesting a potential violation of the parallel trends assumption. Furthermore, in sensitivity analyses that compared different eligible age groups within Oregon and California, Appendix C (available as a supplement to the online version of this article at https://ajph.org) shows that the increases in Medicaid rates among

TABLE 1— Patient Characteristics Among Latinos Aged 50 to 64 Years by Language Preference in States With and Without Medicaid Eligibility Expansion: United States, 2018–2023

Patient Characteristics	Total (n = 40 602), No. (%) or Median (Range)	Latino, No. (%) or Median (Range)	
		Prefers Spanish (n = 32 844)	Prefers English (n = 7758)
Sex			
Female	24 442 (60.2)	20 431 (62.2)	4011 (51.7)
Male	16 160 (39.8)	12 413 (37.8)	3747 (48.3)
First visit year			
2018	20 678 (50.9)	17 192 (52.3)	3486 (44.9)
2019	19 924 (49.1)	15 652 (47.7)	4272 (55.1)
Distinct years of contact			
2	4998 (12.3)	3757 (11.4)	1241 (16.0)
3	8522 (21.0)	6804 (20.7)	1718 (22.1)
4	15 827 (39.0)	12 816 (39.0)	3011 (38.8)
5	11 255 (27.7)	9467 (28.8)	1788 (23.0)
Age at first study visit, y	55 (50–63)	54 (50–63)	55 (50–63)
Total study visits	12 (2–222)	13 (2–112)	12 (2–141)
Single clinic users	23 010 (56.7)	18 945 (57.7)	4065 (52.4)
Last known income			
≤ 138% FPL	28 923 (71.2)	23 785 (72.4)	5138 (66.2)
> 138% FPL	5826 (14.3)	4726 (14.4)	1100 (14.2)
No information	5853 (14.4)	4333 (13.2)	1520 (19.6)
Eligibility expansion state	36 850 (90.8)	30 212 (92.0)	6638 (85.6)

Note. FPL = federal poverty level, as determined by the Department of Health and Human Services. Data from 594 clinics in eligibility expansion states = CA, OR and eligibility nonexpansion states = AK, CT, IN, MN, MT, NC, NJ, OH, WA. Preamendment (2018, 2019) and postamendment (2021, 2022, 2023), among persons aged 50 to 64 years utilizing primary care in both periods. Amendment refers to expansion of Medicaid eligibility regardless of immigration status.

Spanish-preferring Latinas (panel a) and Latinos (panel b) aged 50 to 64 years were not observed among their younger age group counterparts until July of 2023, when Oregon expanded eligibility to all adults regardless of age). Difference-in-difference analyses utilizing the younger age groups within expansion states as the controls shows similar differences as the original analysis between English- and Spanish-preferring Latinos. However, the difference-in-difference estimates in Medicaid rates were greater overall, and, additionally, statistically significant declines in uninsured and privately insured visit rates were also observed beginning in the second-year after the amendment.

Lastly, in these analyses, the difference estimates for the first 6 months of the third-year after the amendment were twice those than in the last 6 months, evidence that the differences between the older and younger groups decreased when the amended eligibility was expanded to the younger age group (Appendix D, available as a supplement to the online version of this article at https://ajph.org).

DISCUSSION

In this early evaluation of 2021 Medicaid eligibility expansion regardless of immigration status, we observed significant increases in Medicaid-insured visits among Spanish-speaking Latina and Latino patients receiving care in CHCs in eligibility expansion states relative to their counterparts in states that did not expand; this was also observed when we compared age groups within Medicaid eligibility expansion states. These results suggest an increase in Medicaid enrollment in these states, which aligns with California enrollment reports.[23] These early findings are promising, especially as both California and Oregon have further expanded eligibility to adults aged 19 to 64 years. In 2024, other states, Washington and Colorado, have expanded eligibility for Marketplace insurance to all adults regardless of immigration status. This study could inform expected increases in Medicaid-insured rates as evaluations

TABLE 2— **Primary Care Insurance Visit Rates by Payment Type and Language Preference, Stratified by Sex, Among Patients Aged 50 to 64 Years in States With and Without Medicaid Eligibility Expansion: United States, 2018–2023**

Payment Type	States Without Eligibility Expansion, Visit Rate[a] (SD)		Eligibility Expansion States, Visit Rate[a] (SD)	
	Preamendment	Postamendment	Preamendment	Postamendment
Latinas				
Medicaid insured				
Prefers Spanish	30.7 (36.7)	31.9 (35.9)	43.0 (29.5)	59.5 (31.5)
Prefers English	43.3 (41.3)	44.8 (40.9)	61.8 (35.4)	63.9 (34.8)
Uninsured				
Prefers Spanish	49.5 (40.2)	42.2 (37.5)	27.3 (29.7)	16.8 (25.0)
Prefers English	17.8 (32.6)	13.0 (30.3)	7.8 (20.8)	4.6 (15.5)
Privately insured				
Prefers Spanish	13.9 (24.7)	19.1 (27.0)	18.5 (25.5)	16.3 (24.3)
Prefers English	21.7 (33.8)	24.1 (34.5)	16.7 (29.6)	15.3 (27.6)
Latinos				
Medicaid insured				
Prefers Spanish	25.0 (33.6)	27.5 (35.4)	36.4 (28.4)	52.4 (32.4)
Prefers English	39.1 (40.6)	43.2 (42.4)	62.3 (35.3)	63.7 (35.8)
Uninsured				
Prefers Spanish	49.0 (40.3)	42.5 (39.5)	28.5 (31.2)	17.8 (25.7)
Prefers English	23.6 (36.5)	13.6 (30.4)	9.2 (21.8)	5.1 (16.3)
Privately insured				
Prefers Spanish	16.4 (26.8)	20.1 (29.0)	18.6 (26.4)	17.1 (25.3)
Prefers English	25.1 (35.5)	28.4 (38.7)	14.1 (27.8)	14.9 (28.0)

Note. Data from 594 clinics in eligibility expansion states = CA, OR and eligibility nonexpansion states = AK, CT, IN, MN, MT, NC, NJ, OH, WA. Preamendment (2018, 2019) and postamendment (2021, 2022, 2023), among persons aged 50 to 64 years utilizing primary care in both periods. Amendment refers to expansion of Medicaid eligibility regardless of immigration status.
[a]Unadjusted rates measured as the number of monthly insured-type visits per 100 visits.

of these policies for these newly expanded states are being performed and assist other states in their decisions to expand their health insurance options regardless of immigration. Evidence shows that if all Latinos were eligible for and enrolled in health insurance, insurance premiums overall would be lower, because Latino communities including immigrants are healthier. Thus, promoting insurance for all would be cost-saving.[24,25]

Findings from the difference-in-difference analyses suggest that the majority of the association between increased Medicaid insurance visit rates and eligibility expansion status among Spanish-preferring Latinos occurs on the third year after the policy expansion. Delays in implementation and dissemination of this policy change and barriers to enrollment likely explain this trend. For instance, immigration-related policies can result in an aversion to enrolling into health insurance, even if eligible.[26] In addition, previous evidence shows that, compared with non-Latino people, Latinos were less likely to be aware of insurance marketplaces during the rollout of the ACA.[27–30] Navigating the health care system, insurance eligibility, and comprehensive benefits can be particularly difficult for those with limited or no English proficiency.[28,31] These barriers may have negatively impacted enrollment of Latino adults. Furthermore, previous evidence shows that Latino patients are more likely to receive assistance from insurance navigators[32] because of these barriers, which could explain a slower uptake. As noted previously, mixed-immigration-status households are at greater risk of being uninsured and may have benefited from this eligibility expansion at a differential rate; future studies are needed to explore the policy impact in this group.

When comparing age groups (expanded Medicaid eligibility aged 50 to 64 years vs not eligible aged 30 to 49 years)

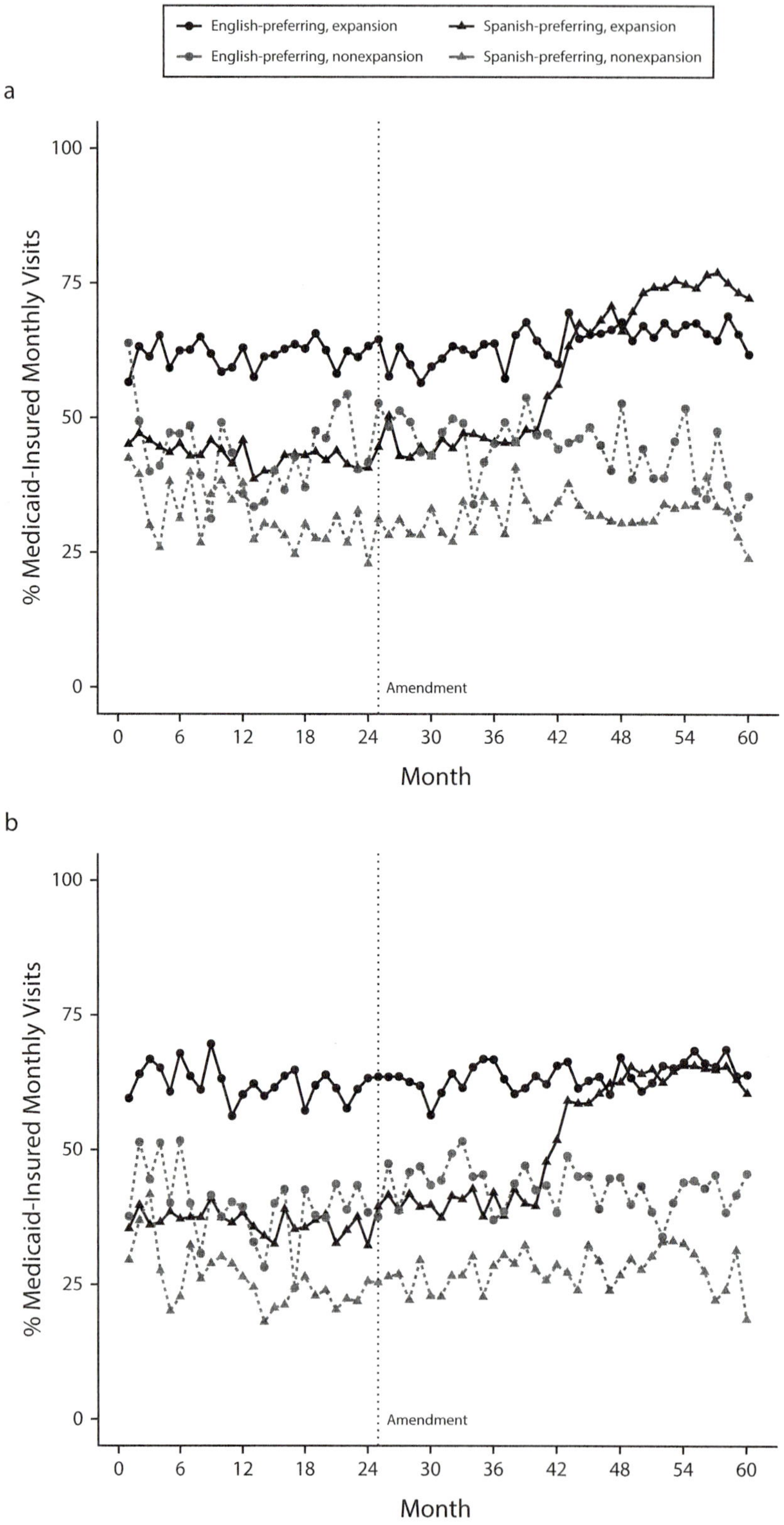

FIGURE 1— Monthly Unadjusted Rates of Medicaid-Insured Visits per 100 Total Visits for (a) Latinas and (b) Latinos Aged 50 to 64 Years by Language Preference and Eligibility Expansion Status: United States, 2018–2023 (Excluding 2020)

Note. Data from 594 clinics in eligibility expansion states = CA, OR; eligibility nonexpansion states = AK, CT, IN, MN, MT, NC, NJ, OH, WA. Preamendment (2018, 2019) and postamendment (2021, 2022, 2023), among persons aged 50 to 64 years utilizing primary care in both periods. Amendment refers to expansion of Medicaid eligibility regardless of immigration status.

TABLE 3— Average Treatment Effect on Treated (ATT) of the 2021 Medicaid Eligibility Expansion on Primary Care Visit Rates by Payment Type and Language Preference, Stratified by Sex, Among Patients Aged 50 to 64 Years in States With and Without Eligibility Expansion: United States, 2018–2023

Payment Type	Postamendment Period, ATT, Percentage Points (95% CI)			
	First Year (2021)	Second Year (2022)	Third Year (2023)	All 3 Years Combined
Latinas				
Medicaid insured				
Prefers Spanish	−5.30 (−12.09, 1.49)	4.19 (−3.56, 11.93)	21.82 (14.04, 29.59)	7.04 (0.10, 13.98)
Prefers English	−5.73 (−14.32, 2.86)	−1.00 (−11.00, 9.00)	4.84 (−5.10, 14.78)	−0.70 (−9.66, 8.26)
Uninsured				
Prefers Spanish	−2.44 (−11.74, 6.86)	−5.42 (−14.66, 3.82)	−15.45 (−24.77, −6.13)	−7.84 (−16.73, 1.06)
Prefers English	3.05 (−4.33, 10.43)	0.15 (−7.25, 7.54)	−0.72 (−8.34, 6.89)	0.86 (−6.27, 7.98)
Private insured				
Prefers Spanish	8.71 (−0.11, 17.53)	4.59 (−3.40, 12.58)	−1.57 (−9.60, 6.45)	3.86 (−4.07, 11.79)
Prefers English	5.49 (−3.41, 14.39)	2.60 (−6.83, 12.03)	−1.11 (−10.91, 8.70)	2.34 (−6.64, 11.31)
Latinos				
Medicaid insured				
Prefers Spanish	5.83 (−2.97, 14.64)	15.44 (6.62, 24.26)	26.56 (16.75, 36.37)	16.08 (7.32, 24.84)
Prefers English	−4.22 (−15.21, 6.76)	−3.69 (−15.82, 8.43)	0.27 (−11.82, 12.36)	−2.58 (−13.72, 8.57)
Uninsured				
Prefers Spanish	−0.81 (−9.93, 8.31)	−7.97 (−18.08, 2.14)	−11.44 (−21.63, −1.26)	−6.81 (−16.26, 2.63)
Prefers English	1.12 (−8.43, 10.67)	−0.38 (−9.66, 8.89)	−0.26 (−10.17, 9.65)	0.17 (−9.13, 9.48)
Private insured				
Prefers Spanish	0.87 (−6.87, 8.60)	0.84 (−7.23, 8.90)	−4.58 (−13.28, 4.12)	−0.98 (−8.72, 6.75)
Prefers English	1.05 (−10.16, 12.26)	2.87 (−8.19, 13.93)	1.11 (−10.01, 12.24)	1.72 (−8.88, 12.31)

Note. CI = confidence interval. ATTs describe the difference-in-difference in insured-type visit rates before to after eligibility expansion (difference 1) between states that did or did not expand eligibility to Medicaid regardless of immigration status (difference 2). Rates were evaluated as the number of monthly insured-type visits per 100 visits and the reported ATT values reflect differences in percentage-point change of insured-type visit rates. ATTs were derived using stabilized inverse probability weighting and ordinary least squares linear regression, adjusted for covariates, and standard error estimates clustered on clinics. Data from 594 clinics in eligibility expansion states = CA, OR and eligibility nonexpansion states = AK, CT, IN, MN, MT, NC, NJ, OH, WA. Preamendment (2018, 2019) and postamendment (2021, 2022, 2023), among persons aged 50 to 64 years utilizing primary care in both periods. Amendment refers to expansion of Medicaid eligibility regardless of immigration status.

within California and Oregon (sensitivity analysis), we found a decrease in private insurance rates among Spanish-speaking Latina and Latino patients. There are several possible explanations for this decrease. First, undocumented Latinos are not eligible for marketplace insurance plans in California and Oregon, so this decline is unlikely to be among those who became newly eligible for Medicaid. Second, it is possible that Latinos eligible for marketplace insurance switched from private insurance to Medicaid by becoming Medicaid eligible or by learning about their Medicaid eligibility, which could have been more frequent in mixed-immigration-status households. Third, marketplace insurance premiums have progressively increased in California and Oregon since 2021,[33] which may lead to less affordable plans and lower enrollment especially among older groups.

Limitations

The study findings should be interpreted in light of key limitations. First, while the 2021 Medicaid expansion aimed to increase Medicaid insurance for low-income undocumented populations, our study does not specifically look at that population. We cannot with certainty estimate the true association among those truly exposed to this policy change. Second, clinics included are part of the OCHIN network, which may not be representative of all primary care clinics in the United States. This visit-based study does not assess changes in patient-level insurance status and does not include individuals who do not seek care or who were not established before the 2021 expansion policy, which may underestimate the association, assuming the effects are stronger for the excluded population. We restricted our sample to those with care before and after the amendment and cannot estimate the impact of the eligibility expansion on patients who sought care only in the postperiod, which also likely underestimates the association. It is also possible that patients in our sample received care outside of our EHR networks; however, previous studies suggest that patients who visit CHCs continue to do so after insurance gain.[34,35] The higher change in Medicaid visits among Spanish-preferring Latinos may be attributable in part to the higher use of insurance navigation programs. The parallel trends assumption may not be satisfied for the private female English-speaking and Medicaid male English-speaking groups (both with null findings), and caution should be used when interpreting the results of these 2 estimates. Lastly, we adjusted for a number of confounders but unmeasured confounding may still exist.

Conclusions

The early findings of this retrospective study suggest that expanding Medicaid eligibility regardless of immigration likely improved access to health insurance for Latino patients receiving care in CHCs. Removing immigration-related restrictions to insurance enrollment could significantly reduce access disparities and improve health for all. AJPH

ABOUT THE AUTHORS

Nathalie Huguet, Jorge Kaufmann, Heather Holderness, Jeremy Erroba, Rachel Springer, John Heintzman, and Miguel Marino are with the Department of Family Medicine, Oregon Health and Science University, Portland. Gretchen Mertes and Anna Steeves-Reece are with the Research Department at OCHIN Inc, Portland.

CORRESPONDENCE

Correspondence should be sent to Nathalie Huguet, PhD, Department of Family Medicine, Oregon Health and Science University, 3181 SW Sam Jackson Park Rd, Portland, OR 97239-3098 (e-mail: huguetn@ohsu.edu). Reprints can be ordered at https://www.ajph.org by clicking the "Reprints" link.

PUBLICATION INFORMATION

Full Citation: Huguet N, Kaufmann J, Holderness H, et al. Medicaid eligibility expansion regardless of immigration status and insurance coverage among Latinos seen in community health centers, 2018–2023. *Am J Public Health*. 2025;115(6): 900–909.

Acceptance Date: January 31, 2025.

DOI: https://doi.org/10.2105/AJPH.2025.308052

ORCID iDs:

Nathalie Huguet https://orcid.org/0000-0002-4064-1553

Jorge Kaufmann https://orcid.org/0000-0002-1516-4636

Jeremy Erroba https://orcid.org/0009-0004-1733-8101

Anna Steeves-Reece https://orcid.org/0000-0001-9740-5079

Rachel Springer https://orcid.org/0000-0002-2633-2180

CONTRIBUTORS

N. Huguet conceptualized the study and drafted the first version of the article. G. Mertes provided the data. J. Kaufmann performed the data processing and analyses. R. Springer and M. Marino provided statistical expertise. All authors provided critically important intellectual content and approved the final version of the article. N. Huguet is the guarantor of this work and takes responsibility for the integrity of the data and the accuracy of the data analysis.

ACKNOWLEDGMENTS

This work was supported by a research grant (RSGI-23-1018762-01-HOPS) from the American Cancer Society and the Silver Family Innovation Fund. The research reported in this work was powered by PCORnet. PCORnet has been developed with funding from the Patient-Centered Outcomes Research Institute (PCORI) and conducted with the Accelerating Data Value Across a National Community Health Center Network (ADVANCE) clinical research network. ADVANCE is a clinical research network in PCORnet led by OCHIN in partnership with Health Choice Network, Fenway Health, University of Washington, and Oregon Health and Science University. ADVANCE's participation in PCORnet is funded through the PCORI award RI-OCHIN-01-MC.

The authors acknowledge the PRIMER (Primary Care Latino Equity Research) Center for their collaboration.

Note. The funding source had no role in design and conduct of the study; collection, management, analysis, and interpretation of the data; preparation, review, or approval of the article; and decision to submit the article for publication.

CONFLICTS OF INTEREST

The authors declare they have no competing interest.

HUMAN PARTICIPANT PROTECTION

Oregon Health and Science University institutional review board (00011858) approved the study.

REFERENCES

1. Cohen RA, Terlizzi EP. Demographic variation in health insurance coverage: United States, 2022. *Natl Health Stat Report*. 2023;(193):1–15.
2. American Cancer Society. Cancer Facts & Figures for Hispanic/Latino People 2021–2023. 2021. Available at: https://www.cancer.org/content/dam/cancer-org/research/cancer-facts-and-statistics/cancer-facts-and-figures-for-hispanics-and-latinos/2024/2024-2026-cancer-facts-and-figures-for-hispanics-and-latinos.pdf. Accessed March 18, 2025.
3. Angier H, Hoopes M, Marino M, et al. Uninsured primary care visit disparities under the Affordable Care Act. *Ann Fam Med*. 2017;15(5):434–442. https://doi.org/10.1370/afm.2125
4. Flores MW, Li L. Lack of access to health insurance for Latinx communities even after Medicaid expansion. *Psychiatr Serv*. 2023;74(6):563. https://doi.org/10.1176/appi.ps.23074010
5. Cha AE, Cohen RA. Demographic variation in health insurance coverage: United States, 2021. *Natl Health Stat Report*. 2022;(177):1–14.
6. US Census Bureau. ACS 1-Year Estimates Selected Population Profiles. 2022; Available at: https://data.census.gov/mdat/#. Accessed December 27, 2023.
7. Baker B. Estimates of the unauthorized immigrant population residing in the United States: January 2015–January 2018. Washington, DC: US Department of Homeland Security; 2021.
8. The Henry J Kaiser Family Foundation. Key facts on health coverage of immigrants. 2023. Available at: https://www.kff.org/racial-equity-and-health-policy/fact-sheet/key-facts-on-health-coverage-of-immigrants. Accessed January 17, 2024.
9. Vargas Bustamante A, Fang H, Garza J, et al. Variations in healthcare access and utilization among Mexican immigrants: the role of documentation status. *J Immigr Minor Health*. 2012;14(1):146–155. https://doi.org/10.1007/s10903-010-9406-9
10. The Henry J Kaiser Family Foundation. State-funded health coverage for immigrants as of July 2023. 2023. Available at: https://www.kff.org/racial-equity-and-health-policy/fact-sheet/state-funded-health-coverage-for-immigrants-as-of-july-2023. Accessed January 2, 2024.
11. Marino M, Angier H, Fankhauser K, et al. Disparities in biomarkers for patients with diabetes after the Affordable Care Act. *Med Care*. 2020;58(suppl 6, suppl 1):S31–S39. https://doi.org/10.1097/MLR.0000000000001257

12. Marino M, Angier H, Springer R, et al. The Affordable Care Act: effects of insurance on diabetes biomarkers. *Diabetes Care*. 2020;43(9):2074–2081. https://doi.org/10.2337/dc19-1571
13. Kaushal N, Muchomba FM. Cost of public health insurance for US-born and immigrant adults. *JAMA Netw Open*. 2023;6(9):e2334008. https://doi.org/10.1001/jamanetworkopen.2023.34008
14. California Legislative Information. Assembly Bill No. 133 Health (2021–2022). Available at: https://leginfo.legislature.ca.gov/faces/billNavClient.xhtml?bill_id=202120220AB133. Accessed March 18, 2025.
15. Oregon Legislative Assembly. House Bill 3352 (2021). Available at: https://olis.oregonlegislature.gov/liz/2021R1/Downloads/MeasureDocument/HB3352/Introduced. Accessed March 18, 2025.
16. Heintzman J, Dinh D, Lucas JA, et al. Answering calls for rigorous health equity research: a cross-sectional study leveraging electronic health records for data disaggregation in Latinos. *Fam Med Community Health*. 2023;11(2):e001972. https://doi.org/10.1136/fmch-2022-001972
17. Heintzman J, Hodes T, Parras D, et al. The role of language in mammography orders among low-income Latinas over a 10-year period. *Prev Med*. 2023;175:107657. https://doi.org/10.1016/j.ypmed.2023.107657
18. Schmidt H, Waltner AM, Muller ST. The Immigrant Health Initiative: A study of health care of recent immigrants in Dutchess County, New York. February 28, 2011. Available at: https://www.dutchessny.gov/departments/dbch/docs/immigrant-health-initiative.pdf. Accessed March 18, 2025.
19. Daniel-Ulloa J, Reyes JA, Morales-Campos DY, et al. Rural Latino men's experiences and attitudes toward health: a pilot photovoice study. *Am J Men Health*. 2023;17(2):15579883231158525. https://doi.org/10.1177/15579883231158525
20. DeVoe JE, Gold R, Cottrell E, et al. The ADVANCE network: accelerating data value across a national community health center network. *J Am Med Inform Assoc*. 2014;21(4):591–595. https://doi.org/10.1136/amiajnl-2014-002744
21. Huguet N, Danna M, Baron A, et al. Delivery of cervical and colorectal cancer screenings during the pandemic in community health centers: practice changes and recovery strategies. *Med Care*. 2023;61(8):554–561. https://doi.org/10.1097/MLR.0000000000001879
22. Sant'Anna PHC, Zhao J. Doubly robust difference-in-differences estimators. *J Econom*. 2020;219(1):101–122. https://doi.org/10.1016/j.jeconom.2020.06.003
23. Centers for Disease Control and Prevention. Leading causes of death and injury. 2021. Available at: https://www.cdc.gov/injury/wisqars/LeadingCauses.html. Accessed December 20, 2023.
24. Brown HS, Wilson KJ, Angel JL. Mexican immigrant health: health insurance coverage implications. *J Health Care Poor Underserved*. 2015;26(3):990–1004. https://doi.org/10.1353/hpu.2015.0102
25. Pourat N, Wallace SP, Hadler MW, Ponce N. Assessing health care services used by California's undocumented immigrant population in 2010. *Health Aff (Millwood)*. 2014;33(5):840–847. https://doi.org/10.1377/hlthaff.2013.0615
26. Touw S, McCormack G, Himmelstein DU, Woolhandler S, Zallman L. Immigrant essential workers likely avoided Medicaid and SNAP because of a change to the public charge rule. *Health Aff (Millwood)*. 2021;40(7):1090–1098. https://doi.org/10.1377/hlthaff.2021.00059
27. Doty MM, Blumenthal D, Collins SR. The Affordable Care Act and health insurance for Latinos. *JAMA*. 2014;312(17):1735–1736. https://doi.org/10.1001/jama.2014.13841
28. Guerrero EG, Legnick-Hall R, Andrews C. Underlying challenges of public health insurance enrollment and use among Latino adults: insights from the largest safety-net institution in Los Angeles. *Public Health*. 2017;152:47–50. https://doi.org/10.1016/j.puhe.2017.06.006
29. Patel MR, TerHaar L, Smith A, et al. Knowledge of health insurance terms and the Affordable Care Act in racially and ethnically diverse urban communities. *J Immigr Minor Health*. 2020;22(3):456–466. https://doi.org/10.1007/s10903-019-00924-3
30. Bustamante AV, Felix-Beltran L, Nwadiuko J, Ortega AN. Avoiding Medicaid enrollment after the reversal of the changes in the public charge rule among Latino and Asian immigrants. *Health Serv Res*. 2022;57(suppl 2):195–203. https://doi.org/10.1111/1475-6773.14020
31. Foiles Sifuentes AM, Robledo Cornejo M, Li NC, Castaneda-Avila MA, Tjia J, Lapane KL. The role of limited English proficiency and access to health insurance and health care in the Affordable Care Act era. *Health Equity*. 2020;4(1):509–517. https://doi.org/10.1089/heq.2020.0057
32. Garcia Mosqueira A, Hua LM, Sommers BD. Racial differences in awareness of the Affordable Care Act and application assistance among low-income adults in three southern states. *Inquiry*. 2015;52:0046958015609607. https://doi.org/10.1177/0046958015609607
33. KFF. Average marketplace premiums by metal tier, 2018–2025. 2025. Available at: https://www.kff.org/affordable-care-act/state-indicator/average-marketplace-premiums-by-metal-tier/?currentTimeframe=0&sortModel=%7B%22colId%22:%22Location%22,%22sort%22:%22asc%22%7D. Accessed January 16, 2025.
34. Huguet N, Kaufmann J, O'Malley J, et al. Using electronic health records in longitudinal studies: estimating patient attrition. *Med Care*. 2020;58(suppl 6, suppl 1):S46–S52.
35. Hatch B, Bailey SR, Cowburn S, Marino M, Angier H, DeVoe JE. Community health center utilization following the 2008 Medicaid expansion in Oregon: implications for the Affordable Care Act. *Am J Public Health*. 2016;106(4):645–650. https://doi.org/10.2105/AJPH.2016.303060

Community Health Worker Influence on COVID-19 Vaccine Uptake in New York City, 2021–2022

Maureen Miller, PhD, Brian G. Weiss, BA, Zoe M. Sakas, MPH, Korin E. Parrella, MPH, Farha Islam, MPH, Julian L. Watkins, MD, and the COVID-19 Equity Program Team

See also Freeman et al., p. 827.

Objectives. To evaluate a community health worker (CHW) intervention to decrease COVID-19 vaccine uptake disparities in historically disinvested communities of color.

Methods. The New York City Health Department partnered with community-based organizations that served 75 zip code–defined communities targeted for rapid response intervention. Analyses used community demographic and COVID-19 vaccine uptake data. Linear regression models evaluated high and low CHW outreach on community vaccine uptake between July 1, 2021, and June 30, 2022.

Results. Of 75 communities, 65 (85%) experienced high CHW outreach, which prioritized trauma-informed engagement with 4.2 million Black and Latino community residents. On average, residents were 70% Black and Latino. Significant differences existed between high and low outreach communities for baseline community COVID-19 vaccine uptake (44% vs 59%; $P < .001$). CHWs provided vaccine information to community residents 18 million times and increased community vaccine uptake from 44% to 76% ($P < .001$) in 1 year.

Conclusions. This research expands the body of evidence documenting the essential role played by CHWs to change population health behaviors.

Public Health Implications. Response readiness during public health crises relies on pre-established trust. When this is lacking, CHW outreach can bridge the gap. (*Am J Public Health*. 2025;115(6):910–919. https://doi.org/10.2105/AJPH.2025.308039)

AJPH June 2025, Vol. 115, No. 6

Achieving health equity in the face of centuries of systemic racism requires legitimately elevating community needs and assets; customizing messaging in terms of both culture and language; investing in a trusted, localized public health workforce; and providing reliable access to accurate information and resources.[1–4] Community-based organizations (CBOs), embedded in the communities they serve, and community health workers (CHWs), who share a concrete historical, cultural, linguistic, and lived experience with community members, are well placed to bridge divides.[5] CHWs have successfully shared medical health information and provided services to navigate an increasingly complex health system for individual community members.[1,4,6,7] CHWs have the adaptive capacity required to tailor community engagement, develop culturally relevant materials, provide connections to care and needed services, and explicitly address the social determinants of health.[2,6]

A major challenge to CHW interventions has been difficulty in demonstrating the impact of the work.[8] Much published CHW scientific research remains descriptive or has focused on tracking the outcomes of individuals with whom CHWs have interacted directly.[6,7,9] Additional analytic challenges exist for CHW-mediated interventions designed to change the behaviors of an entire community. Community interventions include both people who have direct contact with CHWs as well as those who may benefit from subsequent information and resource sharing—even though they themselves do not directly interact with CHWs.[10]

Methods to evaluate interventions explicitly designed to change health behaviors at the population level have existed since the 1990s, when epidemiologists acknowledged that studies that focus solely on individuals cannot account for outcomes seen in populations.[11,12] These methods, which rely exclusively on population-level data, have become the standard of analysis to assess policy impact on populations.[13] They have not been used to evaluate the population impact of community-based CHW interventions, primarily because community-level outcome data have been lacking. Detailed data fully documenting vaccine administration during the height of the COVID-19 pandemic in New York City (NYC) provides complete outcome data at the community level. These data facilitated a novel analysis of a CHW-mediated intervention designed to increase COVID-19 vaccine uptake in a well-defined community.

COMMUNITY HEALTH WORKER VACCINE UPTAKE INTERVENTION

Within weeks of its first COVID-19 case on March 1, 2020, the NYC Health Department released preliminary mortality data. Black and Latino residents had died from COVID-19 at rates twice as high as those of White New Yorkers.[14,15] In anticipation of continued COVID-19 inequities experienced by Black and Latino communities once vaccines became available, the NYC Mayor's Office launched the Taskforce on Racial Inclusion and Equity (TRIE),[16] in partnership with the NYC Health Department in April 2020. The Taskforce analyzed socioeconomic factors, health status, social inequities, and COVID-19 wave 1 morbidity and mortality to identify 75 zip code–defined communities (of 177 total) targeted for CHW intervention to increase community vaccine uptake. The primary goal was to ensure that 70% of all TRIE community residents completed their COVID-19 primary series vaccination within 1 year.

Using a collective impact framework to ensure stakeholder contributions,[17] the Health Department partnered directly with well-established and trusted CBOs to align the COVID-19 vaccine uptake goal with community needs and norms.[18] CHWs were hired by partner CBOs that serve the 75 TRIE communities. CBOs also provided initial training and deployed the CHWs in the community. The number of CBO partners ranged from 66 to 93, and the number of CHWs in the community varied by Health Department funding availability. The Health Department provided continuous resources, both financial and informational, as well as autonomy in developing tailored messaging and community engagement strategies. CHWs formed the core of the intervention effort through community-facing activities. Regular engagement relied on CHWs completing a minimum number of mutually agreed upon, well-defined activities per month in TRIE communities.

Shortly after vaccines became widely available in April 2021, NYC implemented numerous ambitious policies and initiatives, including vaccine mandates,[19] to increase COVID-19 vaccine uptake. To distinguish the influence of the CHW-mediated intervention, which began on July 1, 2021, and additionally addressed social determinants of health from other citywide efforts directed at all New Yorkers, this analysis focused on the 75 TRIE communities where the COVID-19 health equity intervention was implemented. This population-level analysis compares vaccine uptake in TRIE communities where the intervention was implemented with consistency and fidelity (i.e., a minimum number of well-defined activities implemented each month), with TRIE communities where it was not.

METHODS

The 75 TRIE zip codes represent 42% of all NYC zip codes, though they are home to 4.2 million people, more than 50% of New Yorkers. The 75 TRIE communities are distributed across all 5 boroughs: Manhattan (17), Bronx (18), Brooklyn (18), Queens (18), and Staten Island (4).

Population statistics were abstracted for each TRIE community for available demographic data associated with COVID-19 morbidity and mortality in NYC.[1,2] The percentage of residents in TRIE communities who identified as Black or Latino, and population size, were available from the NYC COVID-19 GitHub Web site.[20] Census data were available at the zip code level for mean number of residents per household, median household income, and median age.[21]

Residents in TRIE communities were 32% Black and 38% Latino, for a total representation of 70%. TRIE communities had 2.7 residents per household, on average, a median annual household income of approximately $66 000, and a median age of 37.0 years.

COVID-19 Health Equity Intervention

Through hyperlocal community presence, CHWs prioritized trauma-informed engagement strategies and comprehensive educational efforts in outreach to Black and Latino residents. A multipronged approach included street-level outreach, in-person and multimedia education, referrals and navigation to COVID-19 vaccination and testing sites, personal protective equipment (PPE) and test-kit distribution, and referrals to other health and social services. A deliverables-based funding contract required a monthly minimum number of CHW outreach events and activities in designated TRIE communities. CHWs entered data weekly through a secure, Health Department Web-based data collection tool. Data were analyzed in MS365 Excel (Microsoft, Redmond, WA). Summary slides were presented virtually and in print to community partners on a monthly basis.

A summary variable of the number of times COVID-19 vaccine information was provided to TRIE community residents was created and included all communication methods through which information was shared. To distinguish between education and service provision, all referrals and linkages to COVID-19 vaccine appointments and testing sites, as well as referrals to other health or social services, were excluded. No identifying or health information for individuals with direct CHW contact was collected.

CBO partners and CHWs were supported through frequent structured data sharing, multimedia presentations, and bidirectional communication opportunities coordinated by the Health Department. In addition to Health Department training in trauma-informed engagement strategies, CHWs received regular, mandatory training on topics including up-to-date COVID-19 and vaccine information, de-escalation and safety, and human rights law.

Intervention Outcome

We defined vaccine uptake as the percentage of residents in each TRIE community who completed the COVID-19 primary series vaccination. The primary series included either 2 mRNA vaccinations (Pfizer or Moderna) or 1 Johnson and Johnson vaccination. We abstracted monthly vaccine uptake percentages for each TRIE community from NYC's publicly available COVID-19 GitHub Web site.[20]

Community Health Worker Outreach Intervention

The current population evaluation compared vaccine uptake in TRIE communities with high CHW outreach, defined as engagement in TRIE communities during at least 11 months of the year, and low CHW outreach, defined as engagement in individual TRIE communities conducted for 10 or fewer months. Groups were created based on the bimodal distribution of months of CHW community outreach within each TRIE community.

High CHW outreach was conducted in 65 (85%) TRIE communities. The remaining 10 (15%) TRIE communities received low CHW outreach (Figure 1). On average, high CHW outreach was conducted during all 12 months (range = 11–12; SD = 0.3), while low CHW outreach averaged 6 months (range = 1–10; SD = 2.8) in TRIE communities. Low CHW outreach communities were predominantly located in Manhattan (6 of 10).

Analysis

We hypothesized that TRIE communities with high CHW outreach would experience significantly increased vaccine uptake relative to low CHW outreach within 1 year, even after controlling for population demographics and baseline vaccine uptake.

All population data to evaluate the relationship between intervention consistency and fidelity and vaccine uptake were at the zip code level. We analyzed data using linear regression models and adjusted for each TRIE zip code population size. We used population size to weight zip code–defined community variables (i.e., zip code community data will influence the model results commensurate with population size). In addition, analyses that evaluated zip code–level COVID-19 vaccine uptake on June 30, 2022 (end of study), included July 1, 2021, zip code–level COVID-19 vaccine uptake (baseline). Results are for the first year of program intervention: July 1, 2021, through June 30, 2022. Two-sided *P* values < .05 were considered significant. We conducted all analyses using R software (R Foundation for Statistical Computing, Vienna, Austria) and MASS (Modern Applied Statistics with S) package.[22]

Impact on Vaccine Uptake and Mortality

We made comparisons to determine if the intervention resulted in improvements to COVID-19 vaccine uptake and mortality that were comparable to well-resourced NYC communities (zip code–defined) not in need of intervention. We created COVID-19 vaccine uptake and mortality curves by using publicly available, zip code–level Health Department data.[20,23] We compared data across 3 groups: high and low CHW outreach, and well-resourced communities.

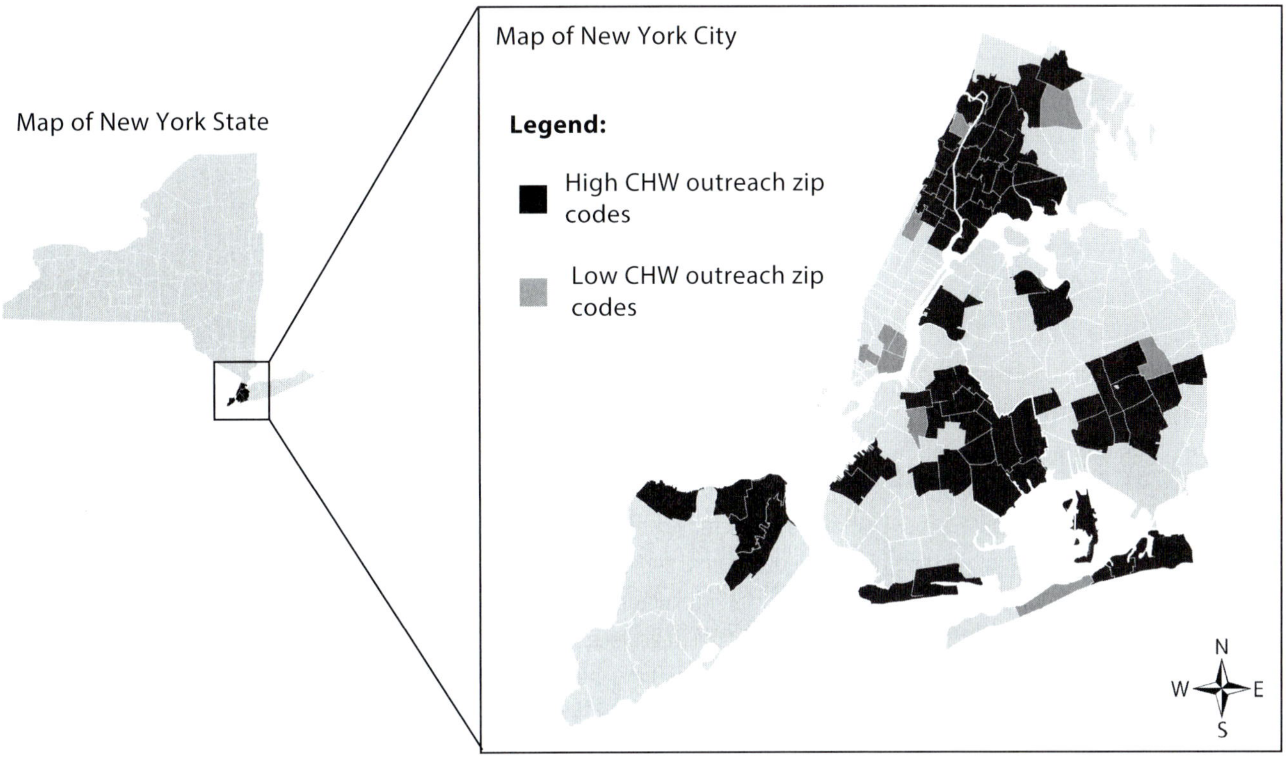

FIGURE 1— **The 75 Taskforce on Racial Inclusion and Equity (TRIE) Zip Code–Defined Communities by High and Low Community Health Worker (CHW) Outreach: New York City, July 1, 2021–June 30, 2022**

Note. High CHW outreach was conducted with consistency and fidelity (i.e., a minimum number of well-defined activities implemented each month). Low CHW outreach was well below this standard.

RESULTS

In 1 year, CHWs provided vaccine information to TRIE community residents more than 18 million times. They participated in 22 621 outreach events that directly engaged TRIE residents 3.1 million times and shared 4 million pieces of educational literature. CBOs regularly tailored multimedia communications to engage and inform the community through flyers, social media, brief videos, and original songs. CHWs provided 800 000 linkages to COVID-19 vaccination appointments and more than 200 000 referrals to COVID-19 testing sites. They distributed 17 million facemasks and 73 000 at-home antigen tests once they became available.

CHWs also made 337 000 referrals to other health and social services that addressed resident priorities, including food insecurity, housing, and financial support. CHWs met and often exceeded the minimum number of contracted deliverables each week.

Over the 1-year period, the Health Department supported CBOs and CHWs through 21 online informational forums, 47 operational guides, and 29 COVID-19 Health Equity newsletters. These multimedia efforts provided up-to-date COVID-19 statistics for NYC; information on vaccination, testing, and treatment; and updates on the changing COVID-19 guidelines. A total of 67 trainings were offered to CHWs.

Taskforce on Racial Inclusion and Equity

COVID-19 vaccine uptake. At the start of the intervention in July 2021, 58% of adult residents and 44% of all residents living in TRIE communities had completed their primary series vaccination. The target 70% vaccine uptake goal was achieved on September 27, 2021, for adult residents and on January 11, 2022, for all residents living in TRIE communities.

Demographics and community health worker outreach. Significant differences existed across all demographics between TRIE communities that received high CHW outreach and those that did not. TRIE communities with high CHW outreach were more likely than those with low CHW outreach to have a higher percentage of Black and Latino ($P < .001$) and younger residents ($P = .02$), more residents per household ($P = .006$), and lower median household incomes ($P < .001$; see Table A, available as a supplement to the online version of this article at https://ajph.org, for additional details).

Outreach Effect on Vaccine Uptake

Figure 2 shows the timeline documenting the dates that high and low outreach communities achieved 70% vaccine uptake. High outreach communities achieved 70% vaccine uptake 2 to 3 months later then low outreach communities. By June 30, 2022, 76% of all TRIE communities had completed their primary vaccination series. When the intervention began in July 2021, high CHW outreach communities had significantly lower vaccine uptake than low CHW outreach communities (44% vs 59%; $P < .001$). One year later, all TRIE communities had exceeded the 70% goal with no significant differences between high and low CHW outreach communities (76% vs 81%; $P = .23$).

Except for median age, bivariable models revealed significant relationships between each TRIE community variable and TRIE community vaccine uptake by June 30, 2022 (Table 1). In the final, multivariable regression model, both high CHW outreach and the percentage of Black and Latino residents for whom the intervention was designed remained independently associated with TRIE community vaccine uptake ($P = .002$ and $P < .001$, respectively). Lower income ($P = .03$), older age ($P = .02$), and higher household density ($P = .008$) in TRIE communities were also independently associated with TRIE community vaccine uptake.

Given significant differences across all TRIE community demographic variables between high and low CHW outreach communities, we conducted a sensitivity analysis. To ensure comparable groups, we created a subsample of TRIE communities with fewer than 50% Black and Latino residents. Although not reflective of the overall sample (40% of TRIE communities were home to > 80% Black and Latino residents), both high CHW outreach and the percentage of Black and Latino residents remained independently associated with TRIE community vaccine uptake in multivariable analyses (see Table B, available as a supplement to the online version of this article at https://ajph.org, for results of sensitivity analysis).

Impact on Vaccine Uptake and Mortality

Figure 3 presents COVID-19 vaccine uptake and mortality curves for high CHW outreach, low CHW outreach, and well-resourced communities. During the January 2022 Omicron peak,

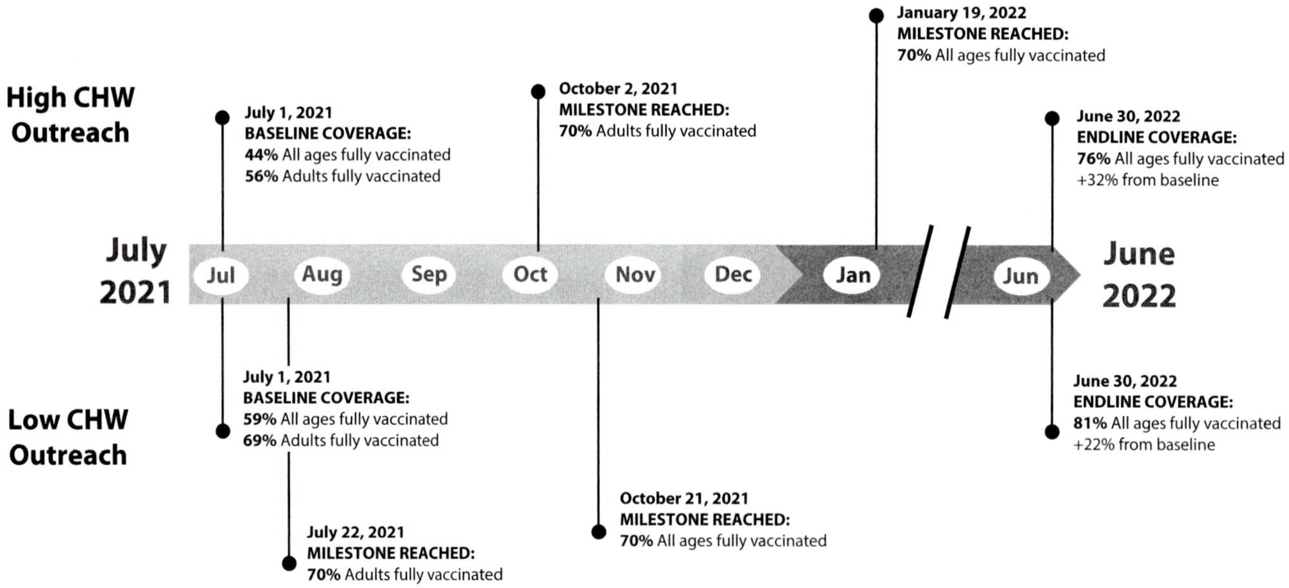

FIGURE 2— Comparison of COVID-19 Vaccine Uptake Milestones for High Versus Low Community Health Worker (CHW) Outreach: New York City, July 2021–June 2022

TABLE 1— Community Health Worker (CHW) Outreach and COVID-19 Vaccine Uptake in Taskforce on Racial Inclusion and Equity (TRIE) Communities: New York City, July 1, 2021–June 30, 2022

	COVID-19 Vaccine Uptake, Bivariable Model			COVID-19 Vaccine Uptake, Multivariable Model		
TRIE Community Variables	b (SE)	*t*	*P*	b (SE)	*t*	*P*
Intervention: CHW outreach	9.0 (2.1)	4.3	<.001	5.6 (1.9)	2.9	.005
Percentage Black and Latino residents	18.1 (3.6)	5.0	<.001	14.8 (3.5)	4.2	<.001
Mean number of residents per household	4.1 (1.6)	2.6	.011	3.5 (1.3)	2.7	.008
Median income	−0.00011 (0.000031)	−3.6	<.001	−0.000065 (0.000029)	−2.2	.028
Median age	0.02 (0.18)	0.1	.91	0.33 (0.14)	2.4	.021

Note. Controlling for July 2021 (baseline) TRIE community COVID-19 vaccine uptake.

mortality rates were 38.6, 37.2, and 32.3 per 100 000 for high CHW outreach, low CHW outreach, and well-resourced communities not in need of intervention, respectively. When compared with NYC zip code–defined well-resourced communities, mortality rates were 17% higher among high CHW outreach communities and 13% higher among low CHW outreach communities.

DISCUSSION

This study provides evidence of high impact for a CHW-mediated intervention explicitly designed to change community health behaviors. Through a combination of multifaceted information exchanges tailored to evolving needs, partnership building, and increased access to vaccines, CHWs helped raise TRIE community vaccine uptake from 44% to 76% in just 1 year. Once the COVID-19 health equity intervention was introduced in July 2021, the differences in vaccine uptake and mortality curves in TRIE communities became more aligned with the vaccination and mortality experiences of well-resourced communities in the rest of NYC. TRIE communities continue to have higher COVID-19 vaccine uptake than communities in the United States overall.[24]

For most TRIE communities, programming was implemented with consistency and fidelity, with active CHW outreach conducted monthly. Notably, high CHW outreach communities differed significantly from low CHW outreach communities. High CHW outreach was consistently conducted in communities that were home to more Black and Latino residents, as well as in communities with lower incomes and fewer resources.[16] Low CHW outreach communities also experienced vaccine uptake levels that consistently tracked with well-resourced NYC communities not in need of intervention.

CBOs may have prioritized outreach in high CHW outreach communities for a variety of reasons, including zip code–defined communities that lumped together wealthy and low-income New Yorkers. Half of low CHW outreach communities were home to both extensive public housing developments, where 1 in 17 New Yorkers reside,[25] and some of the most expensive real estate in the city. In addition, the majority of low CHW outreach communities were in Manhattan, with its greater concentration of vaccination sites and transportation options, which made it easier for residents to access vaccines. The sensitivity analysis supports intervention impact with Black and Latino residents, even within these economically diverse communities.

Over time, CHWs became trusted messengers and helped to address community-level health inequities stemming from mistrust and misinformation[1,26] through hyperlocal, culturally responsive, and place-based outreach that addressed local concerns.[27–31] Trust was built through tailoring educational materials to meet community needs, increasing exposure to vaccine information, and improving access to vaccines, through mobile vaccination vans, vaccination events, and navigation and referrals to vaccination sites.[18,27,28] Research shows that Black and Latino New Yorkers were more likely to get vaccinated against COVID-19 following community-based outreach activities.[4]

While CHWs acted as a bridge to promote the medical necessity of COVID-19 vaccination and testing, they also addressed community members' prioritized needs. Initially, other health and social service referrals were tangential to the goal of COVID-19 vaccine uptake. Through their deep understanding of community,[5] CHWs made more than 300 000 referrals to basic health and

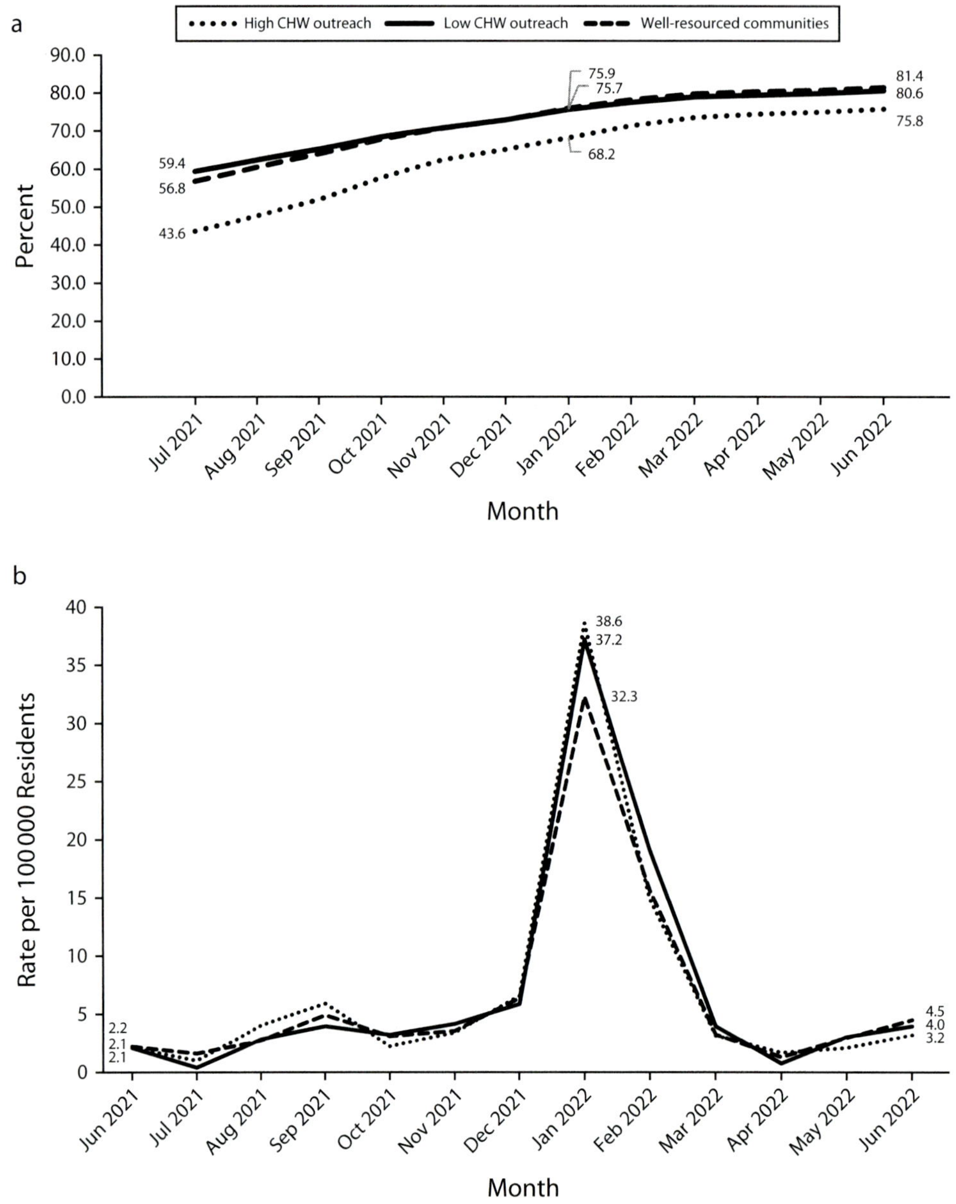

FIGURE 3— COVID-19–Related (a) Vaccine Uptake and (b) Mortality Curves: New York City, June 1, 2021–June 30, 2022

Note. Part a represents the percentage of New York City residents completing COVID-19 primary vaccination series at baseline, during the Omicron peak, and at end of study for high community health worker (CHW) outreach, low CHW outreach, and well-resourced communities not in need of outreach. Part b represents COVID-19 mortality rates per 100 000 residents at baseline, during the Omicron peak, and at end of study for high CHW outreach, low CHW outreach, and well-resourced communities not in need of outreach.

social services. These referrals were key to building trust over time.[18]

A complex relationship exists between COVID-19 vaccine uptake in TRIE communities and subsequent mortality. Mortality data disaggregated by zip code in NYC were first reported on June 1, 2020, when both cases and deaths were nearing a trough after the first deadly wave. By that time, almost 22 000 people had already died. This staggering statistic represents almost half of all New Yorkers who have died from COVID-19 to date.[23] Two thirds of those who died in the first 3 months of the pandemic were Black or Latino, although these 2 groups made up only half of the population.[14]

New Yorkers living in TRIE communities also had higher mortality rates compared with other New Yorkers during the Omicron variant wave. Several factors were at play. Black and Latino New Yorkers were more likely to work in jobs and industries not conducive to work-from-home policies, which increased COVID-19 exposure. These New Yorkers also experienced delays in primary series vaccination and had lower rates of booster doses by winter 2021.[32] Yet, the deadly impact of Omicron was blunted, with differential mortality rates less than 20% higher among TRIE communities than in well-resourced communities that required no intervention—a far cry from the 200% mortality differential at the onset of the pandemic.[14,15] Since the end of the Omicron wave, subsequent inequities in both COVID-19 vaccine uptake and mortality have continued to diminish.

Although the breadth of NYC's response to COVID-19 was substantial after the first traumatic wave, a 1-size-fits-all approach did not immediately engage residents in TRIE communities. High-intensity, hyperlocal programming addressed both COVID-19 concerns and other community priorities to help facilitate population behavior change. By explicitly addressing social determinants of health, such as food insecurity and housing needs, CHWs engaged residents where they needed assistance most. The intervention was designed to build knowledge, respect, and trust, important components in comprehensively addressing persistent inequities. This study also suggests that CHWs based at CBOs with a mission to change community behavior well complement the documented impact of clinically based CHWs who work with individual community members to positively influence their health outcomes.[1,4,6,7]

Limitations

Limitations to the study relate to data quality and availability. Substantial misclassification only allowed for an analysis that combined race and ethnicity,[32] limiting the ability to explore Black and Latino community COVID-19 experiences independently. While COVID-19 policies instituted by the city could have had differential impact on the historically underserved communities that are the subject of this analysis (e.g., job loss because of employee-mandated vaccination in a context of both lack of access and mistrust), once vaccine access, information, and mistrust issues were addressed, inequities in COVID-19 vaccine uptake and mortality decreased substantially. Public health requirements to collect detailed COVID-19 vaccination data provided a rare opportunity to access comprehensive community-level outcome data. In the future, the population impact of CHW-mediated interventions will likely resemble policy analyses because community-level outcome variables, such as vaccine uptake, are more often estimated rather than collected.[33]

Public Health Implications

Response readiness in times of public health crisis relies on preestablished trust. Building trust requires time; honest, accurate, up-to-date information; and a willingness and ability to address the prioritized needs of the community. The time to build trust is not at the moment of crisis, as was the case in many TRIE communities when COVID-19 struck so suddenly. Without trust, the desired public health outcome will always lag, sometimes greatly, and will hit disinvested communities hardest.

Maintaining meaningful relationships between public health institutions and communities, such as those established between the NYC Health Department and TRIE communities during the emergency phase of the COVID-19 pandemic, is essential to ensure a successful and effective rapid response in future health emergencies. Yet, these CHW-mediated relationships may already be threatened. COVID-19 health equity programming, which was foundational to the Health Department Public Health Corps, was predominantly grant funded. Since the COVID-19 national emergency declaration end date, dedicated resources to address the COVID-19 emergency, a major investment in public health infrastructure, have ceased. Inconsistent funding inhibits CBO planning, causes CHW job instability, fuels mistrust in the community, and could diminish Health Department capacity to maintain relationships. Hope exists in New York State's Medicaid 1115 waiver amendment, which recently began funding clinic-based CHWs. Current Health Department efforts aim to expand the waiver to include CBO-based CHWs, as well.[34]

This population analysis provides evidence of the essential role of community-based CHWs in changing community health behaviors. Unlike policy analyses, which require estimations and adjustments to population data because of unknown parameters,[13] this CHW evaluation included all data, unadjusted, from a well-defined population of 4.2 million people. Therefore, this study provides a blueprint for future evaluations of CHW interventions specifically designed to have an impact on population health. AJPH

ABOUT THE AUTHORS

At the time of the study, Maureen Miller, Brian G. Weiss, Zoe M. Sakas, Korin E. Parrella, Farha Islam, and Julian L. Watkins were with the New York City Department of Health and Mental Hygiene.

CORRESPONDENCE

Correspondence should be sent to Maureen Miller, PhD, 250 W 99th St, Suite 3C, New York, NY 10025 (e-mail: mm35@caa.columbia.edu). Reprints can be ordered at https://www.ajph.org by clicking the "Reprints" link.

PUBLICATION INFORMATION

Full Citation: Miller M, Weiss BG, Sakas ZM, et al. Community health worker influence on COVID-19 vaccine uptake in New York City, 2021–2022. *Am J Public Health*. 2025;115(6):910–919.

Acceptance Date: January 20, 2025.

DOI: https://doi.org/10.2105/AJPH.2025.308039

ORCID iDs:

Maureen Miller https://orcid.org/0000-0003-4467-5491

Brian G. Weiss https://orcid.org/0009-0004-8188-0595

Korin E. Parrella https://orcid.org/0009-0005-3859-6713

CONTRIBUTORS

M. Miller made substantial contributions to the conceptualization and design of the work, as well as the acquisition, analysis, and interpretation of data for the work. She also was responsible for drafting the work and revising it critically for important intellectual content. B. G. Weiss made substantial contributions in the acquisition, analysis, and interpretation of data for the work as well as revising it critically for important intellectual content. Z. M. Sakas made contributions to drafting the work and revising it critically for important intellectual content. K. E. Parrella made contributions to revising the work critically for important intellectual content. F. Islam made contributions to drafting the work. J. L. Watkins made contributions to revising the work critically for important intellectual content and provided final approval of the version to be published.

ACKNOWLEDGMENTS

Funding was received from Federal Emergency Management Agency COVID-19 Emergency Response, Centers for Disease Control and Prevention (grants CDCINH750T000036 and CDC6NH23IP922636), National Institutes of Health Office of Minority Health (grant CPIMP 211248), and New York City Tax Levy Dollars in response to a New Needs Request.

Thanks to our community-based partners and the field-based community health workers for changing the health outcomes for millions of New Yorkers. Also, thanks to the insightful and thoughtful comments of reviewers who helped make this a better article.

CONFLICTS OF INTEREST

There are no conflicts of interest from funding or affiliation-related activities for any of the authors.

HUMAN PARTICIPANT PROTECTION

All data used in the study were aggregated at the community level. No individual data were available for this analysis.

REFERENCES

1. Shen AK, Browne S, Srivastava T, Kornides ML, Tan ASL. Trusted messengers and trusted messages: the role for community-based organizations in promoting COVID-19 and routine immunizations. *Vaccine*. 2023;41(12):1994–2002. https://doi.org/10.1016/j.vaccine.2023.02.045
2. Zhang R, Qiao S, McKeever BW, Olatosi B, Li X. Listening to voices from African American communities in the Southern states about COVID-19 vaccine information and communication: a qualitative study. *Vaccines (Basel)*. 2022;10(7):1046. https://doi.org/10.3390/vaccines10071046
3. Dada D, Djiometio JN, McFadden SM, et al. Strategies that promote equity in COVID-19 vaccine uptake for Black communities: a review. *J Urban Health*. 2022;99(1):15–27. https://doi.org/10.1007/s11524-021-00594-3
4. Diaz D, Chacko S, Sperling A, et al. Assessment of digital and community-based outreach interventions to encourage COVID-19 vaccination uptake in an underserved community. *JAMA Netw Open*. 2022;5(6):e2217875. https://doi.org/10.1001/jamanetworkopen.2022.17875
5. American Psychological Association. Situated knowledge. In: *APA Dictionary of Psychology*. 2018. Available at: https://dictionary.apa.org/situated-knowledge. Accessed July 13, 2024.
6. Ingram M, Sabo S, Rothers J, Wennerstrom A, de Zapien JG. Community health workers and community advocacy: addressing health disparities. *J Community Health*. 2008;33(6):417–424. https://doi.org/10.1007/s10900-008-9111-y
7. Witmer A, Seifer SD, Finocchio L, Leslie J, O'Neil EH. Community health workers: integral members of the health care work force. *Am J Public Health*. 1995;85(8 pt 1):1055–1058. https://doi.org/10.2105/AJPH.85.8_Pt_1.1055
8. Rosenthal EL, de Heer H, Rush CH, Holderby L. Focus on the future: a community health worker research agenda by and for the field. *Prog Community Health Partnersh*. 2008;2(3):183–184, 225–235. https://doi.org/10.1353/cpr.0.0025
9. Jack HE, Arabadjis SD, Sun L, Sullivan EE, Phillips RS. Impact of community health workers on use of healthcare services in the United States: a systematic review. *J Gen Intern Med*. 2017;32(3):325–344. https://doi.org/10.1007/s11606-016-3922-9
10. Susser M. The logic in ecological: II. The logic of design. *Am J Public Health*. 1994;84(5):830–835. https://doi.org/10.2105/AJPH.84.5.830
11. Susser M. The logic in ecological: I. The logic of analysis. *Am J Public Health*. 1994;84(5):825–829. https://doi.org/10.2105/AJPH.84.5.825
12. Steel DG, Holt DT. Analysing and adjusting aggregation effects: the ecological fallacy revisited. *Int Stat Rev*. 1996;64(1):39–60. https://doi.org/10.2307/1403423
13. Basu S, Meghani A, Siddiqi A. Evaluating the health impact of large-scale public policy changes: classical and novel approaches. *Annu Rev Public Health*. 2017;38(1):351–370. https://doi.org/10.1146/annurev-publhealth-031816-044208
14. City of New York. *Taskforce on Racial Inclusion & Equity - Progress Report*. 2021. Available at: https://www.nyc.gov/assets/trie/downloads/pdf/TRIE-Report-Final-2020-Recap.pdf. Accessed January 16, 2024.
15. Afzal A, Shariff MA, Perez-Gutierrez V, et al. Impact of local and demographic factors on early COVID-19 vaccine hesitancy among health care workers in New York City public hospitals. *Vaccines (Basel)*. 2022;10(2):273. https://doi.org/10.3390/vaccines10020273
16. City of New York, Task Force on Racial Inclusion and Equity. Neighborhoods. Available at: https://www.nyc.gov/site/trie/about/neighborhoods.page. Accessed January 16, 2024.
17. Kania J, Kramer M. Collective impact. *Stanf Soc Innov Rev*. 2011;9(1):36–41. https://doi.org/10.48558/5900-KN19
18. Ige O, Sakas Z, Kang M, Green C, Brown D. Vaccine confidence in NYC: thematic analysis of community stories. *J Health Commun*. 2023;28(suppl 1):45–53. https://doi.org/10.1080/10810730.2023.2191226
19. Rubenstein BL, Amiel PJ, Ternier A, et al. Increases in COVID-19 vaccination among NYC municipal employees after implementation of vaccination requirements. *Health Aff (Millwood)*. 2023;42(3):357–365. https://doi.org/10.1377/hlthaff.2022.00809
20. New York City Department of Health. COVID vaccine data. GitHub. Available at: https://github.com/nychealth/covid-vaccine-data/tree/main/people. Accessed August 8, 2023.
21. Census Reporter. 2022 American Community Survey (ACS). Available at: https://censusreporter.org. Accessed April 15, 2024.
22. *Modern Applied Statistics With S*. Version 4.2.3. Springer. 2002. Available at: https://www.stats.ox.ac.uk/pub/MASS4. Accessed October 31, 2023.
23. New York City Department of Health. Coronavirus data. GitHub. Available at: https://github.com/nychealth/coronavirus-data/blob/7c1c9ecae394df80de8fa1678d24098fa9f32666/totals/data-by-modzcta.csv. Accessed July 2, 2024.
24. USA Facts. US Coronavirus vaccine tracker. May 10, 2024. Available at: https://usafacts.org/visualizations/covid-vaccine-tracker-states. Accessed March 4, 2025.
25. New York City Housing Authority. About NYCHA. Available at: https://www.nyc.gov/site/nycha/about/about-nycha.page. Accessed October 14, 2024.
26. Best AL, Fletcher FE, Kadono M, Warren RC. Institutional distrust among African Americans and building trustworthiness in the COVID-19 response: implications for ethical public health practice. *J Health Care Poor Underserved*. 2021;32(1):90–98. https://doi.org/10.1353/hpu.2021.0010

27. El-Sadr WM, Vasan A, El-Mohandes A. Facing the new Covid-19 reality. *N Engl J Med.* 2023;388(5): 385–387. https://doi.org/10.1056/NEJMp2213920
28. Ige O, Watkins J, Pham-Singer H, Dresser M, Maru D, Morse M. Embedding health equity in a public health emergency response: New York City's Covid-19 vaccination experience. *NEJM Catalyst.* April 28, 2023. https://doi.org/10.1056/CAT.22.0425
29. Centers for Disease Control and Prevention. How to build COVID-19 vaccine confidence. Available at: https://www.cdc.gov/vaccines/covid-19/vaccinate-with-confidence/building-trust.html. Accessed October 17, 2023.
30. Jarrett C, Wilson R, O'Leary M, Eckersberger E, Larson HJ. Strategies for addressing vaccine hesitancy—a systematic review. *Vaccine.* 2015; 33(34):4180–4190. https://doi.org/10.1016/j.vaccine.2015.04.040
31. McAteer J, Yildirim I, Chahroudi A. The VACCINES Act: deciphering vaccine hesitancy in the time of COVID-19. *Clin Infect Dis.* 2020;71(15):703–705. https://doi.org/10.1093/cid/ciaa433
32. New York City Department of Health and Mental Hygiene. Racial inequities in COVID-19 hospitalizations during the omicron wave in NYC. 2022. Available at: https://www.nyc.gov/assets/doh/downloads/pdf/covid/black-hospitalizations-omicron-wave.pdf. Accessed August 27, 2024.
33. Centers for Disease Control and Prevention. Flu vaccination coverage, United States, 2023–24 influenza season. Available at: https://www.cdc.gov/fluvaxview/coverage-by-season/2023-2024.html. Accessed October 14, 2024.
34. New York State Department of Health. New York 1115 Medical Waiver information page. 2024. Available at: https://www.health.state.ny.us/health_care/medicaid/redesign/medicaid_waiver_1115.htm. Accessed September 8, 2024.

Low HIV Preexposure Prophylaxis Coverage Among Women: Focused, Innovative Strategies Can Increase Use—United States, 2017–2023

Karen W. Hoover, MD, MPH, Weiming Zhu, MD, PhD, Kristen L. Hess, PhD, Pilgrim Spikes, PhD, Ya-Lin A. Huang, PhD, Jeffrey Wiener, PhD, Erica K. Dunbar, MPH, Jerris L. Raiford, PhD, Charles B. Collins, PhD, Elizabeth A. DiNenno, PhD, Athena P. Kourtis, MD, PhD, John T. Brooks, MD, Robyn Neblett Fanfair, MD, and Cari Courtenay-Quirk, PhD

Objectives. HIV preexposure prophylaxis (PrEP) use has increased since its US Food and Drug Administration approval in 2012. Our objective was to describe trends in PrEP use by US women.

Methods. Using national pharmacy and HIV surveillance data, we calculated the PrEP-to-diagnosis ratio (PDR), a measure of PrEP prescriptions each year compared with HIV diagnoses the previous year, for women from 2017 to 2023. We also calculated PDRs in 2023 for the 20 counties with the highest numbers of diagnosed HIV infections among women and reviewed reports of public health activities conducted by recipients of Centers for Disease Control and Prevention HIV prevention funding.

Results. The PDR for women was 1.5 in 2017, and it increased to 5.8 by 2023. In the 20 counties with the highest number of diagnosed HIV infections among women, PDRs ranged from 2.2 to 16.9. Counties with the highest PDRs conducted PrEP activities designed for women.

Conclusions. PrEP is a highly effective HIV prevention intervention that can empower women to protect their health, but its use has been low. Public health and clinical interventions designed for women can increase their PrEP use and support ending the US HIV epidemic. (*Am J Public Health.* 2025;115(6):920–923. https://doi.org/10.2105/AJPH.2025.308056)

AJPH June 2025, Vol. 115, No. 6

Significant progress has been made in reducing HIV transmission in the United States, but systemic factors and long-standing inequities have contributed to ongoing racial and ethnic disparities.[1] In 2022, Black women were 13% of the US female population but accounted for 50% of HIV diagnoses among women. HIV preexposure prophylaxis (PrEP) has been recommended by the Centers for Disease Control and Prevention (CDC) since 2014.[2] PrEP can reduce the risk of sexual HIV acquisition by up to 99%.[3] Although PrEP use has increased among men, its use remains low among women, with only 8% of PrEP prescriptions for women in 2023.[4] The Ending the HIV Epidemic in the US (EHE) initiative includes a goal to increase PrEP implementation and aims to decrease new HIV infections 90% by 2030.[5] It also has an overarching goal to achieve HIV-related health equity with increased implementation of prevention services for disproportionately affected US populations.

The PrEP-to-diagnosis ratio (PDR) is the number of persons prescribed PrEP in a given year for each new HIV diagnosis in the previous year, and it is useful to monitor trends in PrEP use among persons in groups who might benefit.[6] It is an easily calculated measure that can be stratified by demographic characteristics to help increase understanding of PrEP inequities.[7] In this report, we calculated PDRs to understand PrEP use by women.

METHODS

We used the IQVIA Real-World Data—Longitudinal Prescription Database (IQVIA) and the National HIV Surveillance System (NHSS) to calculate PDRs in 50 states; Washington, DC; and

Puerto Rico. We calculated annual PDRs by dividing the number of persons aged 16 years or older who were prescribed PrEP in IQVIA by the number of diagnosed HIV infections in the previous year in NHSS.

We calculated PDRs stratified by year and sex for the United States. We calculated PDRs for US women by age group and geographic location during 2017 to 2023. We also calculated PDRs for women by state; Washington, DC; and Puerto Rico in 2023 and for the 20 US counties with the highest number of HIV diagnoses among women in 2022. For the 10 counties with the highest PDRs, we reviewed 2022 annual progress reports by health department recipients of the programmatic CDC cooperative agreement "PS20-2010: Integrated HIV Programs for Health Departments to Support Ending the HIV Epidemic in the United States" and summarized PrEP activities for women.[8]

RESULTS

The overall PDR increased from 3.9 in 2017 to 13.3 in 2023, indicating that an increasing number of persons were prescribed PrEP compared with persons with diagnosed HIV. The PDR among men increased from 4.5 to 15.0 and among women from 1.5 to 5.8 (Appendix Figure A, available as a supplement to the online version of this article at https://ajph.org).

Among women in 2023, the PDR was highest for those aged 16 to 24 years (8.2) and aged 25 to 34 years (7.1) and was higher in the Northeast (7.3) and West (7.0) compared with the South (5.1) and Midwest (5.6; Table 1). By state, PDRs ranged from 14.7 in Oregon to 0.1 in Puerto Rico (Appendix Table A). Among the 17 US Southern states and Washington, DC, 14 (82%) had PDRs less than the national state median PDR for women of 6.0.

Among the 20 counties with the highest number of women with diagnosed HIV in 2023, PDRs ranged from 2.2 in Dallas County, Texas, to 13.4 in Broward County, Florida, and 16.9 in Miami-Dade County, Florida (Appendix Table B). Health departments in the 10 counties with the highest PDRs reported several programmatic activities focused on women in their annual progress reports (Appendix Table C).[8] These activities included PrEP academic detailing of women's health care providers, PrEP promotion in the community, social media campaigns, PrEP navigation, and PrEP initiation for women who were incarcerated and scheduled for release.

DISCUSSION

PrEP uptake among women has been persistently low in the United States. Among counties with the highest numbers of women with diagnosed HIV infection, PDRs ranged widely, suggesting that some jurisdictions were more successful than others with PrEP implementation for women. Activities conducted by health departments in the 10 counties with the highest PDRs might have contributed to successful PrEP implementation because these counties implemented PrEP activities and service models specifically designed for women. Academic detailing of women's health care providers entailed PrEP experts meeting with individual providers to promote key PrEP messages and to distribute support materials for prescribing PrEP.[8,9] In addition to health department activities in Florida, starting in 2018, Florida provided free PrEP medication in all 67 counties and currently supports the use of PrEP medication assistance programs.[10,11] Navigation service models designed specifically for women coordinate and support PrEP care including to obtain financial access, schedule and attend clinical appointments, and adhere to and persist with PrEP.[8,12] Social media and other community educational campaigns focus on increasing Black women's awareness of PrEP.[8]

Although persistent disparities in PrEP use among racial and ethnic groups are documented,[4] we could not calculate PDRs for women stratified by race and ethnicity because of substantial missing race and ethnicity information in IQVIA data. However, the disproportionate number of HIV diagnoses among Black women underscores that this population is a priority for PrEP implementation. PrEP is a lifesaving biomedical intervention, and its use must be equitable for all disproportionately affected groups, including Black women. Women's use of PrEP empowers them to prevent HIV acquisition regardless of their partners' HIV status or viral suppression. Furthermore, every HIV infection prevented averts a lifetime illness and saves approximately $500 000 for the cost of lifetime treatment.[13]

Women encounter many barriers to PrEP use.[14,15] A key challenge is identifying women who might benefit from PrEP. It was estimated that 177 000 US women had a PrEP indication in 2015,[16] but the US population includes more than 135 million women aged 15 years and older. Clinical encounters provide opportunities for PrEP implementation, yet few women were prescribed PrEP when they presented with objective clinical indications such as a sexually transmitted infection.[17,18] At provider visits, women with indications for PrEP could be identified with clinical decision supports that use information

TABLE 1— Preexposure Prophylaxis (PrEP)-to-Diagnosis Ratios (PDRs) Among Women by Demographic Characteristics and Year: United States; Washington, DC; and Puerto Rico, 2017–2023

Characteristic	Year, PDR						
	2017	2018	2019	2020	2021	2022	2023
Total	1.5	2.1	2.9	3.3	4.9	4.8	5.8
Age group, y							
16–24	1.8	2.0	3.7	3.5	6.7	5.9	8.2
25–34	1.8	2.8	3.8	4.0	5.9	6.3	7.1
35–44	1.5	2.4	2.9	3.5	5.2	4.7	5.7
45–54	1.2	1.7	2.1	2.7	3.7	3.6	4.2
55–64	0.9	1.2	1.5	2.2	2.6	2.6	3.1
≥65	1.1	1.0	1.2	2.2	2.8	2.8	3.1
US geographic region							
Northeast	2.3	3.2	4.2	4.0	5.6	5.9	7.3
Midwest	1.9	2.5	3.1	2.7	4.0	4.4	5.6
South	0.8	1.3	2.1	3.1	4.7	4.1	5.1
West	2.3	3.5	3.9	3.7	5.8	7.0	7.0
Urban or rural location[a]							
Urban	1.5	2.2	2.9	3.3	5.0	4.8	5.8
Rural	1.4	2.2	2.6	2.9	4.8	5.2	5.9
EHE jurisdiction[b]							
EHE county[c]	1.5	2.3	3.1	3.8	5.7	5.6	6.6
EHE state[d]	1.5	2.2	2.9	3.0	4.6	4.6	5.6
Non-EHE	0.8	1.0	1.5	1.5	2.4	2.5	3.1

Note. EHE = Ending the HIV Epidemic in the United States. PDRs were calculated as the number of women prescribed PrEP each year divided by number of women diagnosed with HIV infection in the previous year. Additional information, including the numbers of PrEP prescriptions and HIV diagnoses among women by demographic characteristics and year, is included in Appendix Table A (available as a supplement to the online version of this article at https://ajph.org).
[a]Urban is defined as a metropolitan statistical area with a population ≥ 50 000.
[b]EHE includes 50 US counties and rural areas in 7 states that account for more than half of HIV infections in the United States.
[c]Arizona: Maricopa County; California: Alameda County, Los Angeles County, Orange County, Riverside County, Sacramento County, San Bernadino County, San Diego County, San Francisco County; Florida: Broward County, Duval County, Hillsborough County, Miami-Dade County, Orange County, Palm Beach County, Pinellas County; Georgia: Cobb County, DeKalb County, Fulton County, Gwinnett County; Illinois: Cook County; Indiana: Marion County; Louisiana: East Baton Rouge Parish, Orleans Parish; Maryland: Baltimore City, Montgomery County, Prince George's County; Massachusetts: Suffolk County; Michigan: Wayne County; Nevada: Wayne County; New Jersey; Essex County, Hudson County; New York: Bronx County, Kings County, New York County, Queens County; North Carolina: Mecklenburg County; Ohio: Cuyahoga County, Franklin County, Hamilton County; Pennsylvania: Philadelphia County; Puerto Rico: San Juan Municipio; Tennessee: Shelby County; Texas: Bexar County, Dallas County, Harris County, Tarrant County, Travis County; Washington: King County; Washington, DC.
[d]Alabama, Arkansas, Kentucky, Mississippi, Missouri, Oklahoma, and South Carolina.

in their electronic health record such as sexually transmitted infections or nonoccupational postexposure prophylaxis prescriptions.

Providing more choice in PrEP modalities could increase PrEP use by both men and women. Three PrEP modalities have been proven effective for women: a daily oral pill, a bimonthly injection, and a semiannual injection.[19,20] Additional PrEP modalities in development include a long-acting pill and an implantable device. Research is needed to understand preferences for multipurpose prevention technologies with formulations or strategies designed for combined PrEP and contraception. Research is also needed to develop and evaluate interventions to support PrEP initiation, adherence, and persistence and to identify the best implementation strategies for women, especially Black women.

Limitations

This analysis has 3 limitations. First, IQVIA data were missing race and ethnicity information for two thirds of persons prescribed PrEP, preventing accurate determination of PrEP use by race and ethnicity. Second, IQVIA data do not include information about gender identity, so the sex of transgender persons prescribed PrEP might have been misclassified. Third, PDRs could not be calculated by HIV transmission group. Although NHSS data included information about the transmission group, IQVIA data did not.

Public Health Implications

Despite marked increases in PrEP use in the United States during the more than 12 years since its US Food and Drug Administration approval in 2012, PrEP uptake has been substantially lower among women compared with men. PrEP implementation strategies that are designed specifically for women can be effective to increase use. The goals of EHE will be achieved by preventing HIV acquisition among all persons through increased HIV testing, PrEP use, and sustained viral suppression among persons with HIV. *AJPH*

ABOUT THE AUTHORS

All authors are with the Division of HIV Prevention, Centers for Disease Control and Prevention, Atlanta, GA.

CORRESPONDENCE

Correspondence should be sent to Karen Hoover, 1600 Clifton Rd NE, Atlanta, GA 30329 (e-mail: khoover@cdc.gov). Reprints can be ordered at https://www.ajph.org by clicking the "Reprints" link.

PUBLICATION INFORMATION

Full Citation: Hoover KW, Zhu W, Hess KL, et al. Low HIV preexposure prophylaxis coverage among women: focused, innovative strategies can increase use—United States, 2017–2023. *Am J Public Health*. 2025;115(6):920–923.

Acceptance Date: June 28, 2024.

DOI: https://doi.org/10.2105/AJPH.2025.308056

ORCID iDs:

Karen W. Hoover https://orcid.org/0000-0003-4942-7905

Pilgrim Spikes https://orcid.org/0000-0001-9008-2967

Ya-Lin A. Huang https://orcid.org/0000-0003-3137-8594

Jeffrey Wiener https://orcid.org/0000-0002-3844-1309

Jerris L. Raiford https://orcid.org/0000-0001-8258-3278

Charles B. Collins https://orcid.org/0000-0003-3036-3227

Cari Courtenay-Quirk https://orcid.org/0000-0002-4552-4153

CONTRIBUTORS

All authors contributed equally to the work.

ACKNOWLEDGMENTS

This work was funded by the Centers for Disease Control and Prevention.

Note. The findings and conclusions are solely those of the authors and do not necessarily represent the official position of the Centers for Disease Control and Prevention or the US Department of Health and Human Services.

CONFLICTS OF INTEREST

None of the authors have conflicts of interest.

HUMAN PARTICIPANT PROTECTION

This study was determined to be exempt from institutional review board review because no personally identifying information was collected, and data collections were part of routine clinical care and HIV program evaluation.

REFERENCES

1. Centers for Disease Control and Prevention. Diagnoses, deaths, and prevalence of HIV in the United States and 6 territories and freely associated states, 2022. Available at: https://stacks.cdc.gov/view/cdc/156509/cdc_156509_DS1.pdf. Accessed December 4, 2024.
2. Centers for Disease Control and Prevention. Preexposure prophylaxis for the prevention of HIV prevention in the United States—2014. Available at: https://stacks.cdc.gov/view/cdc/79935. Accessed December 4, 2024.
3. Centers for Disease Control and Prevention. Let's stop HIV together. Available at: https://www.cdc.gov/stophivtogether/hiv-prevention/prep.html. Accessed December 4, 2024.
4. AIDSVu. Deeper look: PrEP. Available at: https://aidsvu.org/resources/deeper-look-prep. Accessed December 4, 2024.
5. US Department of Health and Human Services. What is Ending the HIV Epidemic in the US? Available at: https://www.hiv.gov/federal-response/ending-the-hiv-epidemic/overview. Accessed December 4, 2024.
6. Siegler AJ, Mouhanna F, Giler RM, et al. The prevalence of pre-exposure prophylaxis use and the pre-exposure prophylaxis-to-need ratio in the fourth quarter of 2017, United States. *Ann Epidemiol*. 2018;28(12):841–849. https://doi.org/10.1016/j.annepidem.2018.06.005
7. Sullivan PS, DuBose S, Castel AD, et al. PrEP uptake and equity by race, ethnicity, sex, and region in the United States in the first decade of PrEP: trends in the PrEP equity ratio. *Lancet Reg Health Am*. 2023;33:100738. https://doi.org/10.1016/j.lana.2024.100738
8. *Annual Progress Report for PS20-2010: Integrated HIV Programs for Health Departments to Support Ending the HIV Epidemic in the United States*. Atlanta, GA: Centers for Disease Control and Prevention; 2022.
9. Wahnich A, Gandhi AD, Cleghorn E, et al. Public health detailing to promote HIV pre- and postexposure prophylaxis among women's healthcare providers in New York City. *Am J Prev Med*. 2021;61(5, suppl 1):S98–S107. https://doi.org/10.1016/j.amepre.2021.05.032
10. Miller NS. Local health departments to offer free preventive HIV drug. *Orlando Sentinel*. February 18, 2018. Available at: https://www.orlandosentinel.com/2018/02/01/local-health-departments-to-offer-free-preventive-hiv-drug. Accessed December 4, 2024.
11. Florida Department of Health. PrEP/PEP. Available at: https://www.floridahealth.gov/diseases-and-conditions/aids/PrEP/index.html. Accessed June 3, 2024.
12. Cheek JB, Feldman MB, Montero N, Gambone GF, Hoffman S, Blackstock OJ. Pre-exposure prophylaxis (PrEP) initiation among Black and Latina cisgender women receiving HIV prevention care coordination services in New York City. *AIDS Behav*. 2022;26(10):3174–3184. https://doi.org/10.1007/s10461-022-03661-1
13. Bingham A, Shrestha RK, Khurana N, Jacobson EU, Farnham PG. Estimated lifetime HIV-related medical costs in the United States. *Sex Transm Dis*. 2021;48(4):299–304. https://doi.org/10.1097/OLQ.0000000000001366
14. Hoover KW, Kourtis AP, Smith DKUS. Black women and human immunodeficiency virus preexposure prophylaxis implementation. *Obstet Gynecol*. 2022;140(1):106–109. https://doi.org/10.1097/AOG.0000000000004829
15. Willie TC, Knight D, Baral SD, et al. Where's the "everyday Black woman"? An intersectional qualitative analysis of Black women's decision-making regarding HIV pre-exposure prophylaxis (PrEP) in Mississippi. *BMC Public Health*. 2022;22(1):1604. https://doi.org/10.1186/s12889-022-13999-9
16. Smith DK, Van Handel M, Grey J. Estimates of adults with indications for HIV pre-exposure prophylaxis by jurisdiction, transmission risk group, and race/ethnicity, United States, 2015. *Ann Epidemiol*. 2018;28(12):850–857.e9. https://doi.org/10.1016/j.annepidem.2018.05.003
17. Henny KD, Huang YA, Hoover KW. Low human immunodeficiency virus (HIV) testing rates and no HIV preexposure prophylaxis prescribed among female patients diagnosed with a sexually transmitted infection, 2017–2018. *Obstet Gynecol*. 2020;136(6):1083–1085. https://doi.org/10.1097/AOG.0000000000004148
18. Townes A, Tanner MR, Yu L, et al. Inequities along the human immunodeficiency virus (HIV) pre-exposure prophylaxis services continuum for Black women in the United States, 2015–2020. *Obstet Gynecol*. 2024;143(2):294–301. https://doi.org/10.1097/AOG.0000000000005451
19. Centers for Disease Control and Prevention. Preexposure prophylaxis for the prevention of HIV prevention in the United States—2021 update. Available at: https://stacks.cdc.gov/view/cdc/112360. Accessed December 4, 2024.
20. Bekker L-G, Das M, Karim QA, et al. Twice-yearly lenacapravir or daily F/TAF for HIV prevention in cisgender women. *N Engl J Med*. 2024;391(13):1179–1192. https://doi.org/10.1056/NEJMoa2407001

Crisis Pregnancy Centers in the United States: Post-*Dobbs* Characteristics and Changes

Danielle N. Lambert, PhD, MPH, Nicole Luisi, MPH, MS, Erin R. Johnson, PhD, MPH, Rachel Baugh, MPH, and Andrea Swartzendruber, PhD, MPH

See also Santelli, p. 822, and Daniel, p. 825.

Objective. To enumerate crisis pregnancy centers (CPCs) in the United States in 2024 and examine changes before and after *Dobbs v Jackson Women's Health Organization* and associations with selected state characteristics.

Methods. Repeated cross-sectional analyses used CPC Map data to describe the number of CPCs in the United States after *Dobbs* and examine changes since 2021. We used negative binomial models to compare CPC counts by selected state characteristics.

Results. In 2024, 2633 CPCs operated in the United States, a 3.3% increase from 2021. Nationally, 71.7% offered nondiagnostic ultrasounds, 28.0% advertised sexually transmitted infection (STI) testing, 17.2% STI treatment, 6.8% HIV testing, and 3.8% unproven "abortion reversal" on-site. The total count of CPCs in 2024 was 230% greater in states with a grant program (95% confidence interval [CI] = 148%, 357%; $P < .001$), and the rate of newly identified and re-opened CPCs was 1.81 times (95% CI = 1.15, 2.84; $P = .010$) greater, adjusting for CPCs in 2021.

Conclusions. Despite being largely unregulated and failing to adhere to medical and ethical practice standards, CPCs proliferated and posed risk nationally, particularly in states with CPC grant programs. Health professionals should educate themselves and their communities about local CPCs and risks. (*Am J Public Health*. 2025;115(6):924–935. https://doi.org/10.2105/AJPH.2025.308055)

AJPH June 2025, Vol. 115, No. 6

Crisis pregnancy centers (CPCs) are religious nonprofit organizations that frequently mimic medical clinics to reach their antiabortion, anticontraception, and anti–comprehensive sex education goals.[1–4] CPCs particularly target young people, people of color, and people living in low-income households,[1,2] communities that disproportionately experience barriers to health care, unintended pregnancy, and adverse sexual and reproductive health outcomes.[5–7] Although most CPCs provide limited medical services, they frequently provide inaccurate health information, do not adhere to national medical and ethical practice standards, and are not subject to the Health Insurance Portability and Accountability Act (HIPAA).[1,2,8–10]

The American Public Health Association (APHA) warns, "CPCs often engage in techniques that are coercive, threatening, misleading, and aggressive."[11] National and international public health and medical professional societies warn that CPCs' lack of adherence to medical and ethical standards poses risk.[1,12,13] Potential harms posed by CPCs and their lack of regulation include negative consequences of individual health behaviors resulting from mis- and disinformation; delayed or forgone sexual and reproductive health care, HIV/sexually transmitted infection (STI) services, and other prevention and treatment services; stigma; mistrust of medical providers; and lack of protection of personal information—all of which could negatively affect maternal, infant, and child health.[1,2,14]

Despite APHA's and other major groups' recommendation that governments should only support programs that provide complete, medically accurate, and nondirective information that supports individual informed consent and decision-making,[1,11–13,15]

government funding and support for CPCs significantly increased in the decade before the 2022 *Dobbs v Jackson Women's Health Organization* US Supreme Court decision that overturned the federal right to abortion.[16,17] Since *Dobbs*, some states, particularly Republican-led states that banned or restricted abortion, increased CPC funding and support, including allowing tax breaks for donations to CPCs.[18–26]

Previous research has assessed CPCs' locations, services, characteristics, and spatial proximity to key locations, but no studies, to our knowledge, have examined how the number and locations of CPCs may have changed following the *Dobbs* decision.[3,27,28] Therefore, in this study, we aimed to enumerate and map CPCs operating in the United States in 2024 (after *Dobbs*) and examine changes in the number of CPCs since 2021 (before *Dobbs*) nationally and by region, division, and state. We also examined selected state characteristics associated with total counts of CPCs in 2024 and the proliferation of centers since 2021.

METHODS

CPC Map is an online geocoded directory of CPCs in the United States developed in 2018 using rigorous, scientific methodologies.[3,29] We conducted and released a national update in 2021 (before *Dobbs*)[27] and collected 2024 post-*Dobbs* data between June 2023 and March 2024. Eligible centers provided at least free pregnancy testing in an open brick-and-mortar location. We excluded mobile centers, administrative offices, thrift stores, maternity homes, and adoption agencies. Thus, eligible centers offered free health-related services in a stable location that can be geolocated, with the goals of helping people seeking health services identify CPCs and assessing CPCs' tactics and public health impacts. To identify eligible centers, trained research assistants (1) reviewed the proprietary Web sites of CPCs previously identified in 2021 to identify new locations, (2) used standard state-based keyword Internet searches and reviewed approximately the first 50 Google results per search, and (3) reviewed antiabortion online directories that included CPCs. After identifying possible centers, research assistants reviewed each site's proprietary client-facing Web site to confirm operating status and eligibility, record addresses and contact information, and assess the availability of on-site health-related services including free limited (nondiagnostic) ultrasounds, testing and treatment for at least one sexually transmitted infection (STI), HIV testing, and "abortion reversal." "Abortion reversal" is an "unproven and unethical" procedure using a high dose of progesterone to purportedly "reverse" the effects of mifepristone during a medication abortion.[30,31] Our previous research demonstrated that CPC services advertised on their Web sites approximate services confirmed via telephone calls.[28] We called centers without accessible client-facing Web sites and those that did not advertise free pregnancy testing or nondiagnostic ultrasound services to confirm eligibility. We deemed centers that could not be contacted in five call attempts as ineligible.

Measures

Using data from CPC Map, we report the number of CPCs operating in 2024 nationally and by US census region, division, and state, including the number of CPCs offering free nondiagnostic ultrasounds and advertising on-site STI testing for at least 1 STI, treatment for at least one STI, HIV testing, and "abortion reversal" services. We categorized CPCs as offering limited medical services if they offered nondiagnostic ultrasounds, STI testing, or HIV testing. We categorized the following operational status changes from 2021 to 2024: newly identified, reopened (closed in 2021, open in 2024), permanently or temporarily closed, and no longer eligible. Common reasons centers were no longer eligible included only offering client services in a mobile unit and discontinuation of free pregnancy testing.

To assess associations between state characteristics and counts of CPCs, we categorized for each state and the District of Columbia (DC) the abortion access policy, grant funding for CPCs, tax breaks for CPC donations, and the governor's political affiliation on December 31, 2023. Using Abortion Finder data, we categorized states' post-*Dobbs* abortion policies as either a total ban or restrictions based on gestational limits or no bans or restrictions.[32] We categorized state grant funding for CPCs (yes or no) based on funding enacted through the 2023 fiscal year. Any proposed or enacted tax breaks for CPC donations (yes or no) were assessed through the end of the 2023 calendar year. We recorded the political party affiliations (Democrat or Republican) for each state's governor and the DC mayor from the National Governor's Association's Web site.[33]

Statistical Analyses

In this repeated cross-sectional analysis, we first used descriptive statistics to summarize the total number of CPCs and health-related services available at CPCs in 2024, nationally and by region, division, and state. We identified changes in operating and eligibility statuses since 2021 and calculated the overall net change in CPCs from 2021 to 2024. The total number of CPCs and the number of newly identified or reopened CPCs were not normally distributed; therefore, we compared states in which the total number of CPCs increased versus remained stable or decreased by selected state policies (i.e., abortion policy, CPC grant funding, tax breaks for donations to CPCs, governor political affiliation) using logistic regression models. We used unadjusted negative binomial models with robust standard errors to evaluate differences in the total counts of CPCs in 2024 and rate of newly identified or reopened CPCs in 2021 to 2024 by selected state characteristics. To evaluate the rate of newly identified or reopened CPCs, we used negative binomial models, adjusting for the total number of CPCs operating in 2021 as a covariate. Negative binomial models were selected over Poisson models based on indicators of model fit. We conducted all analyses with R statistical software (version 4.3.1; R Core Team, Vienna, Austria).

RESULTS

Nationally, 2633 CPCs were operating in 2024 (Table 1). By region, the South had the greatest number of CPCs (n = 1043), and the Northeast had the fewest (n = 376). By division, the number ranged from 509 in the South Atlantic to 88 in New England. CPCs operated in every state, ranging from 205 in Texas to 3 in Rhode Island and 2 in DC. Nearly three fourths of CPCs in the United States offered limited medical services (Figure 1).

Advertised Health-Related Services, 2024

Almost three fourths of CPCs offered free nondiagnostic ultrasounds. By region, the South had the highest number and percentage (n = 812; 77.9%), and the Northeast had the lowest (n = 221; 58.8%). By division, the South Atlantic had the greatest number (n = 397), West South Central the highest percentage (79.7%), and New England the lowest of both (n = 48; 58.8%). By state, the number ranged from 169 in Texas to 2 in Rhode Island and 0 in DC.

More than one quarter of CPCs advertised testing for at least one STI, 17.2% STI treatment, and 6.8% HIV testing. By region, the percentage that advertised STI testing ranged from 35.9% to 22.1%, STI treatment from 23.0% to 14.5%, and HIV testing from 10.4% to 4.8%. By division, 37.7% to 14.8% advertised STI testing, 24.3% to 11.4% STI treatment, and 11.7% to 1.1% HIV testing. In 48 states, at least 1 CPC advertised STI testing; in 46, at least 1 advertised STI treatment; and in 37, at least 1 advertised HIV testing. In only 8 states did all the CPCs that advertised STI testing also advertise STI treatment. In no states did all the CPCs that advertised STI testing also advertise HIV testing.

In total, 100 (3.8%) CPCs nationally offered on-site "abortion reversal." By region, the number ranged from 40 in the South to 4 in the Northeast, and the percentage ranged from 5.8% in the West to 1.1% in the Northeast. By division, the number ranged from 21 to 1, and the percentage ranged from 6.5% to 1.0%. CPCs in 31 states advertised on-site "abortion reversal," ranging from 12 in California to 1 in 10 states.

Changes in the Number of Centers, 2021 to 2024

In comparison with 2021, 256 centers were newly identified in 2024, 31 previously closed centers had reopened, 142 centers had closed by 2024, and 58 centers were no longer eligible (Figure 2). The national net change in the number of CPCs was 87 centers (3.4% increase) in 2024. By region, the number of newly identified and reopened centers was highest in the South (n = 116) and lowest in the West (n = 38). The net change ranged from +49 (4.9% increase) in the South to +1 (0.3% increase) in the Northeast. By division, the number of newly identified and reopened centers ranged from 56 in the West North Central to 9 in New England. Net changes by division ranged from +39 (14.7% increase) in the West North Central to –4 (0.8% decrease) in the East North Central. By state, the number of newly identified and reopened centers ranged from 28 in Texas to 0 in 3 states and DC. By state, net changes ranged from +18 (24.7% increase) in Missouri to –6 in Michigan and Pennsylvania (5.7% and 3.8% decrease, respectively). Overall, the number of CPCs in 2024 increased in 26 states, remained stable in 9 states and DC, and decreased in 15 states.

Changes in Number by State Characteristics

In 2024, the number and percentage of CPCs were greater in states with no abortion bans or restrictions after *Dobbs* (52.7% vs 47.3%), with an enacted CPC grant program (55.7% vs 44.3%), without proposed or enacted tax breaks for donations made to CPCs (69.9% vs 30.1%), and in states with a Republican governor (51.2% vs 48.8%; Table 2). We observed no significant

TABLE 1— Number of Crisis Pregnancy Centers (CPCs) and Health-Related Service Availability in the United States, 2024, and Number of CPCs With Status Changes Since 2021

		Health-Related Service Availability, No. (%)						Operating and Eligibility Status Changes Since 2021				
	Total Open CPCs, No.	Offer Limited Medical Services[a]	Offer Free Nondiagnostic Ultrasounds	Advertise STI Testing	Advertise STI Treatment	Advertise HIV Testing	Advertise Abortion Pill Reversal[b]	Newly Identified, No.	Reopened, No.	Closed, No.	No Longer Eligible,[c] No.	Net Change, No. (%)
United States	2633	1892 (71.9)	1888 (71.7)	736 (28.0)	452 (17.2)	178 (6.8)	100 (3.8)	256	31	142	58	+87 (3.4)
Northeast	376	222 (59.0)	221 (58.8)	83 (22.1)	59 (15.7)	18 (4.8)	4 (1.1)	32	8	28	11	+1 (0.3)
New England	88	48 (54.5)	48 (54.5)	13 (14.8)	10 (11.4)	1 (1.1)	1 (1.1)	8	1	4	1	+4 (4.8)
Connecticut	23	9 (39.1)	9 (39.1)	2 (8.7)	2 (8.7)	1 (4.3)	1 (4.3)	3	1	1	0	+3 (15.0)
Maine	12	9 (75.0)	9 (75.0)	2 (16.7)	2 (16.7)	0 (0.0)	0 (0.0)	1	0	0	0	+1 (9.1)
Massachusetts	28	12 (42.9)	12 (42.9)	3 (10.7)	2 (7.1)	0 (0.0)	0 (0.0)	1	0	1	1	-1 (-3.4)
New Hampshire	15	10 (66.7)	10 (66.7)	3 (20.0)	3 (20.0)	0 (0.0)	0 (0.0)	1	0	0	0	+1 (7.1)
Rhode Island	3	2 (66.7)	2 (66.7)	1 (33.3)	1 (33.3)	0 (0.0)	0 (0.0)	1	0	1	0	0 (0.0)
Vermont	7	6 (85.7)	6 (85.7)	2 (28.6)	0 (0.0)	0 (0.0)	0 (0.0)	1	0	1	0	0 (0.0)
Middle Atlantic	288	174 (60.4)	173 (60.1)	70 (24.3)	49 (17.0)	17 (5.9)	3 (1.0)	24	7	24	10	-3 (-1.0)
New Jersey	41	29 (70.7)	29 (70.7)	15 (36.6)	7 (17.1)	3 (7.3)	0 (0.0)	6	0	4	0	+2 (5.1)
New York	93	45 (48.4)	45 (48.4)	17 (18.3)	13 (14.0)	3 (3.2)	3 (3.2)	8	5	10	2	+1 (1.1)
Pennsylvania	154	100 (64.9)	99 (64.3)	38 (24.7)	29 (18.8)	11 (7.1)	0 (0.0)	10	2	10	8	-6 (-3.8)
Midwest	780	550 (70.5)	550 (70.5)	225 (28.8)	142 (18.2)	59 (7.6)	31 (4.0)	86	7	35	23	+35 (4.7)
East North Central	476	350 (73.5)	350 (73.5)	130 (27.3)	76 (16.0)	38 (8.0)	17 (3.6)	35	4	22	21	-4 (-0.8)
Illinois	104	81 (77.9)	81 (77.9)	23 (22.1)	17 (16.3)	2 (1.9)	5 (4.8)	14	0	4	3	+7 (7.2)
Indiana	96	73 (76.0)	73 (76.0)	35 (36.5)	26 (27.1)	18 (18.8)	4 (4.2)	7	1	6	2	0 (0.0)
Michigan	99	68 (68.7)	68 (68.7)	18 (18.2)	10 (10.1)	7 (7.1)	1 (1.0)	5	1	3	9	-6 (-5.7)
Ohio	124	89 (71.8)	89 (71.8)	30 (24.2)	13 (10.5)	7 (5.6)	2 (1.6)	6	1	3	4	0 (0.0)
Wisconsin	53	39 (73.6)	39 (73.6)	24 (45.3)	10 (18.9)	4 (7.5)	5 (9.4)	3	1	6	3	-5 (-8.6)
West North Central	304	200 (65.8)	200 (65.8)	95 (31.3)	66 (21.7)	21 (6.9)	14 (4.6)	51	3	13	2	+39 (14.7)
Iowa	53	33 (62.3)	33 (62.3)	20 (37.7)	12 (22.6)	7 (13.2)	4 (7.5)	11	1	1	1	+10 (23.3)
Kansas	44	31 (70.5)	31 (70.5)	7 (15.9)	6 (13.6)	1 (2.3)	1 (2.3)	9	0	3	0	+6 (15.8)
Minnesota	73	49 (67.1)	49 (67.1)	28 (38.4)	19 (26.0)	7 (9.6)	5 (6.8)	3	1	4	0	0 (0.0)
Missouri	91	58 (63.7)	58 (63.7)	27 (29.7)	21 (23.1)	5 (5.5)	3 (3.3)	20	1	3	0	+18 (24.7)
Nebraska	23	16 (69.6)	16 (69.6)	9 (39.1)	6 (26.1)	0 (0.0)	0 (0.0)	4	0	1	0	+3 (15.0)
North Dakota	10	8 (80.0)	8 (80.0)	2 (20.0)	2 (20.0)	1 (10.0)	1 (10.0)	3	0	0	0	+3 (43.9)
South Dakota	10	5 (50.0)	5 (50.0)	2 (20.0)	0 (0.0)	0 (0.0)	0 (0.0)	1	0	1	1	-1 (-9.1)

Continued

TABLE 1— Continued

	Total Open CPCs, No.	Health-Related Service Availability, No. (%)						Operating and Eligibility Status Changes Since 2021				
		Offer Limited Medical Services[a]	Offer Free Nondiagnostic Ultrasounds	Advertise STI Testing	Advertise STI Treatment	Advertise HIV Testing	Advertise Abortion Pill Reversal[b]	Newly Identified, No.	Reopened, No.	Closed, No.	No Longer Eligible,[c] No.	Net Change, No. (%)
South	1043	812 (77.9)	812 (77.9)	272 (26.1)	151 (14.5)	56 (5.4)	40 (3.8)	105	11	52	15	+49 (4.9)
South Atlantic	509	397 (78.0)	397 (78.0)	142 (27.9)	68 (13.4)	36 (7.1)	21 (4.1)	50	6	25	3	+28 (5.8)
Delaware	5	4 (80.0)	4 (80.0)	0 (0.0)	0 (0.0)	0 (0.0)	2 (40.0)	0	0	0	0	0 (0.0)
District of Columbia	2	0 (0.0)	0 (0.0)	0 (0.0)	0 (0.0)	0 (0.0)	0 (0.0)	0	0	0	0	0 (0.0)
Florida	161	132 (82.0)	132 (82.0)	51 (31.7)	16 (9.9)	12 (7.5)	4 (2.5)	20	3	11	2	+10 (6.6)
Georgia	95	77 (81.1)	77 (81.1)	35 (36.8)	26 (27.4)	11 (11.6)	6 (6.3)	8	2	3	0	+7 (8.0)
Maryland	39	30 (76.9)	30 (76.9)	8 (20.5)	7 (17.9)	6 (15.4)	2 (5.1)	1	0	2	0	−1 (−2.5)
North Carolina	99	79 (79.8)	79 (79.8)	17 (17.2)	4 (4.0)	5 (5.1)	7 (7.1)	14	1	4	1	+10 (11.2)
South Carolina	34	25 (73.5)	25 (73.5)	7 (20.6)	2 (5.9)	0 (0.0)	0 (0.0)	1	0	2	0	−1 (−2.9)
Virginia	57	41 (71.9)	41 (71.9)	20 (35.1)	12 (21.1)	2 (3.5)	0 (0.0)	5	0	2	0	+3 (5.6)
West Virginia	17	9 (52.9)	9 (52.9)	4 (23.5)	1 (5.9)	0 (0.0)	0 (0.0)	1	0	1	0	0 (0.0)
East South Central	199	148 (74.4)	148 (74.4)	42 (21.1)	26 (13.1)	7 (3.5)	4 (2.0)	14	0	9	2	+3 (1.5)
Alabama	56	47 (83.9)	47 (83.9)	9 (16.1)	5 (8.9)	1 (1.8)	1 (1.8)	4	0	0	0	+4 (7.7)
Kentucky	53	35 (66.0)	35 (66.0)	12 (22.6)	7 (13.2)	1 (1.9)	1 (1.9)	3	0	5	0	−2 (−3.6)
Mississippi	29	22 (75.9)	22 (75.9)	3 (10.3)	3 (10.3)	1 (3.4)	1 (3.4)	2	0	1	1	0 (0.0)
Tennessee	61	44 (72.1)	44 (72.1)	18 (29.5)	11 (18.0)	4 (6.6)	1 (1.6)	5	0	3	1	+1 (1.7)
West South Central	335	267 (79.7)	267 (79.7)	88 (26.3)	57 (17.0)	13 (3.9)	15 (4.5)	41	5	18	10	+18 (5.7)
Arkansas	43	32 (74.4)	32 (74.4)	12 (27.9)	5 (11.6)	2 (4.7)	1 (2.3)	3	1	1	0	+3 (7.5)
Louisiana	36	30 (83.3)	30 (83.3)	5 (13.9)	4 (11.1)	1 (2.8)	6 (16.7)	6	0	2	0	+4 (12.5)
Oklahoma	51	36 (70.6)	36 (70.6)	10 (19.6)	8 (15.7)	5 (9.8)	2 (3.9)	7	1	3	1	+4 (8.5)
Texas	205	169 (82.4)	169 (82.4)	61 (29.8)	40 (19.5)	5 (2.4)	6 (2.9)	25	3	12	9	+7 (3.5)
West	434	308 (71.0)	305 (70.3)	156 (35.9)	100 (23.0)	45 (10.4)	25 (5.8)	33	5	27	9	+2 (0.5)
Mountain	187	129 (69.0)	126 (67.4)	63 (33.7)	40 (21.4)	16 (8.6)	9 (4.8)	19	4	15	6	+2 (1.1)
Arizona	45	25 (55.6)	23 (51.1)	9 (20.0)	7 (15.6)	3 (6.7)	4 (8.9)	6	1	5	4	−2 (−4.3)
Colorado	49	36 (73.5)	35 (71.4)	25 (51.0)	20 (40.8)	6 (12.2)	1 (2.0)	3	0	4	1	−2 (−3.9)
Idaho	23	14 (60.9)	14 (60.9)	6 (26.1)	3 (13.0)	1 (4.3)	2 (8.7)	3	1	0	0	+4 (21.1)
Montana	15	11 (73.3)	11 (73.3)	6 (40.0)	4 (26.7)	4 (26.7)	0 (0.0)	0	1	2	1	−2 (−11.8)
Nevada	9	8 (88.9)	8 (88.9)	0 (0.0)	0 (0.0)	0 (0.0)	0 (0.0)	2	0	0	0	+2 (28.6)
New Mexico	27	19 (70.4)	19 (70.4)	11 (40.7)	1 (3.7)	1 (3.7)	0 (0.0)	4	1	2	0	+3 (12.5)

Continued

TABLE 1— Continued

	Total Open CPCs, No.	Health-Related Service Availability, No. (%): Offer Limited Medical Services[a]	Offer Free Nondiagnostic Ultrasounds	Advertise STI Testing	Advertise STI Treatment	Advertise HIV Testing	Advertise Abortion Pill Reversal[b]	Operating and Eligibility Status Changes Since 2021: Newly Identified, No.	Reopened, No.	Closed, No.	No Longer Eligible,[c] No.	Net Change, No. (%)
Utah	8	5 (62.5)	5 (62.5)	1 (12.5)	0 (0.0)	0 (0.0)	0 (0.0)	1	0	1	0	0 (0.0)
Wyoming	11	11 (100.0)	11 (100.0)	5 (45.5)	5 (45.5)	1 (9.1)	2 (18.2)	0	0	1	0	−1 (−8.3)
Pacific	247	179 (72.5)	179 (72.5)	93 (37.7)	60 (24.3)	29 (11.7)	16 (6.5)	14	1	12	3	0 (0.0)
Alaska	9	5 (55.6)	5 (55.6)	3 (33.3)	2 (22.2)	1 (11.1)	0 (0.0)	0	0	1	0	−1 (−10.0)
California	146	102 (69.9)	102 (69.9)	52 (35.6)	37 (25.3)	21 (14.4)	12 (8.2)	7	0	7	2	−2 (−1.4)
Hawaii	7	5 (71.4)	5 (71.4)	3 (42.9)	3 (42.9)	0 (0.0)	0 (0.0)	2	0	1	0	+1 (16.7)
Oregon	41	29 (70.7)	29 (70.7)	9 (22.0)	3 (7.3)	1 (2.4)	0 (0.0)	2	1	0	0	+3 (7.9)
Washington	44	38 (86.4)	38 (86.4)	26 (59.1)	15 (34.1)	6 (13.6)	4 (9.1)	3	0	3	1	−1 (−2.2)

Note. STI = sexually transmitted infection.
[a]Defined as centers that offered free nondiagnostic ultrasounds, testing for at least one STI, or HIV testing.
[b]Abortion pill reversal is an "unproven and unethical" procedure using a high dose of progesterone purportedly to "reverse" the effects of mifepristone during a medication abortion.[30,31]
[c]Includes centers that were eligible for inclusion in the CPC Map database in 2021 but not in 2024. The most common reasons centers were no longer eligible included that they only offered client services in a mobile unit or had discontinued offering free pregnancy testing.

differences by state characteristics in the number of states where CPCs increased between 2021 to 2024 as opposed to states where the number remained stable or decreased.

Examining the total number of CPCs in 2024, the only statistically significant association was between the number of CPCs and states with CPC grant programs. Relative to states without a grant program, the total number of CPCs in 2024 was 2.30 times greater in states with a CPC grant program (95% confidence interval [CI] = 1.48, 3.57; $P < .001$).

When we examined the number of newly identified or reopened CPCs in 2024 relative to 2021, we observed statistically significant associations for state abortion policy and CPC grant funding. In unadjusted analysis, the rate of newly identified or reopened CPCs was 1.77 times greater in states that had banned or restricted abortion (95% CI = 1.02, 3.10; $P = .044$); however, the association did not remain statistically significant in analysis that adjusted for the total number of CPCs in 2021. In states with an enacted CPC grant program, the rate of newly identified or reopened CPCs was 3.08 times as great in the unadjusted model (95% CI = 1.89, 5.05; $P < .001$) and 1.81 times as great in the model adjusted for the total number of CPCs operating in 2021 (95% CI = 1.15, 2.84; $P = .010$). We observed no other statistically significant differences.

DISCUSSION

People at risk for adverse sexual, reproductive, maternal, and infant health outcomes require accurate health information and quality health care.[34–36] Using the sole longitudinal data set of CPCs and first national data about

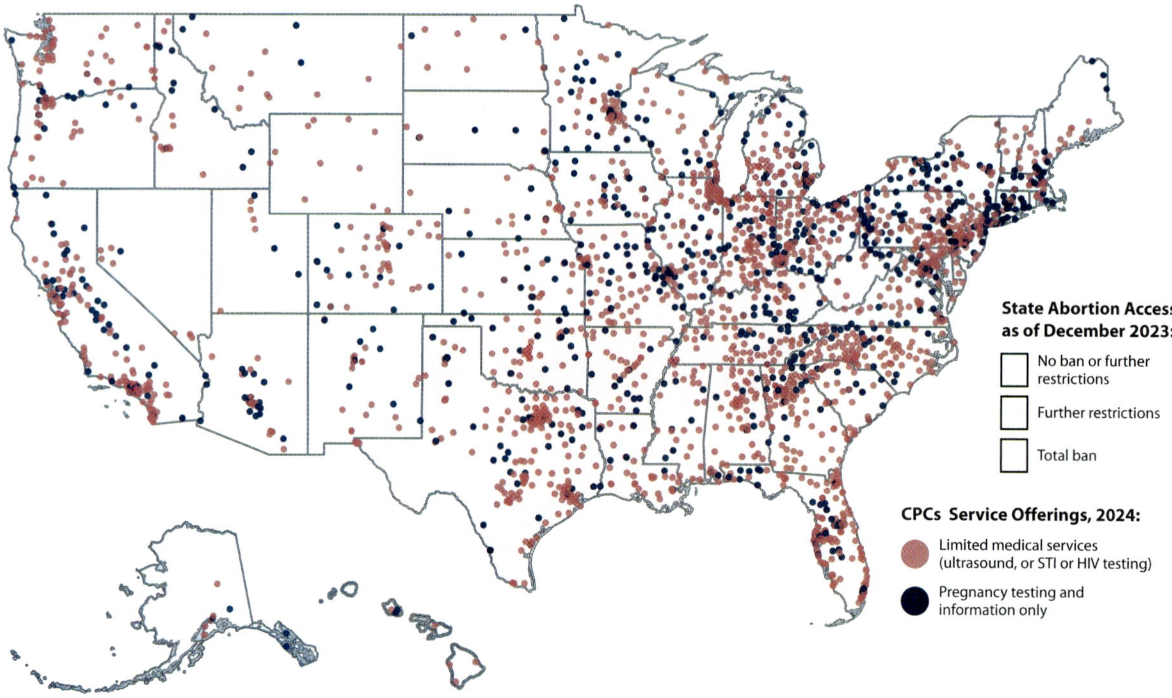

FIGURE 1— Crisis Pregnancy Centers (CPCs) in the United States by Availability of Limited Medical Services in 2024 and State Abortion Policies as of December 2023

Note. STI = sexually transmitted infection.

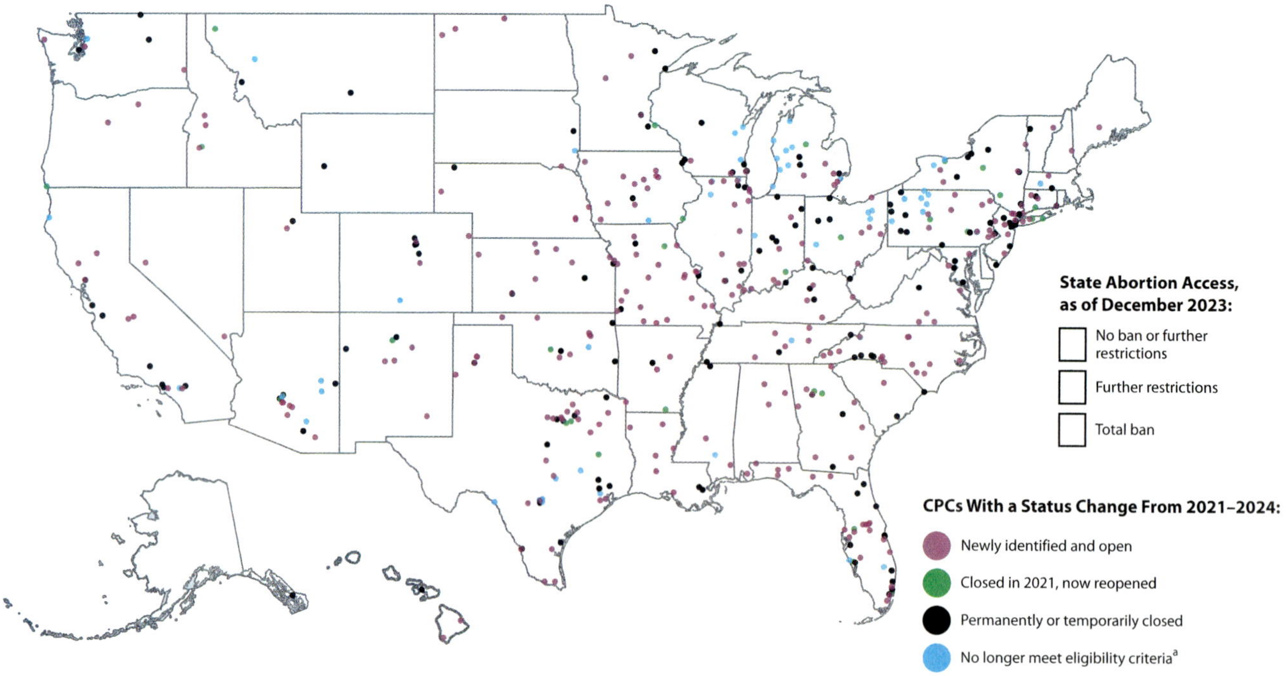

FIGURE 2— Crisis Pregnancy Centers (CPCs) in the United States With Operating and Eligibility Status Changes From 2021 to 2024 and State Abortion Policies as of December 2023

[a]Includes centers that were eligible for inclusion in the CPC Map database in 2021 but not in 2024. The most common reasons centers were no longer eligible included that they only offered client services in a mobile unit or had discontinued offering free pregnancy testing.

TABLE 2— Associations Between Selected State Characteristics and Changes in Numbers of Crisis Pregnancy Centers (CPCs) in the United States From 2021 to 2024

State Characteristics (as of December 2023)	States, No.	State Name Abbreviations	CPCs in 2024, No. (%)	Net Increase in CPCs, 2021–2024, No. (%)	States With No Change or Decrease, 2021–2024, No.	States With Increase in CPCs, 2021–2024, No.	Increase in CPCs vs. No Change or Decrease, 2021–2024, Unadjusted OR (95% CI)	Unadjusted IRR of the Total Count of CPCs in 2024 (95% CI)	Unadjusted IRR of New or Reopened CPCs, 2021–2024 (95% CI)	Adjusted IRR of New or Reopened CPCs, 2021–2024[a] (95% CI)
Post-*Dobbs* abortion policies										
No bans or further restrictions	30	AK CA CO CT DE DC HI IL IA KS ME MD MA MI MN MT NV NH NJ NM NY OH OR PA RI VT VA WA WI WY	1387 (52.7)	+15 (1.1)	17	13	1 (Ref)	1 (Ref)	1 (Ref)	1 (Ref)
Bans or restrictions	21	AL AZ AR FL GA ID IN KY LA MS MO ND NE NC OK SC SD TN TX UT WV	1246 (47.3)	+72 (6.1)	8	13	2.12 (0.69, 6.86)	1.28 (0.78, 2.10)	1.77 (1.02, 3.10)	1.42 (0.95, 2.12)
Enacted state grant funding for CPCs										
No	33	AL AK AZ CA CO CT DE DC HI ID IL KY ME MD MA MI MS MT NE NV NH NJ NM NY OR RI SC SD UT VT VA WA WY	1167 (44.3)	+15 (1.3)	19	14	1 (Ref)	1 (Ref)	1 (Ref)	1 (Ref)
Yes	18	AR FL GA IN IA KS LA MN MO NC ND OH OK PA TN TX WV WI	1466 (55.7)	+72 (5.2)	6	12	2.71 (0.84, 9.50)	2.30 (1.48, 3.57)	3.08 (1.89, 5.05)	1.81 (1.15, 2.84)
Proposed or enacted tax breaks for CPC donations										
No	40	AK AZ CA CO CT DE DC FL GA HI ID IN IA KY ME MA MN MT NE NV NH NJ NM NY NC ND OR PA RI SC SD TN TX UT VT VA WA WV WI WY	1841 (69.9)	+47 (2.6)	21	19	1 (Ref)	1 (Ref)	1 (Ref)	1 (Ref)
Yes	11	AL AR IL KS LA MD MI MS MO OH OK	792 (30.1)	+40 (5.3)	4	7	1.93 (0.50, 8.37)	1.36 (0.88, 2.09)	1.45 (0.82, 2.59)	1.52 (0.94, 2.45)
Governor political affiliation										
Democrat	24	AZ CA CO CT DE DC HI IL KS KY ME MD MA MI MN NJ NM NY NC OR PA RI WA WI	1284 (48.8)	+9 (0.7)	14	10	1 (Ref)	1 (Ref)	1 (Ref)	1 (Ref)
Republican	27	AL AK AR FL GA ID IN IA LA MS MO MT NE NV NH ND OH OK SC SD TN TX UT VT VA WV WY	1349 (51.2)	+78 (5.9)	11	16	2.04 (0.67, 6.39)	0.93 (0.57, 1.53)	1.17 (0.66, 2.07)	1.12 (0.74, 1.69)

Note. CI = confidence interval; IRR = incident rate ratio; OR = odds ratio.
[a]Adjusted for the total number of CPCs in 2021.

CPCs after *Dobbs*, we enumerated CPCs in the United States in 2024, described health-related services advertised by CPCs, assessed changes in CPCs from before to after *Dobbs*, and examined state characteristics associated with the number of CPCs in 2024 and from 2021 to 2024. Nationally, the number of CPCs operating in both 2021 (n = 2546) and 2024 (n = 2633) was greater than the number of local health departments in 2019 (n = 2459) and 2022 (n = 2512).[37,38] Furthermore, the 3.3% increase in CPCs from 2021 to 2024 outpaced increases in the number of local health departments over the past decade.[37–39] The number of CPCs operating in 2024 and the rate of increase in newly identified and reopened CPCs between 2021 to 2024 was significantly greater in the 18 states that provided grant funds to CPCs than in the 33 states that did not.

Nationally, the number and percentage of CPCs offering nondiagnostic ultrasounds slightly decreased from 2021 (n = 1966; 77%).[8] CPCs commonly falsely market their ultrasounds (e.g., purport ultrasounds can predict miscarriage). Over the past 2 decades, maternal mortality rates have been decreasing globally but increasing in the United States.[40] CPC ultrasounds threaten maternal and infant health by delaying or thwarting evidence-based prenatal and abortion care,[1,41] especially after *Dobbs*. The continued lack of regulations for CPCs may risk individual and public health, as highlighted by a recent report documenting failure to adhere to infection control standards and human papillomavirus transmission risk at a Kentucky CPC.[42]

In 2021, 21% of CPCs advertised testing for at least one STI, 12% advertised STI treatment, and 5% HIV testing.[28] Each of these estimates was higher in 2024. HIV and STI services offered at CPCs do not adhere to national medical practice standards.[34–36] The vast majority of CPCs are affiliated with national organizations that oppose contraception, including condoms,[43,44] and CPCs frequently undermine condoms' efficacy to prevent HIV and other STIs.[9,10] Many CPCs advertising STI testing do not offer on-site treatment, as recommended by national clinical guidelines.[28,45] In 2024, STI testing was advertised at CPCs in 48 states and on-site STI treatment at all of the same CPCs in only 6. National guidelines also recommend routine HIV testing for anyone tested for STIs who is not already known to be infected[35]; however, in no state did all CPCs that advertised STI testing also advertise HIV testing. HIV and STI services at CPCs represent missed opportunities for care and may delay or obstruct timely diagnosis and treatment, particularly given the high STI and HIV rates currently in the United States.[6,7] Although major public health and medical organizations urge governments to only support evidence-based programs,[1,11] the Centers for Disease Control and Prevention continues to refer individuals seeking HIV or STI services to CPCs.[46,47]

In 2024, at least 1 CPC in 31 states offered unproven "abortion reversal" on site. In 2021, 14 states required patients to be "informed" about "abortion reversal" before having an abortion.[48] Authors of a 2015 systematic review reported insufficient evidence supporting the efficacy of "abortion reversal" and concluded legislation mandating discussions about "abortion reversal" interferes with patient–physician relationships.[30] In 2023, Colorado passed a law banning "abortion reversal"; however, it is currently blocked while being challenged.[49] In 2024, New York's Attorney General announced a lawsuit against 11 CPCs and Heartbeat International, a CPC umbrella group, for promoting "abortion reversal."[50]

The number of CPCs operating in 2024 and the rate at which new CPCs proliferated since 2021 were significantly greater in states with CPC grant programs. Individuals seeking sexual and reproductive care in these states may represent priority populations for promoting awareness about CPCs. Because of public attention around potential CPC risks, Michigan, Minnesota, and Pennsylvania have defunded their CPC grant programs. We observed no significant differences in the overall number of CPCs in states that banned or restricted abortion after *Dobbs* and those that did not. Although the rate of newly identified and reopened CPCs in 2024 did not remain significantly greater in states with abortion bans or restrictions after *Dobbs* when controlling for the number of CPCs in 2021, our findings confirm that CPCs continued to operate and proliferate in states that banned and restricted abortion after *Dobbs* and those that did not.

Abortion bans and legislation supporting CPCs have been part of the Republican agenda. Eighteen (86%) of the 21 states that banned or restricted abortion were led by Republican governors, nearly three fourths (72%; n = 13) of which were located in the South. Likewise, 72% (n = 13) of states with CPC grant programs and 64% (n = 7) with proposed CPC tax breaks had Republican governors. Six states did not have abortion bans or restrictions but did have active grant programs in 2023. Of these, 2 Democrat-led states (Minnesota and Pennsylvania) defunded their CPC grant programs going forward, and 2 (Kansas and Wisconsin) have not. Of the 2 Republican-led states (Iowa and

Ohio) that did not have bans or restrictions but did have CPC grant programs in 2023, a 6-week ban became effective in Iowa in 2024.[51] However, CPCs operated and proliferated throughout the country, regardless of governors' party affiliation and tax breaks for donations to CPCs. Thus, CPCs are not just a public health concern in "red" states or states where legislators have worked to support them.

Although nearly three fourths offer limited medical services, CPCs operate largely unregulated.[52] APHA supports the enforcement of laws and development of new legislation related to misleading advertising of health services.[11] In recent years, there have been several different attempts at the local, state, and federal level to regulate CPCs. For example, in 2021, Connecticut passed a law regulating CPCs' misleading advertising tactics.[53] In 2022, identical Congressional legislation was introduced in the House and Senate to regulate CPC advertising,[54,55] which, to date, has not passed. In 2023, Illinois passed a law barring CPCs from using misinformation, deception, or misrepresentation[56]; however, the law was ultimately blocked. Some local areas have proposed and passed ordinances restricting CPC locations through zoning laws.[57–59] Given few current regulatory strategies, efforts to increase patient awareness about CPCs and their risks may be particularly warranted.

Strengths and Limitations

This study was subject to multiple strengths and limitations. CPC Map is not continuously updated; therefore, it is possible that CPCs that opened and closed between data collection periods were missed and that centers with name and location changes were misclassified. Nevertheless, CPC Map remains the single scientifically rigorous, national, and longitudinal directory of CPCs. We primarily determined service availability from CPC Web sites, which could have resulted in underestimates, particularly for STI and HIV services. However, our current findings are consistent with previous research that confirmed the availability of STI and HIV services via calls and demonstrated that most CPCs offering STI testing failed to offer treatment and HIV testing.[28] Relatedly, we counted CPCs as advertising STI services if their Web sites mentioned providing services for at least 1 STI. However, previous research shows that CPCs rarely test for or treat a full panel of STIs.[28] In addition, this study was unable to examine the number or credentials of CPC staff and volunteers; client volume; targets, types, and volume of outreach and advertising employed by CPCs; or other factors that might influence CPCs' impact. Lastly, although CPC Map excludes mobile centers, the eligibility criteria represent a public health approach by limiting data to centers that offer free pregnancy testing and options "counseling" at minimum.

Public Health Implications

After *Dobbs*, CPCs continue to operate in every state and increased in number nationally and in 26 states. Health promotion and advocacy campaigns to increase awareness about CPCs and local centers may be useful across the country and particularly in states where CPCs are proliferating. In line with APHA policy,[11] health professionals should educate themselves and patients about local CPCs and their risks, as well as advise people seeking health services about safe sources of health information and care. Medical personnel should refrain from supporting, including serving as medical directors of, any center or organization that uses deceptive practices, provides inaccurate health information, eschews core public health prevention strategies, or otherwise fails to adhere to medical and ethical practice standards. Governments and medical and nursing boards have a responsibility to ensure that health professionals providing services at CPCs adhere to practice standards. Public health and medical professionals can advocate that governments only support evidence-based programs. Since CPCs capitalize on gaps in health care access, advocacy for policies that expand access to quality sexual and reproductive health care may help limit CPC harms. AJPH

ABOUT THE AUTHORS

Danielle Lambert, Nicole Luisi, Erin Johnson, Rachel Baugh, and Andrea Swartzendruber are with the Department of Epidemiology and Biostatistics, College of Public Health, University of Georgia, Athens.

CORRESPONDENCE

Correspondence should be sent to Danielle Lambert, PhD, MPH, B.S. Miller Hall, 101 Buck Rd, Athens, GA 30602 (e-mail: dnl@uga.edu). Reprints can be ordered at https://www.ajph.org by clicking the "Reprints" link.

PUBLICATION INFORMATION

Full Citation: Lambert DN, Luisi N, Johnson ER, Baugh R, Swartzendruber A. Crisis pregnancy centers in the United States: post-*Dobbs* characteristics and changes. *Am J Public Health*. 2025; 115(6):924–935.

Acceptance Date: February 3, 2025.

DOI: https://doi.org/10.2105/AJPH.2025.308055

ORCID iDs:

Danielle N. Lambert https://orcid.org/0000-0002-8787-8013

Nicole Luisi https://orcid.org/0000-0003-4466-7141

Erin R. Johnson https://orcid.org/0000-0003-2643-6534

Rachel Baugh https://orcid.org/0009-0004-9315-9789

CONTRIBUTORS

D. N. Lambert and A. Swartzendruber obtained funding and conceptualized and designed the study. D. N. Lambert, E. R. Johnson, and N. Luisi prepared the data for analysis. N. Luisi conducted the statistical analyses. E. R. Johnson and R. Baugh provided project administration for data collection and validation. All authors contributed to the writing and reviewed and approved the final version of the article.

ACKNOWLEDGMENTS

A portion of this work was funded by the Collaborative for Gender + Reproductive Equity.

Note. The funder had no role in the design and conduct of the study; collection, management, analysis, and interpretation of the data; preparation, review, or approval of the article; and decision to submit the article for publication.

CONFLICTS OF INTEREST

The authors have no conflicts of interest to report.

HUMAN PARTICIPANT PROTECTION

This study used publicly available data and did not involve human participants.

REFERENCES

1. Society for Adolescent Health and Medicine, North American Society for Pediatric and Adolescent Gynecology. Crisis pregnancy centers in the US: lack of adherence to medical and ethical practice standards. Position paper. *J Adolesc Health.* 2019;65(6):821–824. https://doi.org/10.1016/j.jadohealth.2019.08.008
2. Bryant AG, Swartz JJ. Why crisis pregnancy centers are legal but unethical. *AMA J Ethics.* 2018;20(1):269–277. https://doi.org/10.1001/journalofethics.2018.20.3.pfor1-1803
3. Swartzendruber A, Lambert DN. A web-based geolocated directory of crisis pregnancy centers (CPCs) in the United States: description of CPC Map methods and design features and analysis of baseline data. *JMIR Public Health Surveill.* 2020;6(1):e16726. https://doi.org/10.2196/16726
4. Hussey L. *The Pro-Life Pregnancy Help Movement.* Lawrence, KS: University Press of Kansas; 2020. https://doi.org/10.2307/j.ctv11hpv1q
5. Kortsmit K, Nguyen AT, Mandel MG, et al. Abortion surveillance—United States, 2021. *MMWR Surveill Summ.* 2023;72(9):1–29. https://doi.org/10.15585/mmwr.ss7209a1
6. Centers for Disease Control and Prevention. HIV surveillance report: diagnoses, deaths, and prevalence of HIV in the United States and 6 territories and freely associated states, 2022. Available at: https://stacks.cdc.gov/view/cdc/156509. Accessed July 1, 2024.
7. Centers for Disease Control and Prevention. Sexually transmitted infections surveillance, 2022. Available at: https://www.cdc.gov/std/statistics/2022/default.htm. Accessed July 1, 2024.
8. University of Georgia College of Public Health. New data reveals CPCs are spreading, casting wider net to attract non-pregnant clients. April 7, 2022, Available at: https://publichealth.uga.edu/new-data-reveals-cpcs-are-spreading. Accessed June 28, 2024.
9. Swartzendruber A, Newton-Levinson A, Feuchs AE, Phillips AL, Hickey J, Steiner RJ. Sexual and reproductive health services and related health information on pregnancy resource center websites: a statewide content analysis. *Womens Health Issues.* 2018;28(1):14–20. https://doi.org/10.1016/j.whi.2017.10.007
10. Swartzendruber A, Steiner RJ, Newton-Levinson A. Contraceptive information on pregnancy resource center websites: a statewide content analysis. *Contraception.* 2018;98(2):158–162. https://doi.org/10.1016/j.contraception.2018.04.002
11. American Public Health Association. Regulating disclosure of services and sponsorship of crisis pregnancy centers. Available at: http://www.apha.org/policies-and-advocacy/public-health-policy-statements/policy-database/2014/07/22/08/33/regulating-disclosure-of-services-and-sponsorship-of-crisis-pregnancy-centers. Accessed June 28, 2024.
12. American Medical Association. Truth and transparency in pregnancy counseling centers H-420.954. 2022. Available at: https://policysearch.ama-assn.org/policyfinder/detail/pregnancy?uri=%2FAMADoc%2FHOD.xml-0-3697.xml. Accessed June 28, 2024.
13. American Public Health Association. Recommendations for pregnancy counseling and abortion referrals. October 24, 2020. Available at: https://www.apha.org/Policies-and-Advocacy/Public-Health-Policy-Statements/Policy-Database/2021/01/12/Recommendations-for-Pregnancy-Counseling-and-Abortion-Referrals. Accessed June 28, 2024.
14. Warren E, Kissling A, Norris AH, Gursahaney PR, Bessett D, Gallo MF. "I felt like I was a bad person . . . which I'm not": stigmatization in crisis pregnancy centers. *SSM Qual Res Health.* 2022;2:100059. https://doi.org/10.1016/j.ssmqr.2022.100059
15. American Academy of Pediatrics. Options counseling for the pregnant adolescent patient. *Pediatrics.* 2022;150(3):e2022058781. https://doi.org/10.1542/peds.2022-058781
16. Sherman C. Anti-abortion centers raked in $1.4bn in year Roe fell, including federal money. *The Guardian.* February 12, 2024. Available at: https://amp.theguardian.com/world/2024/feb/14/anti-abortion-centers-funding. Accessed June 24, 2024.
17. Kindy K. Partisan battle grows over state funding for antiabortion centers. *Washington Post.* September 14, 2023. Available at: https://www.washingtonpost.com/politics/2023/09/14/gop-lawmakers-crisis-pregnancy-centers-state-funding. Accessed June 24, 2024.
18. Kruesi K. Millions in tax dollars flow to anti-abortion centers in US. *AP News.* February 5, 2022. Available at: https://apnews.com/article/abortion-business-health-nashville-personal-taxes-fffa6f6f86e6eaa448b8ea89087a1c46. Accessed June 24, 2024.
19. Vollers AC. Abortion-ban states pour millions into pregnancy centers with little medical care. *Stateline.* August 24, 2023. Available at: https://stateline.org/2023/08/24/abortion-ban-states-pour-millions-into-pregnancy-centers-with-little-medical-care. Accessed June 24, 2024.
20. Alabama Legislature. Pregnancy Resource Act, HB 356. 2024. Available at: https://alison.legislature.state.al.us/files/pdfdocs/SearchableInstruments/2024RS/HB356-int.pdf. Accessed July 10, 2024.
21. Tennessee Office of the Governor. Gov. Lee launches Tennessee strong families grant program. September 13, 2023. Available at: https://www.tn.gov/governor/news/2023/9/13/gov-lee-launches-tennessee-strong-families-grant-program-. Accessed July 10, 2024.
22. West Virginia Legislature. Support for Mothers and Babies Act, HB 2002. 2023. Available at: https://www.wvlegislature.gov/bill_status/bills_text.cfm?billdoc=hb2002%20intr.htm&yr=2023&sesstype=RS&i=2002. Accessed July 10, 2024.
23. Mississippi Legislature. Pregnancy Resource Act, HB 1685. 2022. Available at: https://billstatus.ls.state.ms.us/documents/2022/html/HB/1600-1699/HB1685IN.htm. Accessed July 10, 2024.
24. Indiana General Assembly Special Session. Senate Bill 2 Fiscal Matters. 2022. Available at: https://iga.in.gov/legislative/2022ss1/bills/senate/2/details. Accessed July 10, 2024.
25. The Florida Senate. Pregnancy and Parenting Support, SB 300. 2023. Available at: https://www.flsenate.gov/Session/Bill/2023/300/?Tab=BillText. Accessed July 10, 2024.
26. Iowa General Assembly. Health and Human Services Appropriations Bill, HF2578. 2023. Available at: https://www.legis.iowa.gov/docs/publications/NOBA/1292077.pdf. Accessed July 10, 2024.
27. Swartzendruber A, Luisi N, Johnson E, Lambert D. Spatial analyses of crisis pregnancy centers and abortion facilities in the United States, 2021: pre-Dobbs cross-sectional study. *JMIR Public Health Surveill.* 2024;10:e60001. https://doi.org/10.2196/60001
28. Swartzendruber A, Solsman A, Lambert DN. The availability of HIV and sexually transmitted infection testing and treatment services at crisis pregnancy centers in the United States. *Sex Transm Dis.* 2021;48(10):738–747. https://doi.org/10.1097/OLQ.0000000000001406
29. Swartzendruber A, Lambert D. Crisis Pregnancy Center Map. 2018. Available at: https://crisispregnancycentermap.com. Accessed June 29, 2024.
30. Grossman D, White K, Harris L, et al. Continuing pregnancy after mifepristone and "reversal" of first-trimester medical abortion: a systematic review. *Contraception.* 2015;92(3):206–211. https://doi.org/10.1016/j.contraception.2015.06.001
31. The American College of Obstetricians and Gynecologists. Medication abortion "reversal" is not supported by science. Available at: https://www.acog.org/advocacy/facts-are-important/medication-abortion-reversal-is-not-supported-by-science. Accessed December 9, 2024.
32. AbortionFinder. State-by-state guide. Power to Decide. Available at: https://www.abortionfinder.org/abortion-guides-by-state. Accessed March 8, 2024.
33. National Governors Association. America's Governors. Available at: https://www.nga.org/governors. Accessed March 8, 2024.
34. Gavin L, Pazol K, Ahrens K. Update: Providing quality family planning services—recommendations from CDC and the US Office of Population Affairs, 2017. *MMWR Morb Mortal Wkly Rep.* 2017;66:1383–1385. https://doi.org/10.15585/mmwr.mm6650a4
35. Centers for Disease Control and Prevention. HIV infection: detection, counseling, and referral.

July 21, 2021. Available at: https://www.cdc.gov/std/treatment-guidelines/hiv.htm. Accessed July 10, 2024.

36. Centers for Disease Control and Prevention. Screening recommendations and considerations referenced in treatment guidelines and original sources. March 22, 2024. Available at: https://www.cdc.gov/std/treatment-guidelines/screening-recommendations.htm. Accessed July 10, 2024.

37. National Association of County and City Health Officials. 2019 National Profile of Local Health Departments. Available at: https://www.naccho.org/uploads/downloadable-resources/Programs/Public-Health-Infrastructure/NACCHO_2019_Profile_final.pdf. Accessed July 22, 2024.

38. National Association of County and City Health Officials. 2022 National Profile of Local Health Departments. Available at: https://www.naccho.org/uploads/downloadable-resources/NACCHO-2022-Profile-Report.pdf. Accessed July 22, 2024.

39. National Association of County and City Health Officials. 2013 National Profile of Local Health Departments. Available at: https://www.naccho.org/uploads/downloadable-resources/2013_National_Profile021014.pdf. Accessed July 22, 2024.

40. World Health Organization. *Trends in Maternal Mortality 2000 to 2020: Estimates by WHO, UNICEF, UNFPA, World Bank Group and UNDESA/Population Division*. 2023. Available at: https://iris.who.int/bitstream/handle/10665/366225/9789240068759-eng.pdf?sequence=1. Accessed July 22, 2024.

41. Cartwright AF, Tumlinson K, Upadhyay UD. Pregnancy outcomes after exposure to crisis pregnancy centers among an abortion-seeking sample recruited online. *PLoS One*. 2021;16(7):e0255152. https://doi.org/10.1371/journal.pone.0255152

42. Morel LC. 'It's a public health risk': nurse decries infection control at US anti-abortion crisis center. *The Guardian*. February 2, 2023. Available at: https://www.theguardian.com/world/2023/feb/02/kentucky-crisis-pregnancy-center-anti-abortion-malpractices. Accessed June 24, 2024.

43. Heartbeat International. Program policies. Available at: https://www.heartbeatinternational.org/about/our-commitment. Accessed June 28, 2024.

44. Care Net. Pregnancy center standards of affiliation. Available at: https://cdn2.hubspot.net/hubfs/367552/Standards%20of%20Affiliation%202019.pdf. Accessed June 28, 2024.

45. Barrow RY, Ahmed F, Bolan GA, Workowski KA. Recommendations for providing quality sexually transmitted diseases clinical services, 2020. *MMWR Recomm Rep*. 2020;68(5):1–20. https://doi.org/10.15585/mmwr.rr6805a1

46. Henderson G. Why won't the CDC kick "crisis pregnancy centers" out of its directories? *Rewire News Group*. May 16, 2023. Available at: https://rewirenewsgroup.com/2023/05/16/why-wont-the-cdc-kick-crisis-pregnancy-centers-out-of-its-directories. Accessed July 1, 2024.

47. Centers for Disease Control and Prevention. GetTested: HIV, STD, and hepatitis testing and vaccines near you. National Prevention Information Network. Available at: https://gettested.cdc.gov. Accessed July 1, 2024.

48. Redd SK, AbiSamra R, Blake SC, et al. Medication abortion "reversal" laws: how unsound science paved the way for dangerous abortion policy. *Am J Public Health*. 2023;113(2):202–212. https://doi.org/10.2105/AJPH.2022.307140

49. Colorado General Assembly Regular Session. Deceptive Trade Practice Pregnancy-Related Service, SB23-190. 2023. Available at: https://leg.colorado.gov/bills/sb23-190. Accessed July 10, 2024.

50. Office of the New York State Attorney General. Attorney General James sues anti-abortion group and 11 New York crisis pregnancy centers for promoting unproven abortion reversal treatment. May 6, 2024. Available at: https://ag.ny.gov/press-release/2024/attorney-general-james-sues-anti-abortion-group-and-11-new-york-crisis-pregnancy. Accessed July 10, 2024.

51. The Iowa Legislature 90th General Assembly, 2023–2024 Session. An Act Prohibiting and Requiring Certain Actions Relating to Abortion Involving the Detection of a Fetal Heartbeat, HF732. 2023. Available at: https://www.legis.iowa.gov/legislation/BillBook?ga=90&ba=HF%20732. Accessed July 10, 2024.

52. Iqbal M. Illinois agrees to stop enforcing a controversial new law cracking down on crisis pregnancy centers. *WBEZ Chicago*. December 13, 2023. Available at: https://www.wbez.org/stories/anti-abortion-activists-claim-victory-in-illinois-over-cpcs/74c93963-aee7-4cab-a298-6cdf0a0f136c. Accessed July 10, 2024.

53. Connecticut General Assembly, Public Health Committee. An Act Concerning Deceptive Advertising Practices of Limited Services Pregnancy Centers, CT SB835. May 26, 2021. Available at: https://www.cga.ct.gov/2021/act/pa/pdf/2021PA-00017-R00SB-00835-PA.pdf. Accessed July 10, 2024.

54. US Senate, 117th Congress sess (Menendez R 2022). Stop Anti-Abortion Disinformation (SAD) Act. S.4469. June 23, 2022. Available at: https://www.congress.gov/bill/117th-congress/senate-bill/4469/text?r=18&s=1. Accessed July 10, 2024.

55. US House of Representatives, 117th Congress (Maloney C 2022). Stop Anti-Abortion Disinformation (SAD) Act, HR 8210. June 22, 2022. Available at: https://www.congress.gov/bill/117th-congress/house-bill/8210/text. Accessed July 10, 2024.

56. Illinois State Government. Gov. Pritzker signs Bill strengthening protections against misinformation at "crisis pregnancy centers." July 27, 2023. Available at: https://www.illinois.gov/news/press-release.26779.html. Accessed July 10, 2024.

57. City of Cambridge, Massachusetts. Crisis pregnancy centers. February 6, 2023. Available at: https://library.municode.com/ma/cambridge/codes/code_of_ordinances?nodeId=TIT5BULIRE_5.64CRPRCE. Accessed July 10, 2024.

58. City of Somerville. Deceptive advertising practices of limited services pregnancy centers, Ordinance No. 2022-03 Ch. 6, Article VI. March 24, 2022. Available at: https://library.municode.com/ma/somerville/ordinances/code_of_ordinances?nodeId=1144192. Accessed July 10, 2024.

59. Hudson M. Mayor Buttigieg vetoes zoning decision for Women's Care Center. *ABC 57*. April 27, 2018. Available at: https://www.abc57.com/news/mayor-buttigieg-vetoes-womens-care-center-zoning. Accessed July 10, 2024.

Health Care, Mortality, and Declining Occupancy Rates in California Prisons, 2013–2023

Jessica L. Adler, PhD, and Weiwei Chen, PhD

See also Goldhaber-Fiebert, p. 819.

Objectives. To assess relationships between changes in population levels, health care access, health care grievances, and mortality in California prisons.

Methods. We examined 30 California prisons using June 2013 to May 2023 data from California Correctional Health Care Services and the California Department of Justice. Associations between prison occupancy rates and care access, health care grievances, and mortality were estimated in linear or generalized linear models controlling for staff vacancies and the characteristics of incarcerated people. Because of the prevalence of COVID-19-specific dynamics in prisons in 2020–2021, baseline models included data up to December 2019; data from January 2022 through May 2023 were added as a robustness check.

Results. Reductions in prison occupancy rates were associated with increased access to care. Associations were more pronounced when postpandemic data were added. However, decreasing occupancy rates were not associated with declines in health care grievances or mortality.

Conclusions. Lowering prison occupancy rates could help ensure better access to care, but it is not a panacea for alleviating varied health-related problems and dangers inside carceral facilities. (*Am J Public Health*. 2025;115(6):936–944. https://doi.org/10.2105/AJPH.2025.308011)

AJPH June 2025, Vol. 115, No. 6

In 2011, the Supreme Court issued its *Brown v Plata* ruling, maintaining that health care in California's prisons was below constitutional standards. The problem could not be remedied, according to the court, without the alleviation of severe prison overcrowding. The decision upheld an earlier ruling that California must decrease the number of people in its prisons from then current levels—about twice the population the facilities were designed to hold—to no more than 137.5% of capacity.[1] The state's 2011 Public Safety Realignment Act enshrined court mandates into law.[2]

California's case, although unique, signified a growing acceptance of the idea that "the number of people behind bars must be reduced."[3(p240),4] Overall, the US prison population decreased 25% between 2010 and 2021; however, the nation's incarceration rate remains staggeringly high in comparison with that of the 1970s, as well as in comparison with other countries.[5] In California, the prison population decreased by 26% between 2006 and 2018, from 173 000 to 128 000.[6] As of 2021–2022, there were slightly under 100 000 people detained in California prisons.[7]

Studies of health care access inside prisons, including how it changes in relation to population declines, are lacking. The National Commission on Correctional Health Care maintains that "large gaps in correctional health care research have hampered policy decision making in all aspects of health care organization, provision, and financing for incarcerated populations," in part because there is a dearth of "standardized reporting networks" and "some correctional administrators may be hesitant to share information about their facilities."[8]

California's publicly accessible and longitudinal health care data dashboard, created in part to satisfy litigation-related requirements, makes it possible to conduct health systems research on one of the largest prison systems in the country and draw conclusions with wide-ranging implications. Analyzing and interpreting data from the dashboard, which includes measure of patient access, utilization, and outcomes, offers a unique opportunity to assess connections between changes in prison populations and health care services.[9]

In addition to considering health care access, we used California Department of Justice data to assess how changes in prison population levels relate to mortality. We contextualize our findings with limited existing data and studies on connections between prison mortality and population levels.

METHODS

We collected California prison data from the Health Care Services Dashboard, made available by California Correctional Health Care Services. The dashboard, launched in 2013, publishes a wide range of measures on health service delivery and characteristics of staff and populations at the state and prison levels. We used monthly data from June 2013 to May 2023, covering 35 prisons that remained operational for the duration of the period. We excluded 4 institutions considered to be specialty treatment or rehabilitation centers housing atypical populations in terms of health characteristics (California Health Care Facility, California Medical Facility, California Rehabilitation Center, and Substance Abuse Treatment Facility and State Prison) and 1 institution with missing data on key variables such as occupancy rates (California City Correctional Facility). A total of 30 prisons were included in our final analyses.

As a complement to the dashboard data, we examined individual mortality data from the California Department of Justice (accessed in December 2023).[10] We extracted information on deaths that occurred among those detained in the same 30 prisons examined via the dashboard data who were under the custody of the Department of Corrections and Rehabilitation Adult Operations and Adult Programs and the Division of Juvenile Justice. We derived the number of deaths per month and institution on the basis of reported dates of death.

Our earliest data observations were from 2013, 2 years after *Brown v Plata* and the passage of the Prison Realignment Act, which fostered a decline in California's incarcerated population.[1] Given that COVID-19 had wide-ranging and unique effects on carceral facilities in 2020 and 2021, we used only prepandemic data (January 2013–December 2019) in our baseline model and added postpandemic data (January 2022–May 2023) in a robustness check.[11]

We plotted trends in the monthly total incarcerated population of the 30 prisons and averaged monthly occupancy rate across prisons from June 2013 to May 2023. We exploited temporal and cross-prison variations in occupancy rates to estimate associations between prison populations and health-related measures.

Variables

Our primary variable of interest was prison occupancy rate, defined as the incarcerated population relative to the prison design capacity on the final day of a reporting month. To examine health-related effects, we assessed access to care, grievances, and deaths. We selected summary measures with the most available observations and minimal changes (in names or definitions) over the study period. We ultimately examined 5 outcomes: access to medical care, access to mental health care, access to dental care, health care grievances (i.e., complaints filed by incarcerated people related to health care) received per 1000 incarcerated people, and deaths per 10 000 incarcerated people (definitions of various measures are provided in the Appendix, available as a supplement to the online version of this article at https://www.ajph.org).

Our covariates included characteristics of incarcerated people and facilities. We considered the percentage of incarcerated people aged 50 years or older; the percentage characterized as high-risk priority 1, high-risk priority 2, medium risk, and low risk (see the Appendix for definitions of risk categories); and the percentage with disabilities. We also considered facility-level supply side factors, specifically vacancies in medical, mental, and dental service staff positions. Because vacancy rates were not reported until January 2017, including them in the regressions considerably reduced the number of observations. We therefore present regressions with and without vacancy rates.

Statistical Analysis

We estimated the association between occupancy rates and each of the health-related outcomes. For the 3 outcomes measured as proportions (medical care access, mental health care access, and dental care access), we estimated generalized linear models with binomial distributions and logit link functions. For the 2 outcomes measured as rates (health care grievances received per 1000 incarcerated people and deaths per 10 000 incarcerated people), we fit linear regression models.

Negative binomial models were also attempted for the latter 2 outcomes in an earlier version of this study. Although the estimates were qualitatively similar, some regressions did not reach convergency. We therefore report the linear regression results.

We show regressions with characteristics of incarcerated people first and then add staff vacancy variables. All of the models included prison, year, and month fixed effects. Standard errors were clustered at the prison level. All of our analyses were conducted with Stata version 18 (StataCorp LP, College Station, TX).

Our baseline analyses included observations from June 2013 to December 2019 (before the pandemic). As a robustness check, we repeated the analyses with additional observations from postpandemic periods (January 2022 to May 2023). We excluded data from 2020 and 2021, when prisons were most heavily affected by the COVID-19 pandemic.

RESULTS

Figure 1 shows monthly total populations and monthly average occupancy rates among 30 California prisons from June 2013 to May 2023 (prison-level trends are presented in Appendix Figure A, available as a supplement to the online version of this article at https://www.ajph.org). Prison populations and mean occupancy rates declined between 2013 and 2015 subsequent to the Prison Realignment Act. They then showed some uptick and fluctuations in the following years, with the mean occupancy rate mostly below 1.375 (or 137.5%), the limit set by the act. The prepandemic trend confirms existing studies regarding changes in California's prison population after legal mandates to reduce the number of people incarcerated in state facilities.[12,13] A deep plummet occurred after the onset of the pandemic in early 2020 as a result of the state's attempt to manage the spread of the virus by reducing occupancy.[14] In 2021, prison populations and occupancy rates started to rise, followed by small fluctuations, but remained at comparatively low levels.

We summarize the statistics of all of the variables used in our analyses in Table 1. Some variables had fewer observations because of missing values for certain months or institutions. Mental health care access measures were discontinued as of February 2020, and vacancy measures became available only as of January 2017. The 3 care access measures all had mean values close to or above 90%, suggesting that about 90% of medical, mental, or dental service requests were completed within the defined time frame. In a given month, there were about 30 health care grievances received per 1000 incarcerated people and about 2 deaths among every 10 000 incarcerated people. More than 20% of the individuals imprisoned were aged 50 years or older, about 6% were disabled, and about half were characterized as medium or high risk, which related to greater medical needs.

Staff shortages—especially among mental health professionals—are widely viewed as a major challenge in prisons, so we considered employee vacancy measures in our analysis.[15] We found that, between January 2017 (when the measures became available) and December 2019, average vacancy rates were above 10% for medical service staff and close to 20% for mental service staff. The mean vacancy rate for

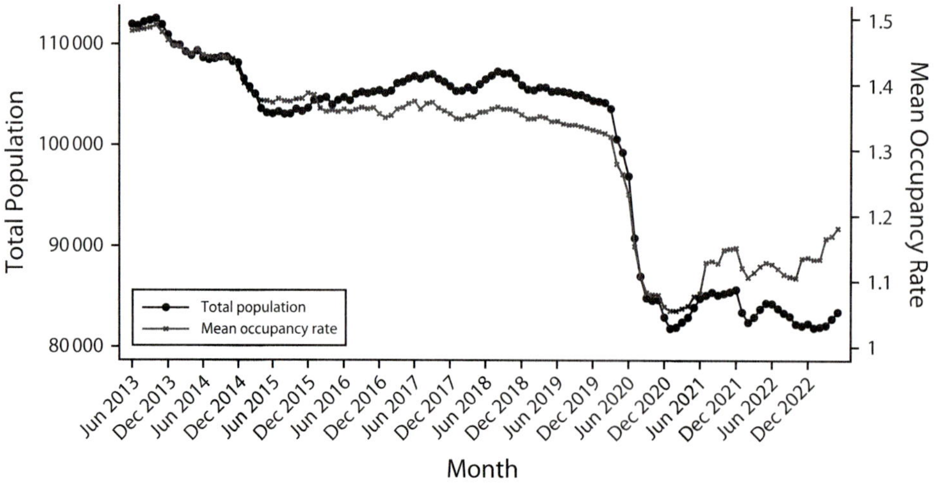

FIGURE 1— Monthly Total Populations and Mean Occupancy Rates of 30 California Prisons: June 2013–May 2023

TABLE 1— Care Access, Grievances, Deaths, and Prison Characteristics During the Prepandemic and Postpandemic periods: California, June 2013–May 2023

Variable	June 2013–December 2019		January 2022–May 2023	
	No.	Mean (SD)	No.	Mean (SD)
Outcome measures				
Medical care access, %	2330	88 (10)	487	88 (10)
Mental health care access, %	2340	92 (8)	0	
Dental care access, %	2322	94 (9)	487	94 (7)
Grievances received, no.	2340	29.94 (20.78)	479	33.11 (29.43)
Deaths, no.	2370	1.62 (2.62)	486	2.24 (12.26)
Independent variables				
Occupancy, no.	2370	1.38 (0.20)	486	1.13 (0.23)
Incarcerated people aged 50 y or older, %	2370	22 (12)	486	26 (14)
Chronic disease burden				
High-risk priority 1, %	2370	4 (5)	486	6 (7)
High-risk priority 2, %	2370	8 (8)	486	10 (8)
Medium risk, %	2370	38 (13)	486	35 (12)
Low risk, %	2370	51 (20)	486	49 (22)
Disabled, %	2370	6 (5)	486	10 (8)
Staff vacancies				
Medical service staff, %	1080	13 (5)	487	20 (9)
Mental health service staff, %	1080	19 (10)	487	28 (12)
Dental service staff, %	1080	5 (5)	487	9 (8)

Note. Observations vary by variable as a result of missing values. Mental health care access measures were discontinued as of February 2020. Vacancy variables were available only as of January 2017. High-risk priority 1, high-risk priority 2, medium risk, and low risk refer to the percentages of patients with different levels of chronic disease burdens; people characterized as high-risk priority 1 were those considered to be at the highest risk level, and people characterized as low risk were those considered to be at the lowest risk level. Grievances received and deaths were monthly counts per 1000 and 10 000 people, respectively. More detailed definitions are provided in the Appendix (available as a supplement to the online version of this article at https://www.ajph.org).

dental service staff was the lowest, at about 5%. We added observations from January 2022 to May 2023 to the regressions in our robustness check analysis. Descriptive statistics for these observations are listed separately.

Tables 2 and 3 present estimates of occupancy rates from the generalized linear models for care access and the linear models for grievances and deaths. For ease of coefficient interpretation, we derived and report marginal effects from the generalized linear models. In the case of the linear models, the reported marginal effects were equivalent to the coefficient estimates. During the prepandemic period (June 2013 to December 2019), variations in occupancy rates showed negative associations with some of our health-related outcomes (Table 2). In the top panel of Table 2 (regressions with controls for characteristics of incarcerated people), 2 of the 3 access measures were significantly negative, indicating less access when the occupancy rate increased. When controls for staff vacancy were added to the regressions (bottom panel), there were still 2 access measures showing significant and negative estimates, although medical care became significant only in the bottom panel and dental care access became insignificant.

For our mental health care access measure, estimates indicated that a 10-percentage-point increase in occupancy rate, for example, was associated with a 1.1-percentage-point decrease in the measure when staff vacancy measures were included (or 0.7-percentage-point decrease when vacancy measures were not included). The number of grievances increased in response to occupancy increases but became insignificant after control for staff vacancy rates. Notably, death rates exhibited no significant change as occupancy rates changed.

The inclusion of additional staff vacancy variables helped control for

TABLE 2— Estimated Associations Between Occupancy Rates, Care Access, Grievances, and Deaths With Prepandemic Data: California, June 2013–December 2019

	Medical Care Access, b (95% CI) or No.	Mental Health Care Access, b (95% CI) or No.	Dental Care Access, b (95% CI) or No.	Grievances Received, b (95% CI) or No.	Deaths, b (95% CI) or No.
Regressions with controls only for characteristics of incarcerated people					
Occupancy	−0.03 (−0.09, 0.03)	−0.07 (−0.12, −0.01)	−0.06 (−0.12, −0.00)	13.61 (3.10, 24.12)	−0.54 (−1.49, 0.42)
No.	2330	2340	2322	2340	2370
Regressions with controls for staff vacancies and characteristics of incarcerated people					
Occupancy	−0.11 (−0.21, −0.01)	−0.11 (−0.19, −0.02)	−0.05 (−0.11, 0.01)	10.31 (−3.46, 24.07)	−0.47 (−2.67, 1.73)
No.	1080	1080	1032	1050	1080

Note. CI = confidence interval. Reported are estimated marginal effects of occupancy rates from 5 regressions based on monthly observations from June 2013 to December 2019. The first 3 regressions are generalized linear models, and the other 2 are linear regressions. The regressions also include characteristics of incarcerated people (percentage who were aged 50 years or older; percentage who were high-risk priority 1, high-risk priority 2, or medium risk; and percentage who were disabled), staff vacancy measures (percentages of vacancies in medical service, mental service, and dental service staff), and prison, year, and month fixed effects. Standard errors were clustered at the prison level. Full regression results are presented in Appendix Table A (available as a supplement to the online version of this article at https://www.ajph.org).

supply side factors that might influence health-related outcomes. However, because of the lack of observations before 2017, adding the vacancy variables also reduced the observations for the regressions by more than half. To compensate for the loss of observations, we conducted a robustness check by including postpandemic years, during which we had more observations for staff vacancies. The results (Table 3) confirmed the reduction in access as occupancy rates increased. All 3 access measures were significantly negative (the estimates for mental health care access remained the same in Tables 2 and 3 because access to mental health care was measured only until February 2020; there were no postpandemic observations). Again, no significant reduction was found in health care grievances or deaths relating to occupancy rate increases.

DISCUSSION

Our study reveals that prison occupancy rates relate to access to health care but not prison mortality or numbers of grievances filed. In the context of the limited literature on prison overcrowding, mortality, and grievances, these findings are not as paradoxical as they may first appear. They suggest that a decline in prison population levels

TABLE 3— Estimated Associations Between Occupancy Rates, Care Access, Grievances, and Deaths With Additional Postpandemic Data: California, June 2013–December 2019 and January 2022–May 2023

	Medical Care Access, b (95% CI) or No.	Mental Health Care Access, b (95% CI) or No.	Dental Care Access, b (95% CI) or No.	Grievances Received, b (95% CI) or No.	Deaths, b (95% CI) or No.
Regressions with controls only for characteristics of incarcerated people					
Occupancy	−0.05 (−0.10, −0.01)	−0.07 (−0.12, −0.01)	−0.05 (−0.08, −0.01)	−7.90 (−30.11, 14.31)	−6.46 (−17.36, 4.44)
No.	2816	2340	2808	2819	2856
Regressions with controls for staff vacancies and characteristics of incarcerated people					
Occupancy	−0.11 (−0.16, −0.06)	−0.11 (−0.19, −0.02)	−0.04 (−0.07, −0.02)	−21.64 (−58.93, 15.66)	−11.68 (−32.21, 8.84)
No.	1566	1080	1518	1529	1566

Note. CI = confidence interval. Reported are estimated marginal effects of occupancy rates from 5 regressions based on monthly observations from June 2013 to December 2019 and January 2022 to May 2023. The first 3 regressions are generalized linear models, and the other 2 are linear regressions. The regressions also include characteristics of incarcerated people (percentage who were aged 50 years or older; percentage who were high-risk priority 1, high-risk priority 2, or medium risk; and percentage who were disabled), staff vacancy measures (percentages of vacancies in medical service, mental service, and dental service staff), and prison, year, and month fixed effects. Mental health care access regressions are the same as in Table 2, because mental health care measures had no observations in the postpandemic periods. Standard errors were clustered at the prison level. Full regression results are presented in Appendix Table B (available as a supplement to the online version of this article at https://www.ajph.org).

could increase the likelihood that an incarcerated person is seen by a health care provider but have muted effects on satisfaction with health care services and chances of death.

Controlling for various factors, we found that in less full prisons, people were more likely to have access to medical, mental, and dental care. Although this is the first study to our knowledge that quantifies the relationship between prison-based access to care and changes in prison occupancy levels, our findings align with previous qualitative research demonstrating that people in overcrowded prisons in and beyond the United States face particular dangers. High prison occupancy rates, studies show, can lead to an increased risk of violence[16] and "late or inadequate medical care."[17] Prison administrators report that "rising populations" make it "harder to manage prisons effectively" because of increased "pressure on resources"; overcrowding has "a wide-ranging impact on prisoner health and wellbeing."[18] Researchers further note that overcrowding can accentuate fears of communicable disease, increase "psychological and emotional burden," and limit access to basic resources.[19] Our study offers quantitative evidence that a decline in access to care is an added cost of overcrowding, one that can further exacerbate its other harms.

In contrast with results suggesting impediments in access to care, we found that higher prison occupancy rates do not relate to higher mortality. Our results correspond with national data suggesting that prison population levels and mortality are not correlated. Data from the Bureau of Justice Statistics reveal that, between 2009 and 2019, the population of people in state or federal prisons fell by 18.9%[20] as the prison mortality rate increased from 259 per 100 000 to 330 per 100 000. Although the number of deaths from drug or alcohol intoxication increased during that period, almost 90% of deaths in prisons were from illnesses such as cancer and heart disease.[21] These findings reflect that a variety of factors relate to deaths in custody, including the demographic characteristics of imprisoned people and widespread health disparities as well as facility characteristics such as turnover rates.[22]

Our findings help explain the results of a 2023 study of California's prison mortality rates between 2011 and 2014 that revealed that crude mortality increased immediately after the implementation of legislation intended to decrease prison populations. The mortality increase had little to do with facility crowdedness, the authors maintained, but instead was related to demographics. During the 3 years of the study, California's decreasing prison population became, on average, older. Age-adjusted mortality rates were lower and showed greater declines in comparison with both unadjusted rates in California and age-adjusted rates in other states. The reason for this declining mortality, according to the study authors, could be that "de-population of California prisons . . . occurred in tandem with dedicated and seemingly effective efforts to improve the quality of medical care provided to prisoners."[13(p14)]

Building on this work, in our assessment of relationships between prison population levels and health-related outcomes, we tracked change over a relatively extended period (2013–2023) in 30 prisons and controlled for incarcerated people's age, medical risk, and disability as well as facility characteristics such as staffing levels.

Our finding that mortality is unrelated to prison occupancy rates underscores that, although lowering prison populations is a positive step forward, it does not alleviate many of the dangers faced by incarcerated people. As noted by Rowe et al., the Supreme Court opinion in *Brown v Plata* stipulated that overcrowding was "the primary reason for healthcare deficiencies," but it also "made clear that resolving overcrowding alone would not be sufficient to improve the quality of care for prisoners."[13(p14)] Incarcerated people are disproportionately likely to have a variety of health problems and, for many, according to a study of immigrant detention centers, "health harms of detention could be mitigated through release."[23(p733),24]

Likewise, our results pertaining to grievances reflect that access to care is but 1 health-related challenge faced by incarcerated people. In one of the few studies assessing the nature and fate of incarcerated people's grievances, Calavita and Jenness note that health-related complaints were by far the most common type of complaint filed in California prisons in the 2000s, accounting for 20% of the 16 kinds of grievances reviewed. Health-oriented grievances, the authors maintained, were related not only to accessing care but also to "contesting the quality of the care" received.[25(p38)] This helps explain why we found that, despite decreasing occupancy and increasing access, rates of grievances remained relatively stable.

In short, decreasing prison occupancy while maintaining staffing levels may improve people's chances of seeing a health professional, but it is not a panacea. It does not change the fact that incarcerated people are generally less healthy than their counterparts in the free world and that prison health systems are riddled with challenges related to, for example, lack of oversight, low staff morale, and profiteering.[26,27] Policies that focus on decreasing the number of people inside prisons should be viewed as potentially effective means of ensuring both that fewer people will experience the many dangers of incarceration and that those who are incarcerated have better access to care. But they are not "magic bullets" that solve all problems related to prison health services and outcomes.

Limitations

Health Care Services Dashboard data were not available until 2013, after the 2011 passage of the Public Safety Realignment Act, making prestudy–poststudy comparisons infeasible. However, we leveraged gradual changes in prison populations after the ruling and examined their association with health care access and outcomes.

Although Health Care Services Dashboard data include a variety of health service measures, they do not contain information on all characteristics of incarcerated people, staff, and prisons. We used panel data to control for time-invariant unobservable variables. With prison, year, and month fixed effects, we controlled for prison-specific and period-specific effects. We considered individuals' age and health status; future studies might explore the possibility of examining additional characteristics.

Although California Department of Justice mortality data are reviewed by the California Criminal Justice Statistics Center with respect to validity, consistency, and completion, the veracity of death statistics from jails and prisons nationwide has been questioned.[10,28]

Our analyses did not reveal statistically significant effects of occupancy rates on mortality rates. Given that deaths are relatively rare events and that occupancy rates vary only within certain levels, such effects may be difficult to detect within our data sets.

The employee vacancy measure we used accounted for positions held or left vacant by civil service staff members. Sources suggest that the California Department of Corrections and Rehabilitation relied on external contractors to provide some medical services in this period, but the extent and exact nature of medical outsourcing are unclear; an audit ordered by the state's legislature in May 2024 is pending.[29]

Finally, our evidence is drawn from a single state, and the generalizability of our findings may thus be limited. However, the changes studied here offer insights into the results of a directed and sweeping effort to reduce prison populations. Experiences in California provide valuable insight into ongoing discussions related to decarceration.

Conclusions and Policy Implications

Our study provides a powerful justification for pursuing decarceration: it can improve access to medical care for imprisoned people. Alongside research demonstrating that lowering incarceration rates does not generate increases in crime[30,31] and that imprisonment (especially in overcrowded facilities) poses various dangers, this should serve as a call to action for policymakers and advocates concerned with improving prison and community health.

Stakeholders must be wary of focusing on alleviating overcrowding rather than the broader goal of decreasing carceral populations. For decades, judges have ordered corrections officials to decrease overcrowding as a means of ensuring the health and safety of people inside prisons. But through the 1990s, litigation related to overcrowding, in fact, had no discernible impact on prison fullness.[32] Corrections officials, politicians, and others used court decisions indicting inhumane and overcrowded conditions as grounds to argue for more funding and more facilities as harsh sentencing laws led to yet higher rates of incarceration. Indeed, at the turn of the 21st century, lawsuits intended to foster decarceration had a paradoxical and unintended consequence: they contributed to the growth of prison systems and populations.[33]

California appears to have avoided that fate; however, to fully assess the health-related implications of policies related to reducing the number of people in prisons, it is necessary to consider their effects on other types of carceral facilities. After *Brown v Plata*, a massive reduction in the prison population was achieved, in part, by detaining people in county jails who would otherwise have been sent to prisons.[34] Notably, health-related conditions in jails are often dire.[35] We found that access to care in California prisons improved as the number of imprisoned people decreased; further studies might examine health-related jail conditions in California in the same period. In the meantime, policymakers aiming to bolster public health should consider decarceration strategies that do not merely shuffle people from one punishment bureaucracy to another but instead enable them to remain in the community.[23]

Our findings related to mortality and grievances underscore that more research is needed on health care quality and outcomes inside prisons. After all, a variety of factors aside from prison occupancy rates influence incarcerated people's health-related experiences. Some of those factors relate to shortfalls in public health and social welfare systems in the free world and others to conditions inside. Sending fewer people to prison, although a step in the right direction, is not a panacea for alleviating the varied health-related problems and dangers inside carceral facilities. AJPH

ABOUT THE AUTHORS

Jessica L. Adler is with the Department of History, Steven J. Green School of International and Public Affairs, Florida International University, Miami. Weiwei Chen is with the Department of Economics, Finance and Quantitative Analysis, Michael J. Coles College of Business, Kennesaw State University, Kennesaw, GA.

CORRESPONDENCE

Correspondence should be sent to Jessica L. Adler, PhD, Florida International University, Department of History, 11200 SW 8th St, SIPA II, Room 302, Miami, FL 33199 (e-mail: jadler@fiu.edu). Reprints can be ordered at https://www.ajph.org by clicking the "Reprints" link.

PUBLICATION INFORMATION

Full Citation: Adler JL, Chen W. Health care, mortality, and declining occupancy rates in California prisons, 2013–2023. *Am J Public Health*. 2025; 115(6):936–944.

Acceptance Date: December 28, 2024.

DOI: https://doi.org/10.2105/AJPH.2025.308011

ORCID iDs:

Jessica L. Adler https://orcid.org/0000-0002-8632-1803

Weiwei Chen https://orcid.org/0000-0002-2162-0941

CONTRIBUTORS

The authors contributed equally to this article.

ACKNOWLEDGMENTS

Funding for this project was made possible by grant G13LM013522 from the National Library of Medicine of the National Institutes of Health.

We thank the reviewers and editors for critical and constructive feedback.

Note. The content is solely the responsibility of the authors and does not necessarily represent the official views of the National Institutes of Health.

CONFLICTS OF INTEREST

The authors have no conflicts of interest to declare.

HUMAN PARTICIPANT PROTECTION

Publicly accessible California prison data and mortality data were used in this study. The former data set provides aggregated information at the facility level, without individual-level information. The latter data set provides deidentified information from deceased individuals. In both cases, the data sets do not meet the regulatory definition of human participant research. Thus, no institutional review board approval was needed for this study.

REFERENCES

1. Newman WJ, Scott CL. Brown v. Plata: prison overcrowding in California. *J Am Acad Psychiatry Law*. 2012;40(4):547–552.
2. Lofstrom M, Martin B. Public safety realignment: impacts so far. Available at: https://www.ppic.org/publication/public-safety-realignment-impacts-so-far. Accessed May 13, 2024.
3. Clear TR. Decarceration problems and prospects. *Annu Rev Criminol*. 2021;4(4):239–260. https://doi.org/10.1146/annurev-criminol-052820-032924
4. Schrantz D, DeBor S. How 5 states achieved substantial prison population decline. Available at: https://www.sentencingproject.org/reports/decarceration-strategies-how-5-states-achieved-substantial-prison-population-reductions. Accessed May 13, 2024.
5. Nellis A. Mass incarceration trends. Available at: https://www.sentencingproject.org/reports/mass-incarceration-trends. Accessed May 13, 2024.
6. Legislative Analyst's Office. How many prison inmates are there in California? Prison populations as of December 31 each year (1986–2018). Available at: https://lao.ca.gov/PolicyAreas/CJ/5_cj_inmates. Accessed May 13, 2024.
7. Petek G. The 2023–24 budget: California Department of Corrections and Rehabilitation. Available at: https://lao.ca.gov/Publications/Report/4686#Trends_in_the_State_Prison.A0and.A0Parole.A0Populations. Accessed May 13, 2024.
8. National Commission on Correctional Health Care. Position statement: health services research in correctional settings. Available at: https://www.ncchc.org/position-statements/health-services-research-in-correctional-settings-2020. Accessed May 13, 2024.
9. California Correctional Health Care Services. Health Care Services Dashboard. Available at: https://cchcs.ca.gov/dashboard. Accessed May 14, 2024.
10. Criminal Justice Statistics Center. Death in custody. Available at: https://data-openjustice.doj.ca.gov/sites/default/files/dataset/2024-07/death-in-custody-context-06062024.pdf. Accessed May 14, 2024.
11. Carson EA, Nadel M, Gaes G. Impact of COVID-19 on state and federal prisons, March 2020–February 2021. Available at: https://bjs.ojp.gov/content/pub/pdf/icsfp2021.pdf. Accessed May 14, 2024.
12. Turner S, Fain T, Hunt SJ. Public safety realignment in twelve California counties. Available at: https://www.rand.org/pubs/research_reports/RR872.html. Accessed May 14, 2024.
13. Rowe CL, Hubbard A, Ahern J. California's Public Safety Realignment Act and prisoner mortality. *PLoS One*. 2023;18(4):e0284609. https://doi.org/10.1371/journal.pone.0284609
14. Chin ET, Ryckman T, Prince L, et al. COVID-19 in the California State Prison System: an observational study of decarceration, ongoing risks, and risk factors. *J Gen Intern Med*. 2021;36(10):3096–3102. https://doi.org/10.1007/s11606-021-07022-x
15. Morris NP, Edwards ML. Addressing shortages of mental health professionals in US jails and prisons. *J Correct Health Care*. 2022;28(4):209–214. https://doi.org/10.1089/jchc.21.08.0072
16. Baggio S, Peigné N, Heller P, Gétaz L, Liebrenz M, Wolff H. Do overcrowding and turnover cause violence in prison? *Front Psychiatry*. 2020;10:1015. https://doi.org/10.3389/fpsyt.2019.01015
17. Zaitzow BH, Willis AK. Behind the wall of indifference: prisoner voices about the realities of prison health care. *Laws*. 2021;10(1):11. https://doi.org/10.3390/laws10010011
18. MacDonald M. Overcrowding and its impact on prison conditions and health. *Int J Prison Health*. 2018;14(2):65–68. https://doi.org/10.1108/IJPH-04-2018-0014
19. Baffour FD, Francis AP, Chong MD, Harris N. Prison overcrowding and harsh conditions: health and human rights concerns to persons in custody, staff, and the community. *Crim Justice Behav*. 2024;51(3):375–400. https://doi.org/10.1177/00938548231219803
20. Carson AE. Prisoners in 2019. Available at: https://bjs.ojp.gov/library/publications/prisoners-2019. Accessed May 14, 2024.
21. Carson EA. Mortality in local jails, 2000–2019: statistical tables. Available at: https://bjs.ojp.gov/content/pub/pdf/mlj0019st.pdf. Accessed May 14, 2024.
22. Adler JL, Chen W. Jail conditions and mortality: death rates associated with turnover, jail size, and population characteristics. *Health Aff (Millwood)*. 2023;42(6):849–857. https://doi.org/10.1377/hlthaff.2022.01229
23. Patler C, Saadi A, Arulanantham A. Looking back: decarcerating immigration prisons as a tool for improved health. *Am J Public Health*. 2023;113(7):732–735. https://doi.org/10.2105/AJPH.2023.307293
24. Patler C, Saadi A, Young MEDT, Franco K. Release from US immigration detention may improve physical and psychological stress and health: results from a two-wave panel study in California. *Ment Health (Lond)*. 2021;1:100035. https://doi.org/10.1016/j.ssmmh.2021.100035
25. Calavita K, Jenness V. *Appealing to Justice: Prisoner Grievances, Rights, and Carceral Logic*. University of California Press; 2015.
26. Puglisi LB, Wang EA. Health care for people who are incarcerated. *Nat Rev Dis Primers*. 2021;7(1):50. https://doi.org/10.1038/s41572-021-00288-9
27. Schmidt JD. See no evil, hear no evil, treat no evil: Centurion and the curse of for-profit prison healthcare. Available at: https://www.prisonlegalnews.org/news/2024/jan/1/see-no-evil-hear-no-evil-treat-no-evil-centurion-and-curse-profit-prison-healthcare. Accessed May 14, 2024.
28. Homeland Security and Governmental Affairs Senate Committee. Uncounted deaths in America's prisons and jails. Available at: https://www.hsgac.senate.gov/subcommittees/investigations/hearings/uncounted-deaths-in-americas-prisons-and-jails-how-the-department-of-justice-failed-to-implement-the-death-in-custody-reporting-act. Accessed May 14, 2024.

29. Jolly V. California to examine medical staffing at state prisons and hospitals. Here's why. Available at: https://www.sacbee.com/news/politics-government/capitol-alert/article288595445.html#storylink=cpy. Accessed May 14, 2024.
30. Lofstrom M, Raphael S. Incarceration and crime: evidence from California's public safety realignment reform. *Ann Am Acad Pol Soc Sci.* 2016;664:196–220. https://doi.org/10.1177/0002716215599732
31. Ghandnoosh N. Fewer prisoners, less crime: a tale of three states. Available at: https://www.sentencingproject.org/reports/fewer-prisoners-less-crime-a-tale-of-three-states. Accessed May 13, 2024.
32. Guetzkow J, Schoon E. If you build it, they will fill it: the consequences of prison overcrowding litigation. *Law Soc Rev.* 2015;49(2):401–432. https://doi.org/10.1111/lasr.12140
33. Schoenfeld H. Mass incarceration and the paradox of prison conditions litigation. *Law Soc Rev.* 2010;44(3/4):731–767. https://doi.org/10.1111/j.1540-5893.2010.00421.x
34. Schlanger M. Plata v. Brown and realignment: jails, prisons, courts, and politics. *Harv Civil Rights Civil Liberties Law Rev.* 2013;48(1):165–216.
35. Huh K, Boucher A, McGaffey F, McKillop M, Schiff M. Jails: inadvertent health care providers. Available at: https://www.pewtrusts.org/-/media/assets/2018/01/sfh_jails_inadvertent_health_care_providers.pdf. Accessed May 14, 2024.

Cigarette and E-Cigarette Use Among LGBT+ Youths and Young Adults According to Strength of State-Level LGBT+ Equality Protections

Elexis C. Kierstead, MPH, Stephanie N. Yoon, MPP, Madison L. Iskra, MPH, Barbara A. Schillo, PhD, and Jennifer M. Kreslake, PhD, MPH

Objectives. To examine whether the state-level LGBT+ (lesbian, gay, bisexual, transgender, and other identities) legal protections where LGBT+ youths and young adults reside are associated with cigarette and e-cigarette use.

Methods. We drew LGBT+ respondents (aged 15–31 years; n = 1255) from a national, probability-based survey conducted from August to December 2023. We scored each state for LGBT+ equality on a scale from restrictive to protective based on the Movement Advancement Project's 2023 policy environment. Using weighted logistic regression models, we examined the relationship between current (past 30-day) cigarette and e-cigarette use and state LGBT+ equality protections, controlling for demographics and state tobacco control expenditure.

Results. LGBT+ individuals in protective policy states had 65% lower odds (odds ratio [OR] = 0.35; 95% confidence interval [CI] = 0.16, 0.78) of current cigarette use, and 56% lower odds (OR = 0.44; 95% CI = 0.25, 0.79) of current e-cigarette use compared with those in restrictive policy states.

Conclusions. LGBT+ individuals living in protective policy environments had lower odds of current cigarette and e-cigarette use, consistent with theoretical relationships between stress, discrimination, and harmful health behaviors.

Public Health Implications. Protective policies may alleviate tobacco use disparities among the LGBT+ community. (*Am J Public Health*. 2025;115(6):945–953. https://doi.org/10.2105/AJPH.2025.308008)

AJPH June 2025, Vol. 115, No. 6

Those who identify as a part of the LGBT+ (lesbian, gay, bisexual, transgender, and other identities) community use tobacco at higher rates than do their heterosexual and cisgender peers.[1] The 2021 National Youth Tobacco Survey identified that 14% of lesbian, gay, or bisexual individuals currently used tobacco compared with 8% of their heterosexual peers.[1] Similarly, 19% of participants who identified as transgender currently used tobacco compared with 8% of those who identified as cisgender.[1] These elevated rates of use may be explained by minority stress theory: the concept that individuals with a minoritized identity experience unique and disproportionate stress because of this identity.[2–4] Some of the drivers of this disproportionate stress are discrimination, lack of acceptance, and lack of familial support.[2,4] Although discrimination can be interpersonal, it can also be structural. Policies that protect LGBT+ individuals can help to attenuate the effect of discrimination on the lives of LGBT+ individuals, whereas policies that are harmful to LGBT+ individuals can amplify discrimination.[5,6] Understanding how these variable policies may influence tobacco use can provide critical information to researchers and policymakers.

Legislation that may harm the LGBT+ community, by limiting their rights or reducing access to important services, is currently on the rise, with 633 such bills considered in 2023 compared with 220 bills that were considered in 2022. Recent examples of proposed policies that harm the LGBT+ community include those that censor school curricula, mandate use of sex assigned at birth in schools, restrict sports participation for transgender athletes, restrict access to health care for LGBT+ youths and adults, and restrict bathroom use based on sex assigned at birth.[7] Meanwhile, in 2023, only 188 policies protecting the LGBT+ community were considered.[8,9] Examples of protective policies include protections of same-sex couples' parental rights, ensuring nondiscrimination based on sexual orientation and gender identity, and protecting access to the ability to change identification documents.[7]

The increase in legislation that may harm the LGBT+ community has concerning implications for the long-term mental and physical health of LGBT+ people. Policies that protect LGBT+ populations are associated with positive mental health outcomes, whereas policies that harm LGBT+ communities are associated with negative mental health outcomes.[10,11] One study found that because of harmful LGBT+ legislation, almost 1 in 3 LGBT+ individuals reported poor mental health most of the time or always.[12] Another study observed that transgender adolescents in states with explicit transgender guidance in antidiscrimination laws were less likely to experience depression.[11] A study found that lesbian, gay, or bisexual adults residing in states with limited protections of LGBT+ people had a higher likelihood of reporting poor physical health than did their heterosexual peers.[13] This evidence indicates that protective LGBT+ policies have the potential to promote positive health outcomes for LGBT+ people.

LGBT+ protections may have a direct impact on tobacco use among LGBT+ individuals. Previous work has indicated that sexual minority adults who experienced high levels of discrimination based on their sexual orientation were more susceptible to tobacco use than were sexual minority adults who had experienced minimal to no discrimination based on their sexual orientation.[14] Another study among LGBT+ people identified that higher levels of discrimination predicted higher rates of poly tobacco use (using multiple tobacco products either concurrently or sequentially), resulting in worse health outcomes.[15] However, that same study found that identity connectedness could predict lower odds of poly tobacco use.[15] Living in a jurisdiction governed by legislation that is either harmful or protective for the LGBT+ community could influence tobacco use among the LGBT+ community. We examined associations between varying state-level LGBT+ legal protections and cigarette and e-cigarette use among LGBT+ youths and young adults covered by those policies.

METHODS

We derived individual-level data from Truth Initiative's longitudinal cohort study. Ipsos fielded the study primarily to assess the effects of Truth Initiative's public education campaign. Truth Initiative collects data from a nationally representative, address-based sample of US youths and young adults aged 15 to 24 years upon enrollment. Further information about sample construction can be found elsewhere.[16] Cohort participants complete online surveys concerning tobacco use knowledge, attitudes, and behaviors, which Ipsos fields every 6 to 12 months.

We studied data of participants aged 15 to 31 years surveyed during the August to December 2023 study wave (n = 5651). Survey respondents provided geographic information, which we used to classify them according to their state-level policy environment. Specifically, we classified participant zip codes by state. We weighted all analyses to national census estimates for gender, age, and race to account for nonresponse, as well as the complex sampling design. Further methodological information about the study is detailed elsewhere.[16]

Measures

Sexual orientation and gender identity. Survey participants were asked if they identified as heterosexual, gay or lesbian, bisexual, another identity, or not at all sure. They were also asked to provide their sex assigned at birth (male or female) and their gender identity (male, female, nonbinary, another identity, or not at all sure). We considered those whose gender identity was the same as their sex assigned at birth cisgender and those who answered with a gender identity different from their sex assigned at birth noncisgender. We considered respondents LGBT+ if they identified as lesbian or gay, bisexual, or another identity other than heterosexual or they were not cisgender (n = 1255).

Cigarette and e-cigarette use. Survey respondents were asked about their cigarette and e-cigarette use. Participants were asked if they had ever tried smoking a cigarette, even 1 or 2 puffs. If they had ever used a cigarette, they were also asked on how many days in the past 30 days they had smoked a cigarette. We considered having smoked a cigarette in the past 30 days current cigarette use. Similarly, participants were asked if they had ever tried using an e-cigarette or vape, even 1 or 2 puffs. They were also asked if they had used an e-cigarette in the past 30 days. We defined current e-cigarette use as having used an e-cigarette in the past 30 days.

Demographic characteristics. Age was collected as a continuous variable and then grouped into 4 categories of 15 to 17, 18 to 20, 21 to 24, and 25 to 31 years. Race and ethnicity were collected as separate measures and combined into 1 measure consisting of 5 categories: non-Hispanic White, non-Hispanic Black/African American, non-Hispanic Asian/Asian American, Hispanic, and non-Hispanic other. The non-Hispanic other category included non-Hispanic Pacific Islander/Native Hawaiian participants, non-Hispanic American Indian/Alaska Native participants, and multiracial participants. Participants were asked how they would describe their overall financial situation. Four response options were combined into a dichotomous variable in which zero represented those who responded "does not meet basic expenses" and "just meet basic expenses with nothing left over" and 1 represented those who responded "meet needs with a little left over" and "live comfortably." This measure is validated for youth and young adult populations.[17,18]

State-level LGBT+ policy score. The Movement Advancement Project is a nonprofit think tank that researches LGBT+ policy, tracks state LGBT-related laws and policies, and uses the information to create a numeric policy score for each state.[7] Negative values are given to policies that are harmful to the LGBT+ community, and positive values are given to policies that protect the LGBT+ community, resulting in a composite score of all LGBT+-related policies for each state. The Movement Advancement Project categorized scores into 5 groups: negative, low, medium, fair, and high. States with a negative score have predominantly restrictive policies for LGBT+ people; states with a low, medium, or fair score have a mix of protective and restrictive policies; and states with a high score have predominantly protective policies. Preliminary analysis showed an unequal distribution of participants across the 5 groups (negative = 328; low = 248; medium = 53; fair = 152; high = 474). To achieve a more equal distribution across groups, we collapsed low, medium, and fair into 1 category, resulting in 3 categories to indicate the policy score: negative (1); low, medium, fair (2); and high (3).

State tobacco control expenditure. We derived state tobacco control expenditure data from the American Lung Association "State of Tobacco Control" 2024 report.[19] This report assesses tobacco control laws and policies at the state and federal levels. The Centers for Disease Control and Prevention determines a recommended expenditure for tobacco control programs, which supplies the actual tobacco control expenditure for each state. We calculated the percentage of the recommended expenditure for each state, and we used the continuous values for analysis. State tobacco control expenditure is significantly negatively associated with both cigarette and e-cigarette use.[20,21]

Analysis

We calculated unweighted frequencies and weighted percentages for all demographic variables, tobacco use variables, and the 3-level policy score among a subsample of LGBT+ youths and young adults (n = 1255). We performed weighted bivariate analyses to assess relationships between current cigarette and e-cigarette use, policy score, race/ethnicity, age, and financial status among the subsample. We used the Pearson χ^2 test to assess statistically significant differences.

We ran weighted multivariable logistic regression models among LGBT+ youths and young adults to examine the relationship between policy score and tobacco use, controlling for covariates. We ran 2 models in which the dependent variables included current cigarette use and current e-cigarette use. Models included the 3-category policy score as the independent variable along with the covariates race/ethnicity, age, income, and percentage of state tobacco control expenditure. We performed the χ^2 goodness of fit test for both models.

After completing primary analyses, we ran additional weighted multivariable logistic regression models among a subsample of non-LGBT+ youths and young adults (n = 4396). Using these models, we also examined the relationship between LGBT+ policy score and current cigarette and e-cigarette use, controlling for race/ethnicity, age, income, and state tobacco control expenditure. We performed the χ^2 goodness of fit test for each model. We performed all analyses in Stata version 18 (StataCorp LP, College Station, TX).

RESULTS

The sample consisted of 1255 LGBT+ youths and young adults. Of these individuals, 11.1% identified as heterosexual, 21.8% identified as gay or lesbian, 51.8% identified as bisexual, 12.6% identified as another sexual orientation not listed, and 2.6% were not sure about their sexual orientation. Approximately 25.1% of participants identified as a gender identity that was not the same as their sex assigned at birth. Additionally, 34.2% identified as male, 55.0% identified as female, 8.6% identified as nonbinary, and 2.1% identified as a gender identity not listed. Approximately 48.2% identified as non-Hispanic White/European American, 10.2% identified as non-Hispanic Black/African American, 5.0% identified as non-Hispanic Asian/Asian American, 20.9% identified as Hispanic or Latino, and 15.8% were considered non-Hispanic other. The participants' ages ranged from 15 to 31 years: 13.8% were 15 to 17 years, 22.7% were 18 to 20 years, 26.3% were 21 to 24 years, and 37.2% were 25 to 31 years. About 69.8% of participants reported that they live comfortably or meet their financial needs with a little left over, whereas 30.2% of the sample do not or just meet basic expenses (Table 1).

Approximately 9.0% of the sample currently smoked cigarettes, whereas

TABLE 1— Characteristics of a US National Sample of LGBT+ Youths and Young Adults: August–December 2023

Characteristic	No. (Weighted %)
Age, y	
15–17	75 (13.8)
18–20	363 (22.7)
21–24	486 (26.3)
25–31	331 (37.2)
Sex at birth	
Male	359 (38.2)
Female	896 (61.8)
Gender identity	
Male	320 (34.2)
Female	764 (55.0)
Nonbinary	147 (8.6)
Another identity	23 (2.1)
Refused	1 (0.0)
Cisgender identity	
Cisgender	902 (74.9)
Noncisgender	353 (25.1)
Sexual orientation	
Heterosexual or straight	148 (11.1)
Gay or lesbian	244 (21.8)
Bisexual	682 (51.8)
Another identity	155 (12.6)
Not at all sure	26 (2.6)
Race/Ethnicity	
Non-Hispanic White/European American	672 (48.2)
Non-Hispanic Black/African American	79 (10.2)
Non-Hispanic Asian/Asian American	53 (5.0)
Hispanic or Latino	218 (20.9)
Non-Hispanic Other	230 (15.8)
Financial status	
Don't or just meet basic expenses	398 (30.2)
Live comfortably or meet with a little left	857 (69.8)
Policy score	
Negative	328 (25.3)
Low, medium, fair	453 (31.0)
High	474 (43.7)
Current cigarette use	
No	1149 (91.0)
Yes	106 (9.0)
Current e-cigarette use	
No	973 (79.9)
Yes	282 (20.1)

Note. LGBT+ = lesbian, gay, bisexual, and transgender, plus other identities. Sample size was n = 1255.

20.1% currently used e-cigarettes. Regarding state LGBT+ policy, 25.3% of participants lived in a state with a negative policy score, indicating that they live in a state where policies predominantly restrict LGBT+ rights; 31.0% lived in a state with a low, medium, or fair policy score, indicating that they live in a state with a mix of protective and restrictive policies; and 43.7% lived in a state with a high policy score, indicating that they live in an environment with predominantly protective policies for LGBT+ people (Table 1).

Bivariate Analyses

Among LGBT+ youths and young adults who lived in a state with a negative policy score, 13.2% (n = 41) had currently smoked cigarettes, compared with 11.3% (n = 42) of those who lived in a state with a low, medium, or fair policy score and 4.8% (n = 23) of those who lived in a state with a high policy score ($P = .02$). Similarly, 23.7% (n = 89) of those who lived in a state with a negative policy score currently used e-cigarettes, compared with 25.5% (n = 114) of those in a state with a low, medium, or fair policy score and 14.2% (n = 79) of those who lived in a state with a high policy score ($P = .015$; Table 2).

Race/ethnicity was significantly associated with current cigarette and e-cigarette use. Financial status was significantly associated with current cigarette use. Approximately 6.3% (n = 53) of non-Hispanic White participants currently used cigarettes, compared with 4.8% (n = 5) of non-Hispanic Black participants, 1.3% (n = 2) of non-Hispanic

TABLE 2— Current Cigarette and E-Cigarette Use by LGBT+ Policy Environment, Race/Ethnicity, Age, and Financial Status Among a US Sample of LGBT+ Youths and Young Adults: August–December 2023

	Current Cigarette Use			Current E-Cigarette Use		
	Yes (n = 106), No. (Weighted %)	No (n = 1149), No. (Weighted %)	χ^2 P	Yes (n = 282), No. (Weighted %)	No (n = 973), No. (Weighted %)	χ^2 P
Policy score[a]			.02			.015
Negative	41 (13.2)	287 (86.8)		89 (23.7)	239 (76.3)	
Low, medium, fair	42 (11.3)	411 (88.7)		114 (25.5)	339 (74.5)	
High	23 (4.8)	451 (95.2)		79 (14.2)	395 (85.8)	
Race/Ethnicity			.01			.74
Non-Hispanic White/European American	53 (6.3)	619 (93.7)		143 (17.4)	529 (82.6)	
Non-Hispanic Black/African American	5 (4.8)	74 (95.2)		21 (18.3)	58 (81.7)	
Non-Hispanic Asian/Asian American	2 (1.3)	51 (98.7)		10 (24.6)	43 (75.4)	
Hispanic/Latino	18 (10.9)	200 (89.1)		50 (21.6)	168 (78.4)	
Non-Hispanic other	27 (16.3)	203 (83.7)		57 (23.4)	173 (76.6)	
Age, y			.01			.74
15–17	2 (3.5)	73 (96.5)		14 (15.9)	61 (84.1)	
18–20	30 (7.9)	333 (92.1)		75 (17.4)	288 (82.6)	
21–24	47 (12.0)	439 (88.0)		124 (25.2)	362 (74.8)	
25–31	27 (9.5)	304 (90.5)		69 (19.7)	262 (80.3)	
Financial status			.004			.025
Don't or just meet basic expenses	53 (14.7)	345 (85.3)		115 (26.3)	283 (73.7)	
Live comfortably or meet needs with a little left	53 (6.5)	804 (93.5)		167 (17.4)	690 (82.6)	

Note. LGBT+ = lesbian, gay, bisexual, and transgender, plus other identities. The sample size was n = 1255. We performed weighted bivariate analyses between policy score, race/ethnicity, age, and financial status as well as current cigarette use and current e-cigarette use. We used the Pearson χ^2 test to assess statistically significant differences.

[a]The Movement Advancement Project tracks LGBT-related laws and policies and uses the information to score each state policy environment from negative (predominantly policies that are harmful to the LGBT+ community); low, medium, and fair (a mix of policies that protect and harm the LGBT+ community) to high (predominantly policies that protect the LGBT+ community).

AJPH June 2025, Vol. 115, No. 6

Asian participants, 10.9% (n = 18) of Hispanic/Latino participants, and 16.3% (n = 27) of non-Hispanic other participants. The relationship between race/ethnicity and current e-cigarette use was not significant.

Approximately 6.5% (n = 53) of those who reported meeting their needs currently used cigarettes compared with 14.7% (n = 53) of those who do not meet their needs. Similarly, 17.4% (n = 167) of those who meet their financial needs currently use e-cigarettes, compared with 26.3% (n = 115) of those who do not. Age was not significantly associated with current cigarette and e-cigarette use in the population.

Regression Analyses

When controlling for race and ethnicity, age, perceived financial situation, and state tobacco control expenditure, LGBT+ youths and young adults living in states with a high policy score had significantly lower odds of current cigarette use (odds ratio [OR] = 0.35; 95% confidence interval [CI] = 0.16, 0.78) and current e-cigarette use (OR = 0.44; 95% CI = 0.25, 0.79) compared with those residing in states with a negative policy score (Table 3). Among the covariates, non-Hispanic other race/ethnicity was a significant predictor of current cigarette use (OR = 2.87; 95% CI = 1.31, 6.28), and a higher perceived financial situation resulted in lower odds of current cigarette use (OR = 0.40; 95%

TABLE 3— The Relationships Between Current Cigarette and E-Cigarette Use and LGBT+ Policy Environment Score, Adjusting for Participant Characteristics and State Tobacco Control Expenditure Among a US National Sample of LGBT+ Youths and Young Adults: August–December 2023

	Current Cigarette Use (n = 106), AOR (95% CI)	Current E-Cigarette Use (n = 282), AOR (95% CI)
χ^2	48.12	27.05
Policy Score[a]		
Negative (Ref)	1	1
Low, medium, fair	0.77 (0.38, 1.58)	1.08 (0.64, 1.83)
High	0.35 (0.16, 0.78)	0.44 (0.25, 0.79)
Race/Ethnicity		
Non-Hispanic White/European American (Ref)	1	1
Non-Hispanic Black/African American	0.59 (0.18, 1.95)	1.00 (0.49, 2.03)
Non-Hispanic Asian/Asian American	0.37 (0.07, 2.05)	2.63 (0.77, 8.93)
Hispanic/Latino	1.94 (0.83, 4.52)	1.48 (0.82, 2.68)
Non-Hispanic other	2.87 (1.31, 6.28)	1.39 (0.75, 2.54)
Age group, y		
15–17 (Ref)	1	1
18–20	2.72 (0.53, 14.10)	1.14 (0.51, 2.53)
21–24	3.97 (0.77, 20.50)	1.75 (0.80, 3.82)
25–31	2.91 (0.56, 15.28)	1.25 (0.53, 2.92)
Financial status		
Don't or just meet basic expenses (Ref)	1	1
Live comfortably or meet with a little left	0.40 (0.21, 0.75)	0.57 (0.36, 0.91)
Percentage of tobacco control expenditure	1.05 (0.25, 4.54)	1.87 (0.65, 5.39)
Intercept	0.06 (0.01, 0.35)	0.25 (0.10, 0.64)

Note. AOR = adjusted odds ratio; CI = confidence interval; LGBT+ = lesbian, gay, bisexual, and transgender, plus other identities. The sample size was n = 1255. We used weighted logistic regression models to examine the relationship between state LGBT+ policy score and current cigarette and e-cigarette use, controlling for race/ethnicity, age, financial status, and tobacco control expenditure. We assessed goodness of fit for each model.
[a]The Movement Advancement Project tracks LGBT-related laws and policies and uses the information to score each state policy environment from negative (predominantly policies that are harmful to the LGBT+ community); low, medium, and fair (a mix of policies that protect and harm LGBT+ community) to high (predominantly policies that protect the LGBT+ community).

CI = 0.21, 0.75) as well as current e-cigarette use (OR = 0.57; 95% CI = 0.36, 0.91; Table 3). The χ^2 goodness of fit test was significant for both models.

Post Hoc Analysis

To support the findings among the LGBT+ subsample, we conducted a post hoc analysis among the excluded, non-LGBT+ sample (n = 4396). These findings are reported in Table A (available as a supplement to the online version of this article at http://www.ajph.org). Regression analyses identified no significant relationship between living in a high policy score state versus a negative policy score state and current cigarette use (OR = 0.87; 95% CI = 0.48, 1.54) or current e-cigarette use (OR = 0.99; 95% CI = 0.67, 1.46). Age and financial status predicted current cigarette and e-cigarette use, and race/ethnicity predicted current e-cigarette use. The χ^2 goodness of fit test was significant for both models.

DISCUSSION

LGBT+ youths and young adults residing in US states with a protective policy environment for LGBT+ people had statistically lower odds of current cigarette use and current e-cigarette use when controlling for individual demographics and state tobacco control expenditure. In post hoc analyses, we did not find these results among a non-LGBT+ sample. The association between a protective policy environment and reduced tobacco use emphasizes the importance of considering the greater policy environment in which a person lives as a key determinant of LGBT+ health.

Those who are exposed to a protective policy environment may be less likely to engage in unhealthy behaviors, such as tobacco use, to manage stress, increasing the likelihood of longer and healthier lives. Studies have shown that some members of the LGBT+ community, specifically sexual minority females and transgender individuals, have an elevated risk of mortality compared with their heterosexual and cisgender peers, respectively.[22–24] Reducing tobacco use could help to extend the longevity and wellness of LGBT+ people, closing the gap in mortality between the LGBT+ community and their cisgender, heterosexual peers. Implementing protective policies could lead to significant progress in reducing disparities in tobacco use and creating more equitable health outcomes for the LGBT+ community.

Restrictive LGBT+ policies can place LGBT+ youths and young adults at increased risk for poor health outcomes attributable to higher tobacco use compared with protective policies. Tobacco use remains the leading cause of preventable death across the country. Tobacco use drastically increases morbidity and mortality from cancer as well as many chronic diseases, including heart disease and chronic obstructive pulmonary disease.[25] Tobacco use can also worsen health outcomes for those with existing conditions such as asthma and HIV.[25] Additionally, using nicotine at a young age can affect brain development and set the pathway for long-term addiction, and heavy use has been associated with symptoms of anxiety and depression.[26–28] Protective policies supporting LGBT+ youths and young adults can lead to lower cigarette and e-cigarette use and reduce the likelihood of these dangerous outcomes, contributing to the reduction of both tobacco use disparities and mortality disparities among the LGBT+ community.

Perceived discrimination on the basis of sexual orientation and gender identity can be a powerful determinant of health.[29] Experiencing discrimination at elevated rates increases the likelihood that LGBT+ individuals will use tobacco products.[14,15,30] Instituting protections against discrimination has a positive effect on overall health and wellness. In a study of US high school students, LGBT+ youths in states with protective policies for LGBT+ youths were less likely to experience discrimination and more likely to perform well in school than were LGBT+ youths in states without these policies.[6] State policies that protect LGBT+ rights may reduce perceived discrimination for LGBT+ people and thus reduce tobacco use.

LGBT+ youths and young adults use tobacco products at disproportionately high rates, contributing to lasting disparities in the long-term health and wellness of the LGBT+ community. Our research supports the implementation of policies that protect the rights and health of LGBT+ communities to lower their cigarette and e-cigarette use. Currently, the Movement Advancement Project estimates that only 40% LGBT+ adults in the United States reside in a protective policy environment.[7] More than half of LGBT+ adults still require substantial policy change in their state to create a protective environment. These policies have the potential to critically change the overall health of this population by reducing unhealthy behaviors directly linked to the disproportionate community stress experienced by LGBT+ people. Policies protecting LGBT+ people not only provide the community with crucial access to health and legal services but have the potential to elicit important downstream effects, such as reducing tobacco use, to improve community longevity.

This work has several limitations. All self-reported data were subject to biases such as recall bias and social desirability bias. Additionally, as this work was cross-sectional, we could not establish causality between variables. It is also possible that unintentionally omitted variables contributed to the relationship between the exposure and outcome variables in unknown ways. Future work should use a longitudinal approach to investigate this relationship and, in a continued effort to understand the relationships between the variables, could also explore interactions between covariates.

In conclusion, LGBT+ youths and young adults who were exposed to policy environments that protected the LGBT+ community had lower odds of current cigarette and e-cigarette use than did those in states with harmful policies. Implementing more local and federal policies that protect the rights of LGBT+ people can help to reduce disparities in tobacco use between LGBT+ and non-LGBT+ youths and young adults. These policies support the long-term health and wellness of LGBT+ people. AJPH

ABOUT THE AUTHORS

All authors are with Truth Initiative's Schroeder Institute, Washington, DC.

CORRESPONDENCE

Correspondence should be sent to Elexis C. Kierstead, MPH, Research Manager, Truth Initiative, 900 G St NW, Washington, DC 20001 (e-mail: lkierstead@truthinitiative.org). Reprints can be ordered at https://www.ajph.org by clicking the "Reprints" link.

PUBLICATION INFORMATION

Full Citation: Kierstead EC, Yoon SN, Iskra ML, Schillo BA, Kreslake JM. Cigarette and e-cigarette use among LGBT+ youths and young adults according to strength of state-level LGBT+ equality protections. *Am J Public Health*. 2025; 115(6):945–953.

Acceptance Date: December 22, 2024.

DOI: https://doi.org/10.2105/AJPH.2025.308008

ORCID iDs:
Elexis C. Kierstead https://orcid.org/0000-0002-8502-0451

Stephanie N. Yoon https://orcid.org/0000-0002-7565-7977

CONTRIBUTORS

E. C. Kierstead conceptualized the study and developed the methodology. E. C. Kierstead, S. N. Yoon, and M. L. Iskra wrote the original draft of the article. S. N. Yoon administered the project. M. L. Iskra performed the formal analyses. B. A. Schillo and J. M. Kreslake supervised the study and contributed writing, review, and editing.

ACKNOWLEDGMENTS

Truth Initiative funded this work.

CONFLICTS OF INTEREST

The authors have no conflicts of interest to declare.

HUMAN PARTICIPANT PROTECTION

The Truth Longitudinal Cohort study was approved by the Advarra institutional review board. All participants provided digital informed consent before data collection.

REFERENCES

1. Centers for Disease Control and Prevention. Tobacco product use and associated factors among middle and high school students—National Youth Tobacco Survey, United States, 2021. *MMWR Surveill Summ*. 2022;71(5):1–29. https://doi.org/10.15585/mmwr.ss7105a1
2. Frost DM, Meyer IH. Minority stress theory: application, critique, and continued relevance. *Curr Opin Psychol*. 2023;51:101579. https://doi.org/10.1016/j.copsyc.2023.101579
3. Mann I, Jenzer T, Miranda R Jr, Mereish EH. Minority stress and nicotine use and dependence among sexual minority youth. *Subst Use Misuse*. 2021;56(14):2264–2268. https://doi.org/10.1080/10826084.2021.1972315
4. Mongelli F, Perrone D, Balducci J, et al. Minority stress and mental health among LGBT populations: an update on the evidence. *Minerva Psichiatr*. 2019;60(1):27–50. https://doi.org/10.23736/S0391-1772.18.01995-7
5. Lombardi E, Sahni H. The impact of anti-discrimination legislation on transgender people within the USA. *Sex Res Soc Policy*. 2024;21:76–85. https://doi.org/10.1007/s13178-023-00851-x
6. Fields X, Wotipka CM. Effect of LGBT anti-discrimination laws on school climate and outcomes for lesbian, gay, and bisexual high school students. *J LGBT Youth*. 2022;19(3):307–329. https://doi.org/10.1080/19361653.2020.1821276
7. Movement Advancement Project. Snapshot: LGBTQ equality by state. Available at: https://www.lgbtmap.org/equality-maps. Accessed May 2, 2024.
8. Trevor Project. Our resolution: defeat anti-LGBTQ bills in 2023. February 1, 2023. Available at: https://www.thetrevorproject.org/blog/our-resolution-defeat-anti-lgbtq-bills-in-2023. Accessed May 2, 2024.
9. Trevor Project. LGBTQ+ legislation heatmap by state. Available at: https://www.thetrevorproject.org/bill-tracker. Accessed May 7, 2024.
10. Taylor CJ. Health consequences of laws and public policies that target, or protect, marginalized populations. *Sociol Compass*. 2020;14(2):e12753. https://doi.org/10.1111/soc4.12753
11. Miller-Jacobs C, Operario D, Hughto JMW. State-level policies and health outcomes in US transgender adolescents: findings from the 2019 Youth Risk Behavior Survey. *LGBT Health*. 2023;10(6):447–455. https://doi.org/10.1089/lgbt.2022.0247
12. Trevor Project. 2023 US National Survey on the Mental Health of LGBTQ Young People. Available at: https://www.thetrevorproject.org/survey-2023. Accessed May 2, 2024.
13. Gonzales G, Ehrenfeld JM. The association between state policy environments and self-rated health disparities for sexual minorities in the United States. *Int J Environ Res Public Health*. 2018;15(6):1136. https://doi.org/10.3390/ijerph15061136
14. McCabe SE, Hughes TL, Matthews AK, et al. Sexual orientation discrimination and tobacco use disparities in the United States. *Nicotine Tob Res*. 2019;21(4):523–531. https://doi.org/10.1093/ntr/ntx283
15. Budenz A, Gaber J, Crankshaw E, et al. Discrimination, identity connectedness and tobacco use in a sample of sexual and gender minority young adults. *Tob Control*. 2024;33(e2):e143–e150. https://doi.org/10.1136/tc-2022-057451
16. Cantrell J, Hair EC, Smith A, et al. Recruiting and retaining youth and young adults: challenges and opportunities in survey research for tobacco control. *Tob Control*. 2018;27(2):147–154. https://doi.org/10.1136/tobaccocontrol-2016-053504
17. Williams VF, Smith AA, Villanti AC, et al. Validity of a subjective financial situation measure to assess socioeconomic status in us young adults. *J Public Health Manag Pract*. 2017;23(5):487–495. https://doi.org/10.1097/PHH.0000000000000468
18. Quon EC, McGrath JJ. Subjective socioeconomic status and adolescent health: a meta-analysis. *Health Psychol*. 2014;33(5):433–447. https://doi.org/10.1037/a0033716

19. American Lung Association. State of tobacco control 2025. Available at: https://www.lung.org/research/sotc. Accessed May 2, 2024.
20. Tauras JA, Chaloupka FJ, Farrelly MC, et al. State tobacco control spending and youth smoking. *Am J Public Health.* 2005;95(2):338–344. https://doi.org/10.2105/AJPH.2004.039727
21. Tauras J, Diaz MC, Schillo B, Vallone D. Examination of the association between state tobacco control spending and the demand for electronic cigarettes by high school students. *Tob Control.* 2023;32(e2):e139–e144. https://doi.org/10.1136/tobaccocontrol-2021-056830
22. Jackson SS, Brown J, Pfeiffer RM, et al. Analysis of mortality among transgender and gender diverse adults in England. *JAMA Netw Open.* 2023;6(1):e2253687. https://doi.org/10.1001/jamanetworkopen.2022.53687
23. Laughney CI, Eliason EL. Mortality disparities among sexual minority adults in the United States. *LGBT Health.* 2022;9(1):27–33. https://doi.org/10.1089/lgbt.2020.0482
24. de Blok CJ, Wiepjes CM, van Velzen DM, et al. Mortality trends over five decades in adult transgender people receiving hormone treatment: a report from the Amsterdam cohort of gender dysphoria. *Lancet Diabetes Endocrinol.* 2021;9(10):663–670. https://doi.org/10.1016/S2213-8587(21)00185-6
25. Centers for Disease Control and Prevention. Cigarette smoking. September 17, 2024. Available at: https://www.cdc.gov/tobacco/about/?CDC_AAref_Val=https://www.cdc.gov/tobacco/data_statistics/fact_sheets/health_effects/effects_cig_smoking/index.htm. Accessed February 8, 2025.
26. Javed S, Usmani S, Sarfraz Z, et al. A scoping review of vaping, e-cigarettes and mental health impact: depression and suicidality. *J Community Hosp Intern Med Perspect.* 2022;12(3):33–39. https://doi.org/10.55729/2000-9666.1053
27. Becker TD, Arnold MK, Ro V, Martin L, Rice TR. Systematic review of electronic cigarette use (vaping) and mental health comorbidity among adolescents and young adults. *Nicotine Tob Res.* 2021;23(3):415–425. https://doi.org/10.1093/ntr/ntaa171
28. Leslie FM. Unique, long-term effects of nicotine on adolescent brain. *Pharmacol Biochem Behav.* 2020;197:173010. https://doi.org/10.1016/j.pbb.2020.173010
29. Pascoe EA, Richman LS. Perceived discrimination and health: a meta-analytic review. *Psychol Bull.* 2009;135(4):531–554. https://doi.org/10.1037/a0016059
30. Caceres BA, Hughes TL, Veldhuis CB, Matthews AK. Past-year discrimination and cigarette smoking among sexual minority women: investigating racial/ethnic and sexual identity differences. *J Behav Med.* 2021;44(5):726–739. https://doi.org/10.1007/s10865-021-00217-x

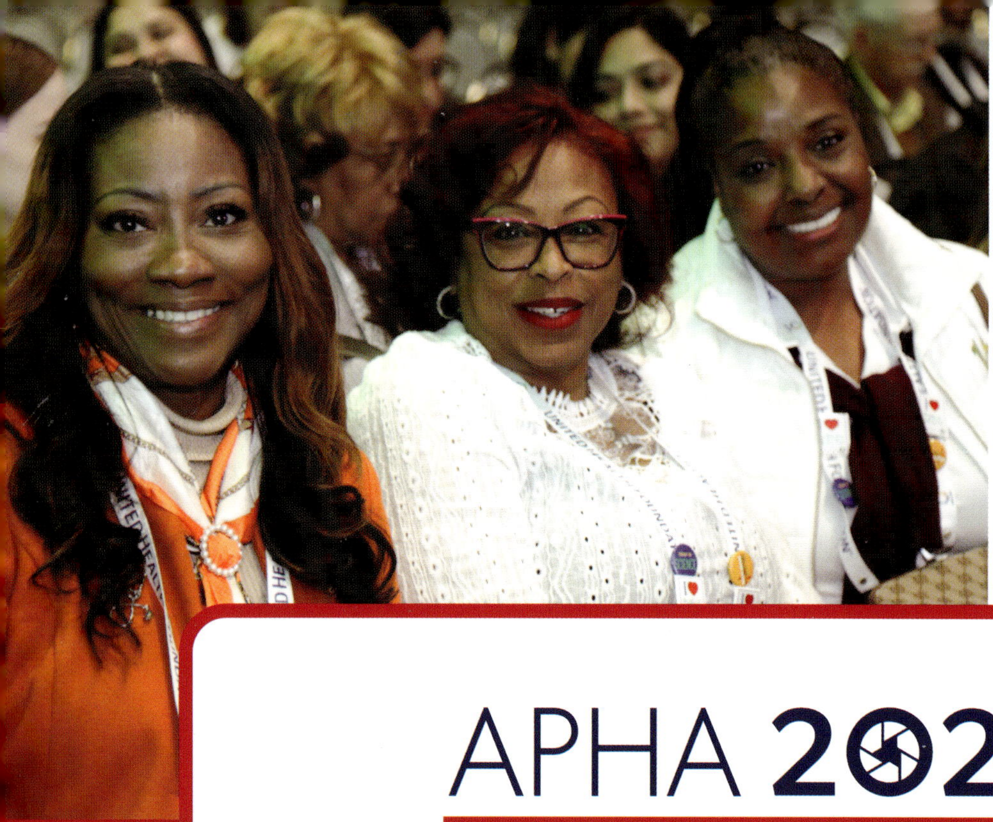

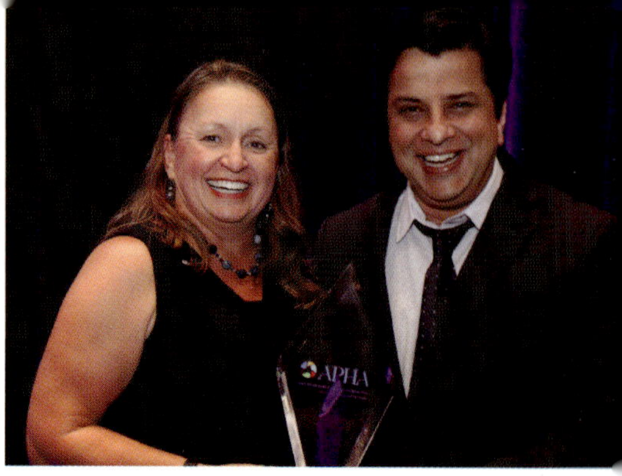

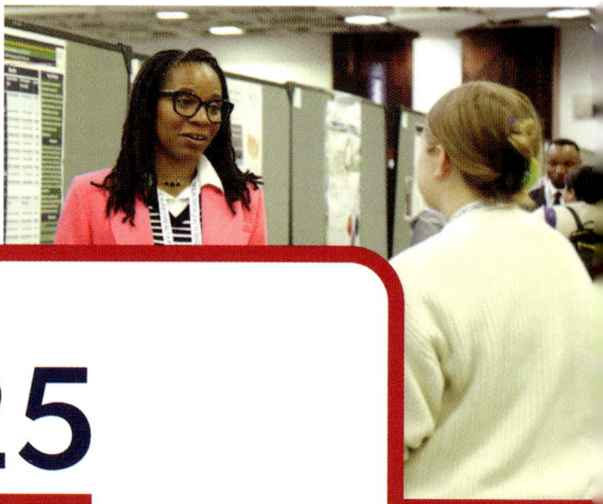

APHA 2025

ANNUAL MEETING & EXPO

NOVEMBER 2-5, 2025 • WASHINGTON, D.C.

Making the Public's Health a National Priority

Registration is Now Open

Early-bird deadline: July 14, 2025

Dive into this experience alongside over 12,000 public health professionals from around the world to share knowledge and advance public health through comprehensive educational sessions and valuable networking opportunities.

APHA
AMERICAN PUBLIC HEALTH ASSOCIATION
For science. For action. For health.

Start your APHA 2025 experience at
APHA.org/AnnualMeeting